**YOUR GUIDE TO**

# Surgical Equipment and Supplies

# LEARN | PRACTICE

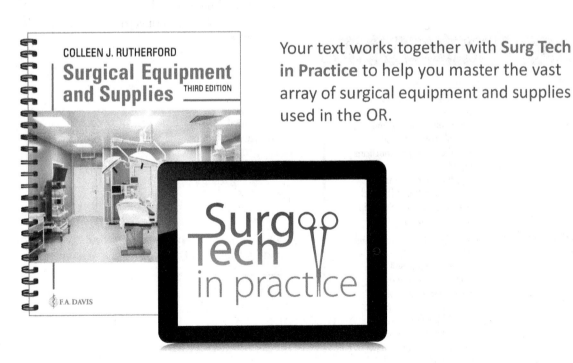

COLLEEN J. RUTHERFORD
**Surgical Equipment and Supplies** THIRD EDITION

F.A. DAVIS

Surg Tech in practice

Your text works together with **Surg Tech in Practice** to help you master the vast array of surgical equipment and supplies used in the OR.

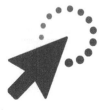

**Don't miss everything that's waiting online to make learning less stressful...and save you time.**

Follow the instructions on the inside front cover to use the access code to unlock your resources today.

# LEARN

## Your go-to guide to the OR.

Over 730 full-color photographs give you an up-close look at common equipment and supplies unique to the surgical setting. Each chapter describes distinct categories of equipment or supplies in detail and how to differentiate between similar supplies.

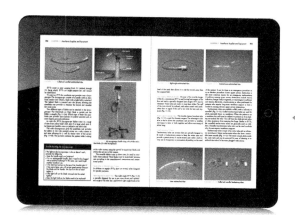

An **eBook version** of your text and online access to **Surg Tech in Practice** make it easy to study on your schedule.

**"Watch Out!" boxes** highlight important, need-to-know information and offer practical advice.

## WATCH OUT! Epidural Anesthesia

- Accidental puncture of the dura during needle insertion could result in total spinal anesthesia. Signs of total spinal anesthesia include bradycardia, respiratory paralysis, and vasodilation.
- Continuous monitoring of vital signs is necessary during insertion of an epidural.
- *Remember:* Watch what is said in the room; the patient is awake!

## Tourniquet Troubleshooting Tips

| PROBLEM | WHAT TO LOOK AT |
|---|---|
| The surgical field suddenly starts to fill with blood | ■ Has the cuff come loose or off?<br>■ Is the tubing still connected to both connections?<br>■ Are the tubing connections tight?<br>■ Are the connections still attached to the cuff? (Did one of the connections rip out of the cuff?) |
| The cuff doesn't inflate | ■ Is the pressure reading still where you set it?<br>■ Is the machine on?<br>■ Is the cuff securely connected to the tubing?<br>■ Are you using the inflati control for the correct cuff? (Most machines allow you to connect tw tourniquets, but each is connected to separate tubing and controlled b separate controls.)<br>■ Is there a hole or leak ir the cuff? |

**"Troubleshooting" boxes** identify common equipment malfunctions and offer potential solutions.

**"Surgical Session Review" questions** help you assess your understanding and apply what you're learning to practice.

### Q&A Surgical Session Review

1) The purpose of _____ is to absorb carbon dioxide in the anesthesia machine breathing circuit.
   a. Soda lime
   b. Limestone
   c. Soap stone
   d. Soda pop

2) _____ is the medication used in the treatment of malignant hyperthermia.
   a. Decadron
   b. Lasix
   c. Dantrolene
   d. Digoxin

3) A reading of below _____ on the BIS monitor means the patient is unconscious.
   a. 80
   b. 90
   c. 70
   d. 60

4) A _____ _____ is a type of blanket that blows warm air over the patient's skin surface to help prevent hypothermia.
   a. Bear Hugger
   b. Bair Hugger
   c. Bare Hugger
   d. Bear Blanket

# PRACTICE

**Practice. Practice. And more practice.**
Interactive recall and application activities help you learn to identify key equipment and supplies, while applying your knowledge in a safe setting.

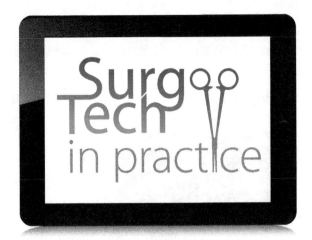

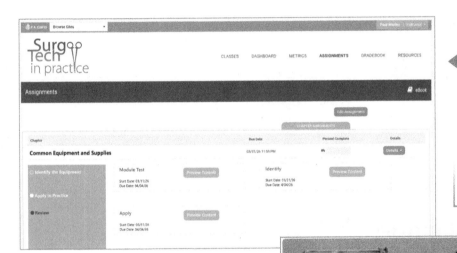

**Modules** within Surg Tech in Practice let you build your knowledge and advance your understanding.

A **chapter overview video** for each module provides a comprehensive summary of important concepts.

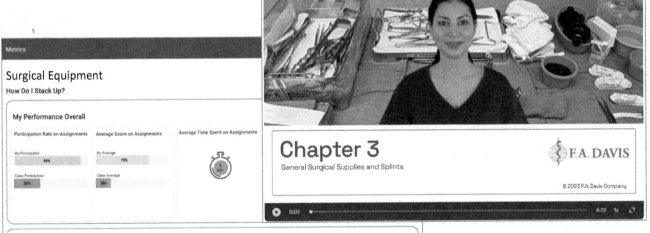

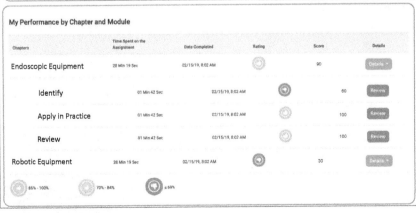

**Your personal dashboard** lets you track your progress every step of the way. You'll know exactly how you're doing and where you need to focus your studies.

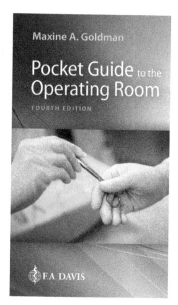

# SURGICAL EQUIPMENT and SUPPLIES

## THIRD EDITION

Colleen J. Rutherford, RN, MSN

Retired Faculty and Hospital Supervisor

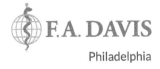

F.A. DAVIS

Philadelphia

F. A. Davis Company
1915 Arch Street
Philadelphia, PA 19103
www.fadavis.com

Copyright © 2023 by F. A. Davis Company

Printed in the United States of America

Last digit indicates print number: 10 9 8 7 6 5 4 3 2 1

*Publisher, Health Professions:* Christa Fratantoro
*Director of Content Development:* George W. Lang
*Content Project Manager:* Megan Suermann
*Design and Illustrations Manager:* Carolyn O'Brien

As new scientific information becomes available through basic and clinical research, recommended treatments and drug therapies undergo changes. The author and publisher have done everything possible to make this book accurate, up to date, and in accord with accepted standards at the time of publication. The author, editors, and publisher are not responsible for errors or omissions or for consequences from application of the book, and make no warranty, expressed or implied, regarding the contents of the book. Any practice described in this book should be applied by the reader in accordance with professional standards of care used regarding the unique circumstances that may apply in each situation. The reader is advised always to check product information (package inserts) for changes and new information regarding dose and contraindications before administering any drug. Caution is especially urged when using new or infrequently ordered drugs.

**Library of Congress Cataloging-in-Publication Data**

Names: Rutherford, Colleen J., author.
Title: Surgical equipment and supplies / Colleen J. Rutherford.
Other titles: Differentiating surgical equipment and supplies
Description: Third edition. | Philadelphia, PA : F.A. Davis Company [2023] |
    Includes index.
Identifiers: LCCN 2022037277 (print) | LCCN 2022037278 (ebook) | ISBN
    9781719648417 (spiral bound) | ISBN 9781719648790 (ebook)
Subjects: MESH: Surgical Equipment | Operating Rooms—organization &
    administration | Atlas
Classification: LCC RD755  (print) | LCC RD755  (ebook) | NLM WO 517 | DDC
    617.9—dc23/eng/20220824
LC record available at https://lccn.loc.gov/2022037277
LC ebook record available at https://lccn.loc.gov/2022037278

This book is dedicated to all the surgical technology instructors who are teaching, or have taught, in programs throughout the world. Through your hard work and dedication, the next groups of surgical technologists are being educated to provide the best practices and safest care to their patients.

To all of the practicing operating room personnel—the care you provide to patients on an everyday basis helps to make the miracle of modern surgery a reality.

Thank you.

# PREFACE

Entering the operating room for the first time can be intimidating; it is like entering a foreign country. The clothes are different (scrubs, masks, and hats), the culture is different, the temperature is cold, and there is a lot of unfamiliar equipment and supplies not used anywhere else except in surgery. What is a "lap pad," for example? What is the difference between a "Chromic" and "Vicryl" suture? What safety precautions are necessary when the laser is in use? This book answers those questions and many more. Its objectives are to:

- Describe common equipment and supplies unique to the surgical setting
- Highlight important information using boxes
- Serve as a reference for students or personnel new to the operating room environment

Each chapter describes different categories of equipment or supplies in detail and helps differentiate between similar supplies (e.g., types of sutures). In some cases, the equipment and supplies require less narration; on those pages you will find pictures of the item and a short description that includes its use.

*Watch Out* boxes provide key points and hazards to remember when aiding in patient care or handling equipment and supplies. *Guideline* boxes focus on important skills and information. *Troubleshooting* boxes provide aid for getting equipment working properly.

Each chapter ends with a surgical session review, quizzes students can use to test their knowledge and identify areas in which they may need extra study. The answers are in the back of the book.

## NEW TO THIS EDITION

Those of you familiar with the second edition will find that I have kept much of the same format. I have changed or added content based on updated OR procedures and technology as well as feedback from reviewers of the previous edition. Some changes you will see include the following:

- Aseptic techniques and sterilization are the foundation of what we practice in the OR environment, so that content appears in Chapter 1. The section can be referenced as needed.

- The medication section has been shortened and updated to include only the most commonly used medications in the surgical field, in emergencies, or by the anesthesia provider.
- Microscopes and robotics have their own chapters (Chapters 6 and 9) because their usage has become more common.
- Lasers are now covered in Chapter 7, before endoscopic equipment and robotics. This organization acknowledges the fact that lasers are used in many endoscopic surgeries, and thus students should be aware of laser safety first.
- Specialty Equipment (Chapter 10), has been expanded to include more updated information.
- The information on post-op splints is now in Chapter 3 to improve the flow of the chapters.
- The *Surgical Session Review* questions at the end of each chapter have been revised and updated, and new questions have been added where needed.

Educators who adopt this book for use in their classrooms will receive access to the following supporting materials, which are housed on F. A. Davis's website at www.fadavis.com: a test generator with more than 500 questions; PowerPoint presentations; a digital image bank of the supplies and equipment that can be inserted into their own tests or presentations; and an instructor's guide with ideas for lessons, homework assignments, and lectures.

As with the third edition of *Differentiating Surgical Instruments* (2020, F.A. Davis Company), the purchase of this textbook also includes free access to "Surg Tech in Practice"—a dynamic array of electronic learning content, specific to this text. This content can be assigned as homework, used to review material, or used as an in-classroom adjunct to enhance learning.

The operating room is an exciting and dynamic foreign land, full of joy and some sorrow, but most of all a wonderful opportunity to learn and make a difference for patients. It is my hope that you find this book a valuable aid in navigating the world of surgery!

# ACKNOWLEDGMENTS

No one writes a book alone. It is through the efforts of many special people that this book has come into being.

First, I would like to give a special acknowledgement to Christa Fratantoro, publisher of F.A. Davis Publishing Company. You have been there to guide me, give me good advice, and "cheer me on" since I started writing my first book in 2003. Your faith in me and my materials has motivated me to keep writing.

To George Lang from F.A. Davis—you have been here since the beginning of my author journey. Thank you for your involvement and good advice.

To Megan Suermann—thank you for your work on this edition. Keeping track of all the changes is not an easy task.

Jeanne Rieger—thank you for providing some of the photographs for this edition when, due to COVID-19 restrictions, we could not take a professional photographer into the hospital. Your help was valuable and appreciated.

To the marketing department at F.A. Davis Publishing—your job often goes unheralded, but you provide a vital service by promoting my materials. I attend the Association of Surgical Technologists convention yearly to meet users and talk about my materials, but you are out there promoting them on an everyday basis. Thank you.

I have used numerous websites and surgical supply catalogs to double-check facts and information on the equipment and supplies in this book.

And last but most importantly, thank you to my family and friends. You enrich my life on a daily basis. I am very blessed to have each and every one of you in my life.

# REVIEWERS

**Stephanie Allen,** CST, FAST, CRCST, CIS, CHL, MBA

Surgical Technology Program Director
Michigan Community College Association
West Branch, Michigan

**Tammy Allhoff,** B.L.S., CST, CSFA

SUT Program Director
Surgical Technology Department
Pearl River Community College
Hattiesburg, Mississippi

**Mel Angelisanti,** CSFA, CST

Program Chair
Health and Human services
Central Piedmont Community College
Charlotte, North Carolina

**Sylvia C. Bache,** CST

Surgical Technology and Allied Health Instructor
Surgical Technology
Lanier Technical College
Gainesville, Georgia

**Jacqueline R. Bak,** R.N. MSN CNOR CST

Program Director & Professor
Perioperative Programs
Delaware County Community College
Media, Pennsylvania

**Dana Bancer,** CST

Program Director
School of Health Careers
Daytona State College
Daytona Beach, Florida

**Renee Bridges,** CST, AGE

Program Director
Surgical Technology/Central Sterile Processing
Davidson County Community College
Thomasville, North Carolina

**Vicki Bushey,** CST, BS Ed.

Program Director/Instructor
Surgical Technology
Metro Technology Centers
Oklahoma City, Oklahoma

**Kathy Cabai,** EdD

Program Director
Perioperative Programs
College of DuPage
Glen Ellyn, Illinois

**Melissa Carnahan,** BS, CST

Program Director and Professor
ST Program
Allied Health
Kirkwood Community College
Cedar Rapids, Iowa

**Toni Choy,** RN, CST

Program Director
Nursing
Kapiolani Community College
Honolulu, Hawaii

**Raetta S. Coleman,** CST, FAST, BS

Program Director
Surgical Technology
Robeson Community College
Lumberton, North Carolina

**Shea Coleman,** CST

Surgical Technology Instructor
Career/Technical
Holmes Community College
Ridgeland, Mississippi

**JoLane Collins,** CST, ATC, MA Ed., CBSPD, FAST

Surgical Technology and Sterile Processing Program Director
Health Science
Technical College of the Lowcountry
Beaufort, South Carolina

**Danielle Cook,** MS, CST

Surgical Technology Program Director/Instructor
Surgical Technology
Moraine Park Technical College
Fond du Lac, Wisconsin

**Howard Coverdale,** CST, BSHS

Program Director
Surgical Technology
Pennsylvania College of Heath Sciences
Lancaster, Pennsylvania

**Debra M. Crews,** RN, CNOR, KCSA, CST/CSFA, FAST
Assistant Professor/Program Coordinator (Retired)
Surgical Technology/Allied Health
Southcentral Kentucky Community & Technical College
Bowling Green, Kentucky

**Terri Crosson,** CST
Instructor
Surgical Technology
Ogeechee Technical College
Statesboro, Georgia

**Melanie Croucher,** CST, CRCST
Instructor, Program Director
Surgical Technology
Delcastle Technical High School
Wilmington, Delaware

**Jessica A. Elliott,** RN, CST, FAST
Program Director/ Instructor
Surgical Technology
Holmes Community College
Grenada, Mississippi

**Marsha Eriks,** BA/CST
Program Chair
Surgical Technology
Ivy Tech Community College
Lawrenceburg, Indiana

**Alice R Erskine,** CST, MSN, RN, CNOR
Professor
Surgical Technology
Skyline College
San Bruno, California

**Javier Espinales,** CST, M.Ed.
Surgical Technology Program Director
Academics
Concorde Career College
San Antonio, Texas

**Kristine Flickinger,** MAOM, RN, CNOR, CST
Program Director
Surgical Technology
Odessa College
Odessa, Texas

**Marsha D. Flowers,** BS. CST
Assistant Professor/Clinical Coordinator
Surgical Technology Program
Ivy Tech Community College
Indianapolis, Indiana

**Richard Fruscione,** MA, CST, FAST
Program Director
Surgical Technology
Kingsborough Community College
Brooklyn, New York

**Christine L. Gardner,** CST
Program Director
Surgical Technology
College of Eastern Idaho
Idaho Falls, Idaho

**Kathryn General,** CST, M.Ed
Clinical Coordinator/Instructor
Surgical Technology
Central Piedmont Community College

**Debi Gipson,** CST, BA
Surgical Technology Director
Surgical Technology
Academy of Careers & Technology
Beckley, West Virginia

**Dana Grafft,** CST, BOE, FAST
Program Director
Surgical Technology
Iowa Lakes Community College
Spencer, Iowa

**Roselynn Graham,** CST, AAS
Surgical Technology Instructor
Concorde College
San Antonio Texas

**Rhonda Green,** CST
Clinical Coordinator
Health Science-Surgical Technology
Collin College
McKinney, Texas

**Renee Guillory,** CST, CSPDT, MBA
Director of Surgical Technology
Health Sciences
Louisiana State University Eunice
Lafayette, Louisiana

**Jia Hardimon-Eddington,** MS, CST
Health Sciences
Ivy Tech Community College
Kokomo, Indiana

**Mildred J. Hill**, CST, RN, BSN, CNOR, RNFA

Instructor
Surgical Technology
Tulsa Technology Center, HSC
Tulsa, Oklahoma

**Julia Hinke**, RN MHS, CNOR

Program Chair
Surgical Technology
Ivy Tech Community College
Evansville Indiana

**Douglas J. Hughes**, MAE-CI, CSFA, CST, CRCST

Dean for Health Sciences
Associate Professor for Surgical Technology
School of Health Sciences
Columbia Basin College
Pasco, Washington

**Teri Junge**, MEd, CSFA, CST, FAST, CSPDT

Surgical Technology Program Coordinator
Health Careers
Triton College
River Grove, Illinois

**Amy L. Kennedy**, MSN, RN, CNOR

Program Director
Health and Public Service
Harrisburg Area Community College
Harrisburg, Pennsylvania

**Colleen Leard**, TS-C

Perioperative Education Consultant

**Jayne MacPherson**, CST PhD FAST

Professor
Surgical Technology
Bunker Hill Community College
Boston, Massachusetts

**Jennifer Mazey**, CST, AAS

Program Director
Allied Health-Surgical Technology
Cisco College
Abilene, Texas

**Meloney McRoberts**, CST

Assistant Professor
Allied Health-Surgical Technology
Southern West Virginia Community & Technical College
Mount Gay, West Virginia

**Amanda Minor**, CST, BS

Chairperson
Department of Surgical Technology
Mount Aloysius College
Cresson, Pennsylvania

**Joyce Moyer**, RN, CST, CRCST

Retired Department Head
Surgical Technology and Sterile Processing Technology
Greenville Technical College
Greenville, South Carolina

**Rosemary Nagler**, MSNed, RN, CNOR

Administrator
Health Careers
Western Suffolk BOCES
Northport, New York

**AnneMarie O'Shea**, CST, BS

Health Science Instructor
Surgical Technology
Delaware County Community College
Media, Pennsylvania

**Kathy Patnaude**, CST, BS, FAST

Surgical Technology Program Director
School of Health Science
Midlands Technical College
West Columbia, South Carolina

**Kristi Pair**, CST, BS

Clinical Faculty Specialist
Surgical Technology
Cabarrus College of Health Sciences
Concord, North Carolina

**Tina Putman**, CST

Director of Surgical Technology
Lord Fairfax Community
Middletown, Virginia

**Raeann Quintana**, CST

Instructor
Surgical Technology
Pueblo Community College
Pueblo, Colorado

**Robert Sanchez**, CST, ADN, BSN, RN

Program Chair
Surgical Technology
Texas State Technical College
Harlingen, Texas

Rita Schutz, RN
Program Director
Surgical Technology
Anoka Technical College
Anoka, Minnesota

Suzi Shippen-Wagner, CST, BS
Program Chair
Surgical Technology
Edgecombe Community College
Rocky Mount, North Carolina

Shannon E. Smith, M.H.Sc., CST, CSFA, CDEI
Program Chair
Surgical Technology
Vincennes University
Vincennes, Indiana

Renona Smutny, CST BAS
Adjunct/Clinical Instructor
Surgical Technology
Oakland Community College
Southfield, Michigan

Theresa A. Sorgen-Burleson, CST, MBA
Program Director and Assistant Professor
Surgical Technology
University of Saint Francis
Fort Wayne, Indiana

Toni Steward, BS, CSR
Accreditation Liasion
Surgical Technology
Iowa Western Community College
Council Bluffs, Iowa

Beth D. Stokes, BFA, AAS, CST, CPSDT
Program Director
Surgical Technology and Sterile Processing
Cuyahoga Community College
Cleveland, Ohio

Lenette Thompson, CST
Surgical Technology Clinical Coordinator/Instructor
Health Care Division
Piedmont Technical College
Greenwood, South Carolina

Jamey D. Watson, BAS, CST
Program Chair
Surgical Technology
Athens Technical College
Athens, Georgia

Eddy R. Wenzel, CST, RN, BSN, CNOR
Department Chair
Surgical Technology & Imaging Sciences
Ivy Tech Community College-Columbus
Columbus, Indiana

Erin White-Mincarelli, PhD, MS, CST
Program Coordinator/ Assistant Professor
Surgical Technology
Montgomery County Community College
Blue Bell, Pennsylvania

Alison M. Wilson, CST, AAS, BSHA. MoA
Corporate Director of Education
Academics
Brookline College
Tempe, Arizona

Andrea Winslow, BS, CST
Program Director
Surgical Technology
National American University
Overland Park, Kansas

Brenda Young, RN CNOR
Program Director
Surgical Technology
Gadsden State Community College
Anniston, Alabama

# CONTENTS

# 1 | Aseptic Technique, Sterilization, OR Attire, National Time Out, and Hand Hygiene

You may wonder why a chapter on aseptic technique and other basic operating room information is included in a book on surgical equipment and supplies. In my past experience as the director and instructor of a surgical technology program, I found that students and new operating room (OR) personnel cannot be exposed to this information too many times. These concepts are critically important to understand; it is how we protect our patients. Please read and reread this chapter and be sure you understand the concepts. It is the least you can do for your future patients, who will place their lives in your hands and trust you will do your very best for them.

## ASEPTIC (STERILE) TECHNIQUE

Aseptic technique is the foundation of all that goes on in the OR. No matter what else happens, failure to practice proper aseptic technique increases the patient's risk of infection, injury, or even death.

*Asepsis* means "without infection," but the generally accepted definition is "absence of all microbes." In surgery, an inanimate object (e.g., instrument or supply) is considered sterile (aseptic) only after it has been exposed to a process that kills all microbes, including spores. Sterilization processes can use steam, gas, chemicals, hydrogen peroxide, or radiation to render an item free of microbes. The skin can never be rendered *sterile* (i.e., free of all microbes); therefore, aseptic technique dealing with skin (e.g., scrubbing or prepping) is aimed at reducing microbes to an absolute minimum.

This section of the book covers principles of aseptic technique and provides an overview of sterilization methods. It is imperative that ALL personnel working in the OR have a thorough understanding of aseptic technique in order to protect their patients.

### WATCH OUT! Surgical Conscience

- Surgical conscience is the ethical motivation to practice proper aseptic technique. ALL personnel must be willing to police themselves and each other, be willing to admit to a break in technique, and be ready to take corrective action. The willingness to police oneself, whether there is anyone else around to notice the break in technique, is imperative. Anyone who is not willing to admit to a break in technique should NOT be working in the OR.
- ANY break in sterile technique, no matter how minor it may seem, puts the patient at increased risk of infection.
- There is no such thing as "slightly contaminated" or "almost sterile." Sterility of an item is an absolute— either an item is sterile or it is not. If there is ANY doubt about an item's sterility, DO NOT use it—dispose of it and get a new one.

## Principles and Guidelines of Aseptic Technique

The principles listed here are adapted from various OR textbooks as well as the Association of Operating Room Nurses (AORN) guidelines and standards of practice. Although some of these principles and guidelines may be practiced and enforced to varying degrees, depending on institutional policies, they have a solid foundation in patient care and safety.
- Only sterile (scrubbed) personnel handle sterile items. Only nonsterile personnel handle nonsterile items.
- Sterility of an item is an absolute—either an item is sterile or it is not. If there is ANY doubt about an item's sterility, DO NOT use it—dispose of it and get a new one.
- Proper attire must be worn by all personnel. This includes scrub suits, masks covering the mouth and nose, hats or caps that cover hair and scalp, eye protection, and shoe covers if contamination of shoes is reasonably expected or if needed as personal protective equipment (PPE). Beards should be covered when entering a restricted area or when packaging and assembling equipment in the clean area of sterile supply. Waist ties and scrub tops should be tucked inside the pants to prevent inadvertent contamination of the field.
- Long-sleeved jackets may be worn by nonsterile personnel but need to be buttoned to avoid opening out and possibly contaminating the field. Fleece jackets are not recommended because they release large amounts of lint particles into the air. Jackets should be laundered daily or when visibly soiled. Jackets that are hung in lockers and reused are potential sources of contamination.

*Continued*

## Principles and Guidelines of Aseptic Technique—cont'd

- The wearing of cloth hats or caps depends on institutional policy. Cloth caps should be thrown into the laundry at the end of the day and when they become visibly soiled. Cloth hats that are worn for more than 1 day without being laundered become sources of increased microbial contamination.
- Jewelry is a potential source of microbes.
- Nonsterile persons must stand a minimum of 12 inches away from any sterile area (e.g., the sterile field, sterile tables, or ring basins). Nonsterile items should be kept a minimum of 12 inches away from sterile items.
- The draped patient is the center of the sterile field, and all other components of the sterile field (e.g., Mayo stand, back tables, and ring stand) should be placed close to and around the patient. Nonsterile items or personnel should not be in this area.
- The sterile field should be created as close to the time of surgery as possible. The longer sterile items are left out, the greater the chance of contamination.
- Talking in the sterile field should be kept to a minimum. Excessive, nonessential talking increases the amount of airborne microbes.
- Movement (including traffic in and out of the room) should be kept to a minimum during the surgical procedure. Doors should be kept closed. Opening of doors and movement of personnel stir up air currents that can lead to increased microbial contamination.
- Handling and moving drapes and linen should be kept to a minimum to prevent the spread of lint and dust.
- The only part of the surgical table that is considered sterile is the TABLETOP. Sterile items should NOT hang over the table edge.
- Once placed, table drapes and patient drapes should be left in place. Repositioning drapes could cause a part of the drape that previously had been below tabletop or patient level (therefore unsterile) to be brought back into the sterile field.
- Tubing that falls below the level of the patient is considered contaminated. If the electrosurgical hand unit or suction tip falls below the patient level, it must be discarded and replaced with a new one.
- The only parts of the sterile gown that are considered sterile are the front of the gown from waist up to midchest and the sleeves to 2 inches above the elbow (Fig. 1–1). The stockinette cuffs are NOT considered sterile because they are not impervious to perspiration, which can wick upward through the stockinette, bringing microbes with it.
- Scrubbed personnel should NOT place their hands in their axillary (armpit) area. Even though scrubbed personnel are wearing sterile gowns, strike-through contamination could occur from perspiration wicking microbes up through the gown from the axillary area.
- Only an item that has been processed using an approved method is considered sterile. Check sterilization indicators on all items to make sure they have been exposed to the proper conditions to render them sterile.

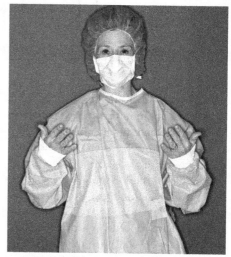

FIGURE 1–1 Areas of the gown considered sterile.

- Before introducing an item into the sterile field, inspect it for any breaks in the integrity of the wrapper (Fig. 1–2). If the wrapper has a hole (no matter how small), a tear, or a break in the integrity of the seal or if the wrapper is wet or the sterilization indicator is missing or has not turned color, the item is NOT considered sterile and CANNOT be used.
- Store sterile items in a clean, dry area. Sterile items should NOT be stored in a dirty work area or with unsterile items. They should NOT be stored under sinks or any place they may be exposed to moisture.
- Once scrubbed and properly attired, sterile personnel should remain within the immediate area of the sterile field. Sterile personnel should NOT leave the sterile field or the room to retrieve items; needed items should be brought to them by nonsterile personnel. The farther sterile personnel move away from the sterile field, the greater the chance of contamination.

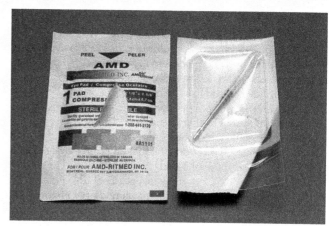

FIGURE 1–2 These items should NOT be used.

## Principles and Guidelines of Aseptic Technique—cont'd

- If sterile personnel must change positions during the procedure, they must move around each other either by moving front to front or back-to-back. The unsterile back of one person's gown should NOT be facing the sterile front of the other person.
- Nonsterile personnel should NOT walk between two sterile surfaces (e.g., the circulating nurse should not walk between two sterile tables that are next to each other).
- Nonsterile personnel should NOT reach over the sterile field to deliver an item to the sterile field. The item should be flipped onto the field from the package, or the open package presented to the scrub person so that he or she can retrieve the item without contamination.
- When pouring solutions into basins on the sterile field, the nonsterile person should pour slowly to minimize splash onto the sterile field. Unless the drape is impervious, moisture can draw microbes up from the unsterile surface (it acts as a "wick"). This is known as strike-through contamination.
- Basins, graduates, or medication cups should be held outward by the scrub person or placed at the edge of the table (Fig. 1–3) to receive fluids or medication. This allows the nonsterile person to pour the solution without reaching over the field.

- Materials used for drapes and barriers should be strong, moisture resistant, and low linting.
- A 1-inch margin around the edge of a sterile wrapper or covering is considered unsterile. Care must be taken not to allow a sterile item to drag over the edge of the wrapper when distributing it to the sterile field (Fig. 1–4).
- When opening a sterile package, the nonsterile person should protect his or her hand underneath the wrapper to avoid having it contact the sterile item.
- If towel clips puncture the drapes, the tips of the instrument are considered contaminated. The towel clips must be left in place until the end of the procedure.
- When retrieving a sterile item from a package, the scrub person should reach straight into the package and pull the item straight upward, making sure not to touch the item on the unsterile edge of the wrapper.
- All PPE (e.g., gowns, gloves, and masks) should be properly removed at the end of the case and discarded.
- All sharps must be discarded into a puncture-proof sharps bucket in the OR at the end of the case. Sharps should NOT be transported to the dirty work room to be disposed. Transporting the sharps increases the chance that someone could get stuck or injured.
- At the beginning of the day and between each case, all furniture surfaces (including lights, tables, beds, and so on) are cleaned with a disinfectant and the floor mopped according to institutional policy. Bed padding should be lifted and cleaned underneath if there is ANY chance that blood or body fluid may have gotten under it.

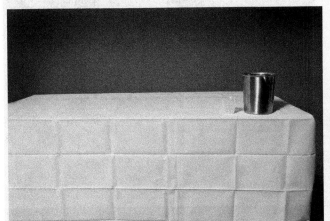

FIGURE 1–3  Place graduate and medicine cup near the edge of the table.

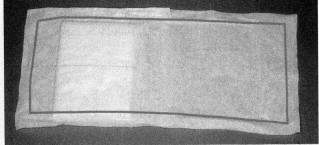

FIGURE 1–4  A 1-inch margin around the perimeter is considered to be NOT sterile.

## Opening Sterile Supplies

Opening supplies and distributing them to the sterile field is not difficult to learn, but it does require some practice. It also requires vigilance on the part of the entire surgical team. As I stated previously, there is NO compromise to sterile technique. If any item is contaminated (no matter how "minor" the contamination may seem), it must be discarded and replaced with a new one. Failure to follow strict standards of asepsis places the patient at risk!

### Opening a Pack Onto a Table

The large pack is the first thing opened when you are preparing a room for surgery (Fig. 1–5). Opening the large pack first creates a sterile field on which other sterile items can be distributed.

Before placing the large pack on the table, the outer plastic cover (i.e., dust cover) should be inspected for any tears or holes. If there are *any* tears or holes, DO NOT use the pack; get another one. Once the dust cover has been inspected, remove it and inspect the outer wrapping of the pack (Fig. 1–6). Again,

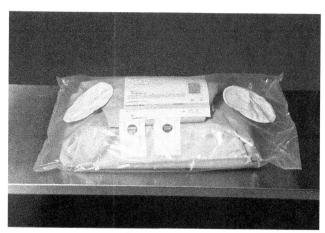

FIGURE 1-5 Large pack.

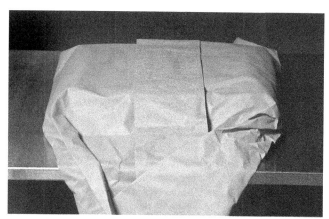

FIGURE 1-8 Pack on the table with both ends unfolded.

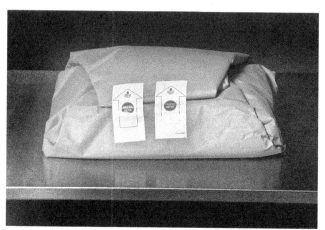

FIGURE 1-6 Pack in the middle of an instrument table.

Unfold the layers outward so that they cover the entire surface of the table. Remember: handle the layers by their edges and pull the layers toward you so that you are not reaching over the sterile area (Fig. 1–9A and B). Once the pack has been unfolded onto the table, DO NOT readjust it; only the tabletop is considered sterile, and readjusting it will bring a part of the drape that has been below tabletop level (therefore unsterile) up into the sterile field.

if there are any holes or tears, DO NOT use it. If the seal is broken, DO NOT use it: The seal should be intact until you break it.

To open a large pack, you can place it in the center of the table (it should have a label that says which side of the pack faces the back of the table). Break the seal on the pack and fold the long ends of the pack outward to cover the table (Figs. 1–7 and 1–8).

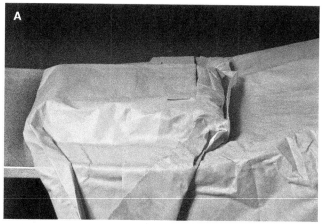

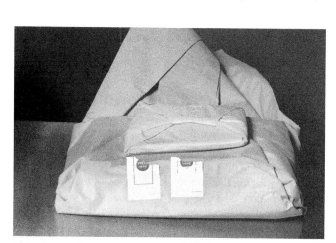

FIGURE 1-7 Pack with one end unfolded.

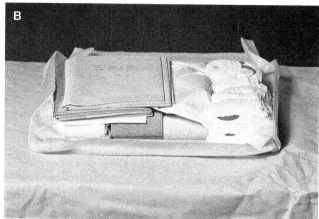

FIGURE 1-9 (A) Edge layers of the pack being unfolded. (B) The unfolded pack.

## Opening a Peel-Pouched Item

Many sterile items come in a peel pouch (Fig. 1–10). The item is placed in a pouch, the edges are sealed, and the item is put through sterile processing. The edges are sealed in such a way that when a person grabs one side of the top in each hand and pulls outward in opposing directions, the pouch peels apart, making it easy to access the item inside.

Peel-pouch items that are small (e.g., sutures and peanut sponges) can be opened and distributed to the sterile field by "flipping" them onto the field. Items that are large or awkward could potentially puncture the sterile drape if flipped onto the field (e.g., instruments) and should be opened and presented to the scrub person for him or her to take from the package (Fig. 1–11A and B).

## Opening an Envelope-Style Package

Items that come wrapped in an envelope-style package include linens, some drapes, gowns, basin sets, and some individual instruments or small instrument sets. To open this type of package, you need to grasp the package in one hand so that the flap farthest from you is opened first.

*Note:* These same steps can be used to open an envelope-wrapped instrument tray on a small table. Instead of grasping the tray in your hand, set it on the table with the first flap to be opened farthest away from you (Fig. 1–12A and B). This same method is also used to open the basin set into the ring stand.

Open the flap farthest away from you first. Pull the flap downward and away from the sterile item. If you are holding the item, secure this flap by holding it in your hand underneath the package (Fig. 1–13A and B).

Open each of the side flaps by pulling them out and downward away from the sterile item (Figs. 1–14A and B and 1–15).

Open the flap closest to the body last. Pull the flap toward your body and downward, securing it so that it does not flap back and contaminate the item (Fig. 1–16A and B). If you are holding the item, it can now either be flipped into the sterile field or presented to the scrubbed person for him or

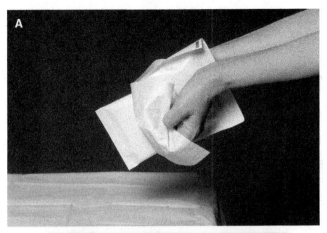

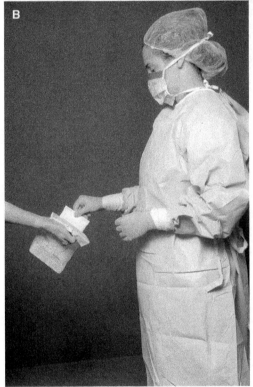

FIGURE 1–11 (A) Item is being "flipped" onto the sterile field. (B) The sterile package opened and presented to the scrub person taking the item.

her to take. If the item is on a table, the tabletop is now covered by the inside of the wrapper and is considered a sterile field. Care needs to be taken not to contaminate the tabletop.

## Opening an Instrument Pan

Some institutions assemble and sterilize their larger instrument sets inside an instrument pan. Before opening the instrument pan, look at both sides to determine the location of the handles used to open it. There should be plastic indicators on it inserted through holes in the handle system (Fig. 1–17). This ensures that the indicators will be broken when the pan is opened. DO NOT use the instrument set if *either* of the

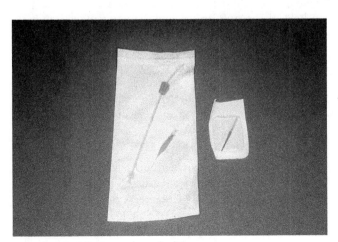

FIGURE 1–10 Two peel-pouched items.

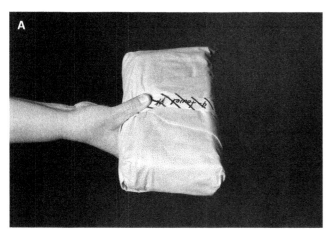

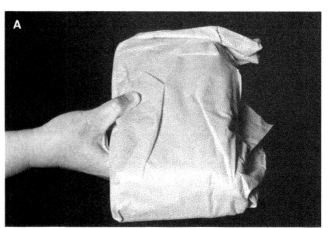

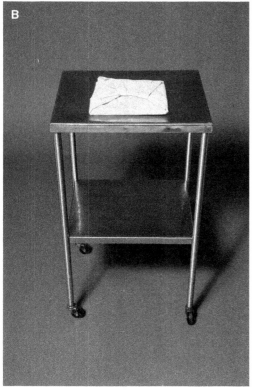

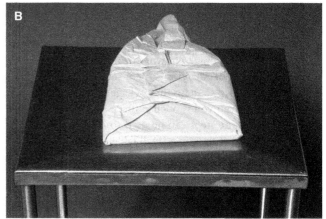

FIGURE 1–13 (A) Hand holding an item with first flap unfolded and secured. (B) Item on a table with the first flap unfolded.

FIGURE 1–12 (A) Hand grasping an envelope-style wrapped package. (B) An envelope-style package on a small table.

indicators is missing or broken or if the sterility indicators have not turned black.

Look at the top of the pan to make sure you can see a filter showing through the holes in the top of the lid. If the filter is missing, DO NOT use the instrument set.

If both indicators are present and unbroken, the sterility indicators are black, and the filter is present in the lid, insert your fingers under the handles and lift upward to break the seal and remove the lid. Remove the lid by lifting straight up and then away from the instrument pan. DO NOT reach over the inside of the pan. Once the lid has been removed, take the filter out of the lid of the tray and inspect it to make sure there are no holes in it or that it is not wet. If the filter is wet or has holes, DO NOT use the instrument set.

Look at the instrument tray inside the pan. There should be a piece of chemical indicator tape on the tray (Fig. 1–18). Look at the tape to make sure it has turned color; usually it will have black stripes on it. If the location of the tape is not obvious, the scrubbed person may have to move instruments in the tray to look for it.

If the indicator tape is present and has turned the proper color, the scrub person removes the instrument set from the pan by lifting it straight out and away from the pan. The scrub person holds the instrument set until the nonsterile person has a chance to look at the bottom of the pan to make sure that there is a filter present, that the filter is not wet and does not have any holes in it, and that the bottom of the pan does not contain water (Fig. 1–19). Once the nonsterile person is satisfied that the bottom of the pan is dry and the filter intact, the scrub person may place the instrument tray on his or her back table.

## Distributing Fluids to the Field

Fluids should only be distributed into a sterile container that is placed close to the edge of the sterile field or held in the hand of the scrub person. The nonsterile person should NOT reach over the sterile field to pour fluid into a container. Fluid should be distributed by pouring the entire container (or desired amount) all at once into the receptacle without

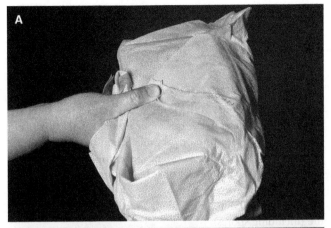

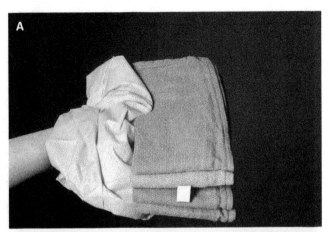

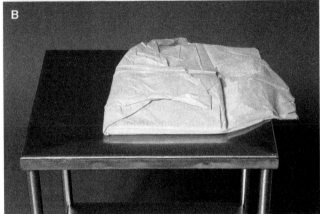

FIGURE 1-14 (A) Hand opens side flap keeping the open side flap secure. (B) Second flap opened and covering the edge of the table.

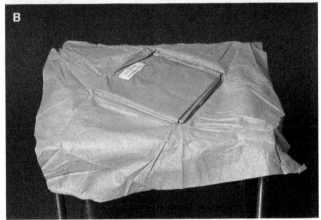

FIGURE 1-16 (A) Handheld item completely opened. (B) Completely open item on table.

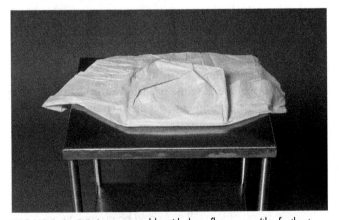

FIGURE 1-15 Item on a table with three flaps open (the farthest one and both side flaps).

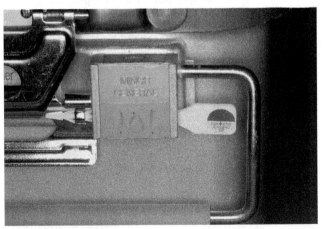

FIGURE 1-17 The sterility indicator should be black.

stopping. Care should be taken to hold the lip of the container close enough to the receptacle to avoid splashing the fluid on the field, but the lip *cannot* be so close as to touch the rim of the receptacle and contaminate it (Fig. 1–20).

*Important:* Before the distribution of any fluid onto the sterile field, the type and strength of the solution as well as the expiration date MUST be verified by BOTH the

person pouring the solution and the scrub person. BOTH parties must visualize the label as well as verbally acknowledge what is being poured into the receptacle. The scrub person must then *immediately* label the receptacle with the type and strength of fluid it contains. Unmarked fluids on the sterile field are an *unacceptable* practice because of the potential to harm the patient.

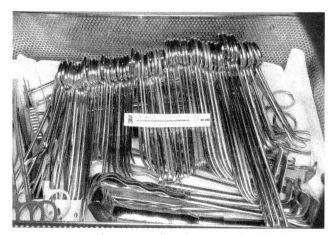

FIGURE 1-18 The stripes on the indicator tape should be black.

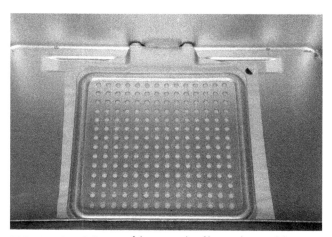

FIGURE 1-19 Bottom of the pan with a filter in place and the bottom dry.

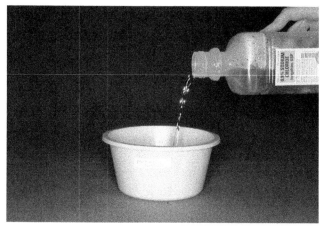

FIGURE 1-20 Saline fluid being distributed into a container.

## TYPES OF STERILIZATION

All items that are distributed to and used within the sterile field have to undergo a sterilization process before being used. There are several different methods available, all of which have the potential to render an item sterile. The method used usually depends on the item that is being sterilized. This section is an overview of the different types of sterilization processes available and when each type is used.

### Steam Sterilization

Steam under pressure is the most common and cost-effective method of sterilization but cannot be used for items that could be damaged by moisture or pressure. Steam by itself is not an effective sterilization method. The steam must be under pressure for a specific amount of time before it can render an item sterile. The pressure is used to raise the temperature of the steam up to 250°F to 270°F, high enough to kill all microbial life (including spores).

The steam sterilizer is an enclosed chamber that pressurizes the steam to specific levels. The pressure needed to raise the temperature of the steam to 250°F is 15 psig (pounds per square inch gauge). Raising it to 270°F requires a pressure of 27 psig. It is important to note that these settings are for sea level atmospheres. If your institution is located at a higher elevation, the pressure inside the chamber needs to be increased to achieve levels adequate for sterilization. Generally, this means an increase of 0.5 psig for every 1,000 feet above sea level.

There are two basic types of steam sterilizers: gravity displacement and prevacuum (also known as a dynamic air removal sterilizer). In a gravity displacement sterilization chamber, the air is pushed downward (by gravity) and out through a valve by the pressurized steam. All of the air is removed from the chamber, leaving the pressurized steam to sterilize the items. In this type of sterilizer, it is important that items be loaded properly, because improperly placed items can trap air, which will act as an insulator against the steam. Any items in these air pockets will not be sterile. Minimum exposure time (at 250°F) depends on the items in the load and can vary from 15 to 45 minutes or more. These times do not include the time needed for the chamber to fill with steam, for the chamber to get up to temperature, and for

> **WATCH OUT!**   Sterilization and Bioburden
>
> - Bioburden is any blood, tissue, or body fluid (e.g., pus, vomit, feces, or skin oil) that could be present on an instrument or item.
> - ALL bioburden MUST be removed before placing an item in the sterilizer either to flash it or to send it through a full cycle. Bioburden may be removed by washing all visible contaminants from the instrument as well as by sending the instrument through a washer.
> - If you open a tray and there is blood or dirt on an instrument, DO NOT use it! There is NO such thing as "sterile blood" or any other "sterile contaminant!" Sterilants cannot penetrate bioburden; therefore, the area under the bioburden is NOT sterile.

the chamber to cooldown after exposure to the steam. The complete sterilization cycle is about 2 hours, which must be considered in turnaround time for items needed for subsequent cases.

The prevacuum sterilizer does not rely on gravity to remove the air. In the prevacuum sterilizer, the air is pulled out of the chamber using a built-in vacuum, which enables a greater steam penetration in a shorter period of time. Prevacuum sterilizers operate at 270°F, and the exposure times are much shorter than those required by gravity displacement sterilizers. The minimum exposure for most items in a prevacuum sterilizer is 3 to 4 minutes. Again, this does not take into account the time for the air to leave the chamber or to cool down at the end; planning ahead is essential for items needed for subsequent cases.

## Immediate Use Sterilization

Immediate use sterilizers are used in the OR to quickly resterilize an item that has become contaminated but is needed to finish the surgical procedure (Fig. 1–21). This type of sterilization should *only* be used when there is no other alternative. Before using this method, make sure there is not another of the same item available that is already sterile (e.g., in a rack or cabinet of peel-pouched items or from central sterile supply). Items that are to be sterilized using this method are unwrapped and *must* be washed (and free of visible bioburden) before they are placed in the sterilizer. The item or items should be placed in a pan with a mesh-type bottom to allow for the steam to reach all surfaces. A piece of indicator tape must be placed in the pan with every load. Failure to include the indicator tape means that there will be no visible monitor to indicate that proper sterilization conditions occurred; therefore, the item cannot be used and the cycle would need to run again.

Immediate use sterilizers heat the steam to 270°F to 275°F. The minimum exposure time in a gravity displacement flash sterilizer for metal items without a lumen is 3 minutes and for items with a lumen is 10 minutes. Minimum exposure times for prevacuum flash sterilizers are 3 minutes for metal items without a lumen and 4 minutes for items with a lumen or those that are porous. Remember the complete cycle is longer, usually 10 to 20 minutes.

## Cold Chemical Sterilization

The most common form of cold chemical sterilization used in the OR is peracetic acid (Steris system; Fig. 1–22). This method of sterilization provides chemical irrigation of the item for 30 to 45 minutes at temperatures of 122°F to 133°F. This method can be used only for items that can be fully immersed in fluid (e.g., some cameras, scopes, and cords).

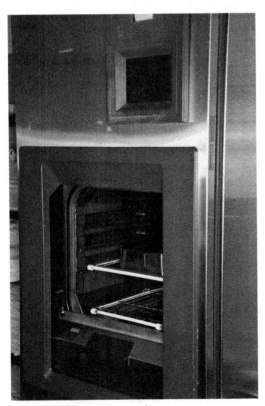

FIGURE 1–21 Immediate use sterilizer.

> ### A Few More Guidelines for Immediate Use (Flash) Sterilization
>
> - Cameras, scopes, power equipment, or other delicate items should NOT be flash sterilized unless you have thoroughly read the manufacturer's instructions and found that they indicate it is safe to do so.
> - Implants should NEVER be flash sterilized. IF you HAVE NO OTHER CHOICE in an emergency, a rapid read-out biological monitoring device (not a piece of indicator tape) must be placed in the pan with the implant.
> - Immediate use sterilizers need to be located in an area outside the OR room but close to the doorway so that items can be quickly and directly transported to the sterile field.
> - Items to be sterilized are unwrapped unless the manufacturer's instructions indicate otherwise.

> ### WATCH OUT!   Handling of Chemical Sterilants
>
> - When handling the sterilant chemicals used in the Steris machine, remember that the sterilant contains 35% peracetic acid, which can cause severe burns and blindness if it comes into contact with unprotected skin or eyes. Personal protective attire such as eyewear, gloves, and long sleeves (gown or jacket) should be worn when removing the cup from the package and placing it into the machine. The same attire should be worn when removing the used cup from the machine at the end of the cycle.

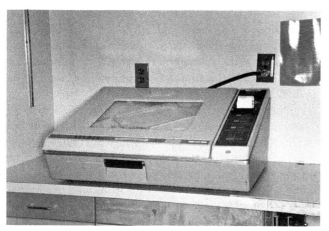

FIGURE 1–22 Steris machine.

Manufacturer's instructions for use of the Steris system must be followed to ensure that the items are properly sterilized. All items must be cleaned, and all visible bioburden removed before being placed in the Steris pan. A special chemical indicator and a sterilant containing 35% peracetic acid must be placed inside the pan with every load that is run. When the load has finished its cycle, the indicator must be checked before the items are placed on the sterile field. The items must be used immediately after processing and should not be stored for later use (sterility cannot be ensured with storage).

Another cold chemical that can be used to sterilize immersible items is glutaraldehyde (Cidex or Cidex OPA). The problem with using glutaraldehyde as a sterilant is that, for an item to be deemed sterile, it must be soaked for about 10 hours in the solution (Fig. 1–23). This long soaking time makes it impractical to use in most cases in the OR. It is, however, used as a high-level disinfectant for endoscopes. *Caution:* Before placing any scope in the solution, make sure it is *clean* and *dry*. Any bioburden or water left on the item can negatively affect the concentration of the solution, rendering it less effective.

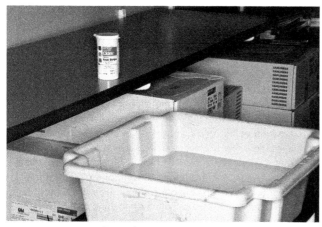

FIGURE 1–23 Cidex soaking tub.

## Gas Plasma Sterilization

Gas plasma sterilization uses low-temperature hydrogen peroxide gas plasma technology. Items that are heat or moisture sensitive can be safely sterilized using gas plasma.

Gas plasma technology came about as an alternative to ethylene oxide (EO) sterilization, which is discussed in the following section. The by-products of gas plasma sterilization are oxygen and water, making it safer to use than EO sterilization. There is no exposure to hazardous materials. This system does not require aeration or ventilation procedures; therefore, the cycle time is shorter than with EO (1 hour for gas plasma versus up to 24 hours for EO). Gas plasma does have some limitations; it cannot sterilize linens, liquids, and cellulose. With some of the Sterrad systems, there may be limits on the length and diameter of lumened instruments that can be effectively sterilized. *Always* refer to manufacturer's instructions before sterilizing any equipment or supplies.

## Ethylene Oxide (Gas) Sterilization

Ethylene oxide is a flammable, toxic liquid that is combined with inert gas to produce sterilization. This type of sterilization is used for delicate items (i.e., those that cannot withstand heat, pressure, or moisture). EO penetrates wrappers and other materials that other sterilization methods may not. As with all sterilization methods, items must be thoroughly cleaned before sterilization.

The main disadvantage to EO is the toxicity. Any sterile processing center that uses EO must have devices throughout the area that monitor for leaks or unsafe levels of EO. If a leak is detected, the area must be evacuated and a hazardous materials team called to deal with the problem. Exposure to EO has been associated with leukemia, respiratory damage, possible birth defects, and neurological damage.

Items that have been sterilized with EO must be aerated to rid them of any residual gas. Aeration time varies item to item and can be anywhere from 2 to 32 hours.

The long cycle time and the toxicity of the gas, as well as the expense of monitoring and maintaining the system, are causing some institutions to stop using EO sterilization completely and replace it with gas plasma systems.

## Radiation Sterilization

The use of ionized radiation to sterilize equipment and supplies is extremely expensive. Medical device manufacturers are the primary users of radiation sterilization. This type of sterilization has strict guidelines and standards that must be followed to ensure the safety of personnel as well as the sterility of items.

## OPERATING ROOM ATTIRE

When you work in the OR you are asked to surrender your street clothes and wear special attire. The purpose of this attire is threefold:

1. To protect the patient and OR from contamination that you could have brought in on your street clothes

2. To contain any of your body's shedding skin or hair
3. To protect you from contact with body fluids or soil

The basic OR attire consists of a scrub suit, mask, hat or cap, eye protection, and, in some instances, shoe covers. The circulator or other nonscrubbed personnel also may wear a cover jacket. Additional attire for scrubbed personnel includes sterile gown and sterile gloves.

Although institutional policies may vary, it is recommended that OR personnel wear only attire that has been laundered at a hospital (or institution), not attire laundered at home. Institutional laundering of scrub attire helps ensure that it has been subjected to consistent and specialized cleaning standards that aid in keeping bacterial counts low.

Scrub attire should be stored in clean, enclosed carts or cabinets that are disinfected regularly or in vending machines. They should NOT be stored in lockers that contain personal items from the outside, as this increases the chances of contamination.

*Note:* It is a recommended practice that NO jewelry be worn in the OR unless it is completely contained within the scrub suit (institutional policies may vary). Jewelry has been found to harbor microorganisms, making it a potential source of contamination. Earrings or necklaces that are not fully contained under the scrub attire could come loose and fall into the surgical field or the wound. Jewelry could become contaminated with blood or other particles and pose a risk to personnel wearing it or others who contact it.

## Scrub Suit

Most scrub suits consist of a top and pair of pants (Fig. 1–24), although some institutions also offer the option to wear scrub

dresses. This attire is made of lint-free material that can stand up to the rigors of institutional laundering.

Scrub suits should be close fitting to keep the material from "blousing" out, which could contaminate the sterile field, but they should not be so tight that they produce chafing or are offensive to others. Tunic-style tops should be tucked into the pants to avoid potentially contaminating the field by hanging loose. If the pants have drawstrings at the top, the strings should be tucked into the pants to avoid any potential contact with sterile items.

Scrub suits should be changed daily or whenever they become contaminated with blood or body fluids (including excess perspiration). Institutional policy also may dictate that they be changed following certain isolation cases (e.g., methicillin-resistant *Staphylococcus aureus*); be sure to know the policies of your OR.

## Masks

Masks are worn to protect the operative area from the airborne contamination that everyone generates when they breathe, talk, cough, or sneeze. Masks are worn whenever you enter a restricted area of the OR suite, when you are near a scrub sink where personnel are scrubbing in preparation for entering the sterile field, or when you are in an area where sterile instruments are processed and stored. Institutional policies vary about which areas of the OR suite are "restricted"; it is imperative to know the layout and policies of your OR.

An additional function of a surgical mask is to protect the wearer from any spraying blood, body fluids, and pieces of matter during the surgical procedure. The mask must be worn properly in order to do its job correctly—namely, block droplets and filter the air. The mask should cover *both* the mouth and nose because both are potential sources of airborne contamination. It should fit snugly, and the wearer should mold the pliable insert over the bridge of the nose to ensure a good fit. The ties should be tied at the top of the head and around the back of the neck to prevent unfiltered breath from escaping out the sides. The mask should be worn correctly or taken off and discarded; it should not be worn dangling around the neck. Masks should be changed *after each case.* The mask should be removed by handling it by the strings, not the face part (this is the most contaminated part of the mask and therefore handling it should be avoided). Hands should be washed after removing the mask and disposing of it in the trash.

Masks come in several styles (Fig. 1–25A and B), including those that have a built-in face shield to protect the eyes from splash. There are special masks that need to be worn during procedures that involve the use of lasers (Fig. 1–26). Laser use produces smaller particles when it destroys tissue cells, thus necessitating the use of a higher filtration mask (particle filtration of 0.1 μm) to protect the wearer from possibly inhaling these smaller particles. Some institutions recommend or require the use of a laser mask for specific procedures (e.g., electrosurgical removal of condylomata).

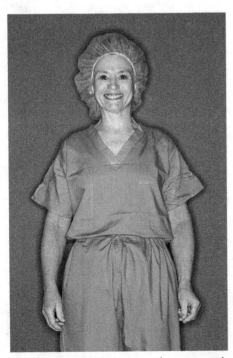

FIGURE 1-24 Operating room personnel wearing scrub attire— shirt and drawstrings tucked inside the pants and cap on.

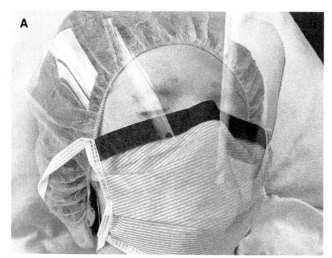

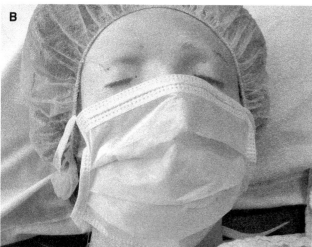

FIGURE 1-25 (A) Fluid shield mask. (B) Regular mask.

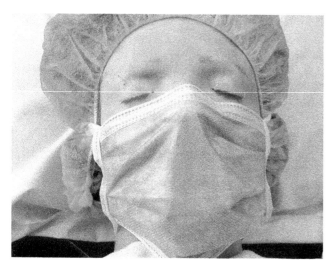

FIGURE 1-26 Laser mask.

## Hats and Caps

A hat or cap that covers the hair and scalp must be worn in the restricted and semirestricted areas of the OR. The purpose of the hat is to reduce contamination from hair or dander. There

are several styles of cap or hat (Fig. 1–27A and B) that can be worn, but the important thing is that it completely covers the hair and scalp.

Operating room hats are made of disposable, lint-free material. They should be changed daily or when they become grossly contaminated or wet. Some institutions allow the wearing of individual cloth hats or caps in the OR, but others do not. This is an institutional decision; you need to check the policies of your OR before assuming it is acceptable to wear a cloth cap or hat. Cloth caps should be placed in the hospital laundry at the end of the day (or if grossly contaminated) to be cleaned; a cap that is worn for multiple days without being laundered is a source of contamination.

Recommended practices state that the cap or hat should be put on before donning your scrub suit to help prevent shedding of hair and dander onto clean scrub attire.

## Eye Protection

The personnel who are required to wear eye protection varies by institutional policy. Some institutions require *everyone* in the OR to wear eye protection during a procedure, but others may require only scrubbed personnel to wear eye protection and nonscrubbed personnel to don it only when there is

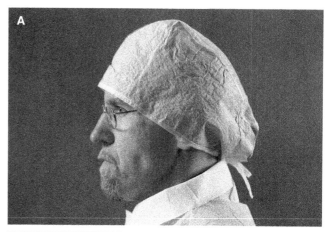

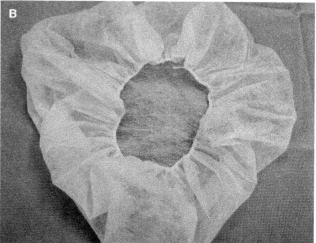

FIGURE 1-27 (A) Cap. (B) Hat.

a chance they could contact blood, body fluid, or tissue. Make sure to check your institution's policy regarding the wearing of eye protection.

Eye protection (Fig. 1–28) must cover the eyes from the top of the eyebrows to the top of the surgical mask and wrap around the sides of the face along the temples. (Covering the temples protects the eyes from splash or tissue coming in around the sides.) Regular eyeglasses DO NOT meet standards for eye protection because they do not provide protection along the sides of the eyes. In order to make eyeglasses meet the requirements, eye shields made for this purpose can be purchased and attached to them. Goggles and surgical masks with face shields are other acceptable types of eye protection. The type of eye protection that one wears depends on personal preference, comfort, ability to see to perform duties, availability, and cost.

## Cover Jacket

Nonscrubbed personnel may choose to wear a cover jacket or "scrub jacket" (Fig. 1–29). The jackets should be close fitting, with the front buttoned or snapped closed. Jackets that are very loose or are flapping open in the front may pose a contamination risk by brushing up against sterile items. Jackets should be made of material that does not shed (e.g., in most places, fleece jackets are not acceptable because they shed fibers, thus increasing contamination). There are currently no recommendations for the wearing of a long-sleeved jacket except during the performance of preoperative skin antisepsis. Check your institutional policy before you assume it is acceptable to wear a jacket.

## Shoe Covers

Institutional policy varies on the wearing of shoe covers. Even if your institution does not require you to wear shoe covers, you may want to consider doing so, especially during procedures when there is a high likelihood of your shoes becoming wet (e.g., arthroscopy or cesarean section). The covers help to protect your shoes, socks, and feet from becoming contaminated

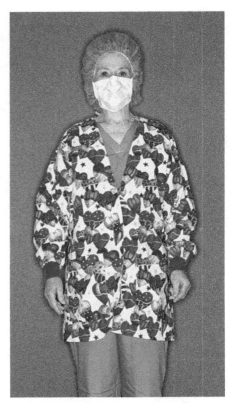

FIGURE 1–29 Scrub jacket.

with water, blood, and body fluids. If you wear shoe covers, they need to be changed daily or when they become soiled, torn, or wet. They must be removed when you are leaving the OR area.

Shoe covers are available in two lengths (Fig. 1–30A and B). One length comes up to the ankle and covers the foot and shoe. This length is worn in most cases. The second length extends up the leg to the knees. This longer length is worn during arthroscopies and other surgeries in which there is a potential for a large amount of water and body fluid to make its way onto the floor.

## Nonsterile Gloves

Although not necessarily considered part of OR attire, nonsterile gloves are an important part of personal protective attire. These gloves are worn by nonsterile personnel whenever there is any chance of contact with blood, body fluids, or tissues (e.g., handling specimens or specimen containers, performing intubation, handling soiled linen or instruments). Gloves must be worn by all personnel when cleaning the room between cases.

After you use the gloves, discard them in the trash (being careful not to touch the contaminated part with your bare skin) and wash your hands. Gloves are not impervious to all contaminants; therefore, wearing gloves does not mean that your hands are clean after you remove the gloves. *Wearing gloves is NOT a substitute for handwashing!*

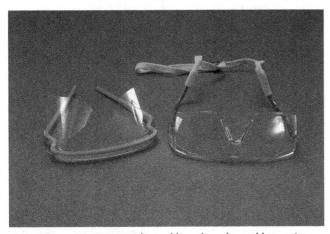

FIGURE 1–28 Eyewear (disposable and nondisposable types).

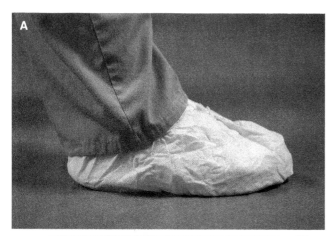

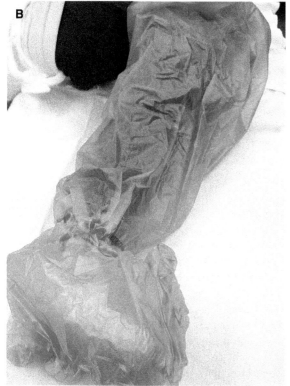

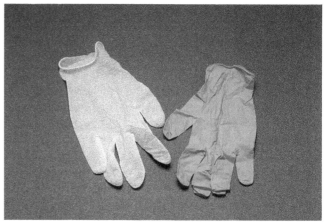

FIGURE 1–31 Nonsterile gloves.

FIGURE 1–30 (A) Short shoe cover. (B) Long shoe cover.

Nonsterile gloves are available in sizes small, medium, large, and extra large (Fig. 1–31). They are made from latex and non-latex materials. Many institutions have switched to nonlatex gloves to lessen health-care workers' exposure to latex.

## X-Ray Gowns (Lead)

Another piece of attire that OR personnel are required to wear during certain procedures is a lead apron (also referred to as a *lead gown*). The apron should have an attached thyroid shield. If the thyroid shield is not attached to the gown, then a separate thyroid shield should be used. The lead apron and thyroid shield are put on over the scrubs but underneath the sterile gown of scrubbed personnel. They are also put on over the scrubs of nonsterile personnel.

The lead apron is used whenever personnel are going to be exposed to radiation (i.e., x-rays or fluoroscopy) during the procedure. There are several styles of lead aprons: one and two piece (vest and skirt), those that completely wrap around the body, and those that cover only the person's front and sides. Which style you choose depends on the procedure being done and the type of x-ray machinery being used. For example, the lead aprons worn when the mini C-arm is being used have a thinner lead lining because exposure to radiation is minimal. These aprons cannot be used when other types of x-ray machinery are in use because they do not offer enough protection.

Whenever possible, lead shields or aprons and thyroid shields are placed on the patient to protect the reproductive organs and thyroid from radiation exposure.

## Sterile Attire

Sterile attire is worn by scrubbed personnel during the surgical procedure. Sterile attire consists of sterile gown and gloves. Some institutions may require that sterile hoods be worn during joint replacement surgery.

Sterile Gown: The sterile gown is designed to cover the body of the scrubbed person from the base of the neck to below the knees. This provides a sterile barrier between the person's unsterile scrub attire and the sterile field.

The gown is only sterile if the integrity of the package is not compromised. If the package has a hole, is torn, or is wet or if the package seal is compromised, the gown is no longer sterile and must be discarded.

Once donned, the only parts of the gown that are considered sterile are the front of the gown from the waist up to midchest level, and the sleeves up to 2 inches above the elbow. The stockinette sleeve cuffs are NOT considered sterile because they are not impervious; therefore, the sleeve cuffs must be completely covered by the cuff of the sterile gloves at all times. The reason that only these limited areas are considered sterile is because they are the only parts of the gown that

## Guidelines for the Care of Lead Aprons

- Before use, lead aprons should be checked to make sure they are not cracked or torn. Cracks or tears can compromise the integrity of the shield and decrease its effectiveness.
- Lead aprons should be hung up on appropriate hangers when not in use; they should not be folded or heaped in piles (Fig. 1–32A and B).

- Lead aprons should be x-rayed at least yearly to check for breaks in the integrity of the lead.

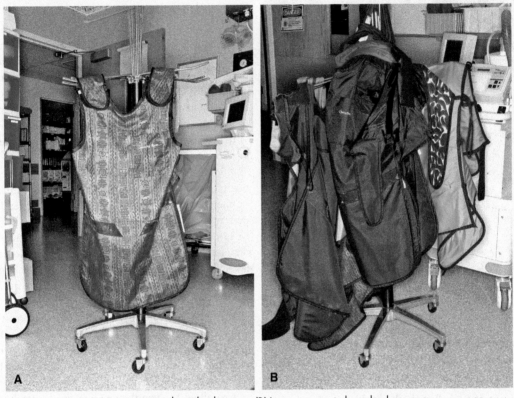

**FIGURE 1–32** (A) Proper way to hang lead aprons. (B) Improper way to hang lead aprons.

the scrubbed person can see and therefore ensure that they have not been inadvertently contaminated.

Sterile gowns are available in cloth or paper (Fig. 1–33). Which type of gown a person uses is based on personal preference and availability. Most gowns are available in sizes large and extra large, and some styles are available in sizes up to triple extra large.

**Sterile Gloves:** Sterile gloves have been specially processed to render them microbe free. They come in sealed packages, the inside of which is considered sterile (except for a 1-inch margin around the edges). Sterile gloves can be made of latex or nonlatex material (Fig. 1–34A and B). They come in half sizes, generally ranging from size 5½ to 9. Most sterile gloves are now powder free, but special care must be taken if your institution is still using powdered gloves.

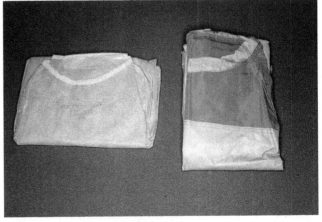

**FIGURE 1–33** Paper and cloth gowns.

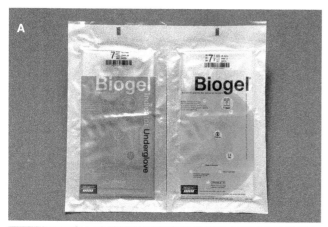

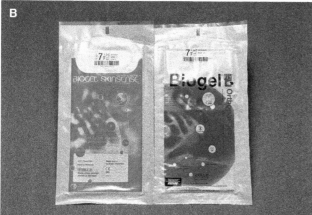

FIGURE 1–34 (A) Latex glove package. (B) Nonlatex glove package.

It is generally recommended that scrubbed personnel double glove—that is, *put on a colored underglove and top it with an outer glove. Double gloving provides many advantages:*

- In the event of a needlestick, the health-care provider is exposed to less contamination from the needle. It has been shown that fewer microbes are left on the needle point after puncturing through two layers; microbes are wiped off as the needle passes through each layer.
- If the scrubbed person touches a contaminated instrument or tray or the patient's unprepped skin, only the outer glove(s) need to be changed. The scrub person can change the outer glove(s) him- or herself without waiting for assistance.
- Wearing a pair of colored undergloves has been shown to make it easier to detect a hole in the outer gloves. The outer gloves can be changed immediately, thus decreasing chances of contamination through an unnoticed hole.
- If the outer gloves become torn or have a hole, there is still a protective barrier between the patient and the scrub person. The patient is not accidently exposed to microbes from the scrub person's skin, and the scrub person is not exposed to blood or body fluid from the patient.

## Guidelines for Powdered Gloves

- Gloves that contain powder have the potential to cause adhesions at the surgical site. Powdered sterile gloves should be rinsed in sterile saline or wiped with a sterile saline-soaked sponge before beginning surgery.
- Discard the sponge used to wipe the gloves into the kick bucket or other proper sponge receptacle.

What size glove combination a person wears is a matter of personal preference and comfort. Each person should try a different combination of glove sizes for both inner and outer gloves until a combination is found that allows for the performance of duties without restriction on the nerves or blood flow. *Hint:* If you get numb fingers, try an inner glove that is ½ to 1 size larger. If you still have problems, increase the outer glove size.

Gloves come in a variety of materials: heavier for "orthopedic" gloves, softer for those with sensitive skin, and latex and nonlatex material. The type of glove used depends on personal preference and patient and personnel allergy history. Whether or not you can use latex gloves and when they can be used depend on institutional policy. Some ORs are latex free, and latex gloves are not allowed at all. Make sure you know your institution's policy regarding the use of latex gloves.

Sterile Space Suit: The so-named sterile space suit consists of a regular sterile gown and a sterile hood that completely covers the head and face (Fig. 1–35). The hood has a convex clear full-face shield and resembles a hood used by astronauts. The hood has a self-contained, battery-operated fan in the top to allow for ventilation. The fan is attached to a plastic headpiece that is placed on the scrub personnel's head before scrubbing. The battery pack is worn on the person's waistband.

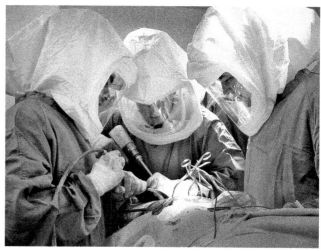

FIGURE 1–35 Sterile space suit hood. © imageofsurgery.com

The sterile hood is placed over the plastic frame when the person gowns and gloves.

This type of attire is required in some institutions during total joint replacement surgery. The theory behind this attire is that it cuts down on contamination from respiratory droplets and uncovered hair.

## NATIONAL "TIME OUT"

Unfortunately, mistakes involving surgical procedures can and have happened. Some of the most common but most preventable mistakes involve misidentification of patients and wrong site or type of surgery. To prevent these types of errors, institutions have implemented "time out" protocols that must be done *before* any invasive procedure is performed. The Association of Surgical Technologists (AST) has developed the *Standards of Practice for Patient Identification, Correct Surgery Site and Correct Surgical Procedure,* which is outlined here:

1. "The patient should have at least two corroborating patient identifiers as evidence to confirm identity."

The following are deemed acceptable identifiers by AST standards; please check your institutional policy for acceptable identifiers.

- Name
- Date of birth
- Telephone number (not generally used as it could change)
- Assigned identification number
- Social Security number
- Address (not generally used as it could change)
- Photograph

NEVER use the room number as a patient identifier because patients are often moved to different rooms. The two most commonly used identifiers are the patient's full name (NOT just first or last) and date of birth.

2. "All patients undergoing a surgical procedure should wear an identifying marker."

Wrist bands with complete, correct information should be on all patients undergoing surgical procedures.

3. "All patients undergoing a surgical procedure must be properly identified by the surgical team members before transporting the patient to the surgery department."

It is recommended that confirmation of the patient's identity takes place:

- When the surgery is scheduled
- When the patient is admitted to the health-care facility
- Any time the patient is transferred to another caregiver
- Before sedation
- Before the patient goes into the operating room

4. "Verifying the correct surgical procedure and site is the responsibility of the surgical team members."

Methods of confirmation should include but are not limited to:

- Oral confirmation
- The patient's identification marker (wrist band)
- The surgery schedule
- The patient's chart (consent, history, and physical)
- The marking of the surgical site (by the surgeon and the patient, if possible). The mark must be placed so it will be visible after placement of the drapes. The marking must be done with the patient alert, oriented, and able to indicate the surgery site. Use a permanent marker that will *not* wash off with surgical prepping

5. "Before the start of any surgical procedure, a 'time out' should be completed to verify the correct patient, correct surgical procedure, and correct surgical site."

The time out serves as a final confirmation of the correct patient, procedure, and site. It should be performed according to hospital policy just before the surgeon makes the first skin incision.

REMEMBER: The "time out" is done to improve patient safety and cut down on preventable medical errors. It is the responsibility of *every* team member to make sure that the correct policy is followed. This is NOT a step that can be skipped or glossed over.

6. In order to ensure that the correct procedure is followed for each and every patient undergoing any invasive procedure, the institution should have a standardized checklist that is followed and properly documented.

## HAND HYGIENE

Proper hand hygiene has always been a hot topic in health care but even more so because of the COVID-19 pandemic. Although hand washing may seem a simple and basic part of life, studies have shown that it is often forgotten in the busy and stressful health-care environment. This is one procedure that cannot be ignored for the safety of our patients, ourselves, and others.

Following are some generally accepted times when staff should perform hand hygiene. Please check your institution's policy for any additional institutional requirements.

- After being exposed to blood or body fluids
- After using the restroom
- When hands are visibly soiled
- When caring for patients with spore-forming organisms (e.g., *Clostridium difficile, Bacillus anthracis*) or norovirus
- Before and after touching a patient
- After touching an inanimate object that is possibly contaminated

■ Upon entering or exiting the room
■ Before donning or after removing gloves
■ Before or after eating

Each institution's infection control department should issue written procedures for hand hygiene, including proper hand washing. Although an institution's procedure may vary, here are some general guidelines for proper hand washing (adapted from the AORN Standard of Hand Hygiene and Centers for Disease Control [CDC] Standard for Hand Washing).

■ Remove all jewelry from the hands and wrist.
■ Wet the hands thoroughly with warm (not hot) water.
■ Apply the amount of soap needed to cover all surfaces of the hands.

■ Rub hands together covering all surfaces of the hands and fingers for at least 20 seconds.
■ Rinse with water to remove all soap.
■ Dry hands thoroughly with a disposable paper towel.
■ When hand-free controls are not available on the sink, use a clean paper towel to turn off the water to avoid contaminating your clean hands.

Alcohol-based hand rub may be used as a substitute for soap and water in certain circumstances, such as when the hands are NOT visibly soiled or dirty. In these circumstances, apply the hand rub following the manufacturer's instructions and your institution's hand hygiene policies.

 **Surgical Session Review**

1) All of the following statements are true about masks *except:*
   a. They should be changed after each case
   b. They help to protect the wearer from blood spray and other body fluids
   c. They have to be worn in unrestricted areas of the OR
   d. They must be worn so that they cover the mouth and the nose

2) Which of the following statements is *false* regarding OR attire?
   a. Caps or hats must cover the hair and scalp
   b. Cloth caps or hats can be worn for 3 consecutive days without laundering
   c. Tunic-style scrub tops should be tucked into scrub pants
   d. Regular eyeglasses alone do not meet the standards for protective eyewear

3) Unsterile personnel should stand a minimum of _____ inches from the sterile field.
   a. 8
   b. 12
   c. 20
   d. 24

4) Principles of aseptic technique include:
   a. Talking is kept to a minimum at the field
   b. Only sterile (scrubbed) personnel handle sterile items
   c. Creating the sterile field as close to the time of surgery as possible
   d. All of the above

5) All of the following are true about sterile drapes *except:*
   a. They should be made of a low-linting material
   b. Once in place, they should not be moved
   c. Handling should be kept to a minimum
   d. The part of the drape that falls below the level of the tabletop is sterile

6) Surgical conscience is the:
   a. Legal motivation to practice proper aseptic technique
   b. Ethical motivation to practice proper aseptic technique
   c. Institutional policies governing the practice of proper aseptic technique
   d. Financial motivation to practice proper aseptic technique

7) Asepsis means:
   a. Absence of all viruses
   b. Absence of all bacteria
   c. Absence of all flagella
   d. Absence of all microbes

8) Which of the following is considered sterile on a sterile gown?
   a. The stockinette cuffs
   b. The back
   c. The front between the waist and midchest
   d. The entire front of the gown

9) If scrubbed (sterile) personnel need to change positions during surgery, they must move:
   a. Back to side
   b. Side to side
   c. Front to side
   d. Back-to-back

10) A _____-inch perimeter around an open peel pack is NOT considered sterile.
    a. ½
    b. 1
    c. 1½
    d. 2

11) Immediate use sterilizers use _____ to render sterilized instruments.
    a. Steam
    b. Cold chemicals
    c. Radiation
    d. Gas

12) You may be asked to wear a "sterile space suit" for which type of surgery?
    a. Exploratory laparotomy
    b. Shoulder arthroscopy
    c. Total joint replacement
    d. Endoscopic abdominal aortic aneurysm repair

13) Which of the following is an example of an acceptable patient identifier?
    a. Mr. Jones
    b. Room 213
    c. Robert R. Jones
    d. May 20

14) Who can ask for a "time out" to be done before skin incision?
    a. The circulator
    b. The surgeon
    c. The surgical technologist
    d. Any of the above

15) Gas plasma sterilization uses _____ gas plasma technology.
    a. Hydrogen peroxide
    b. Ethylene oxide
    c. Hydrogen sulfide
    d. Ethylene sulfide

16) After applying soap to your hands during hand washing, hands should be rubbed together, covering all surfaces for at least _____ seconds.
    a. 10
    b. 20
    c. 30
    d. 45

17) The surgical technologist just finished eating his/her lunch. What does he/she need to do before they go to the scrub sink to prepare to go back into the OR?
    a. Brush their teeth
    b. Comb their hair
    c. Wash their hands
    d. Put on a clean scrub suit

18) While setting up for a case, the surgical technologist bumps the back table and a couple of lap pads fall onto the floor. They are in the room by themselves. Count has already been done. What should he/she do?
    a. Pick them up and put them back on the table
    b. Pick them up, walk across the room, and place them on the counter
    c. Pick them up and toss them in the trash
    d. Leave them, and when the circulator returns, ask him/her to pick them up and place them in the sponge collection bag so they can be included in the count later

# 2 Common Equipment and Supplies

## OPERATING ROOM TABLE

The operating room (OR) table (also referred to as the OR bed) is the central focal point of the OR suite. It is the most important piece of furniture in the room; this is where the patient is placed and the procedure takes place. The table is located near the center of the room so that there is enough room to move equipment, instrument tables, and personnel around the patient on both sides and at the bottom. The head of the bed is reserved for anesthesia personnel, supplies, and machinery.

Operating tables come in a variety of styles. Most tables are electrical and are operated using remote controls (Fig. 2–1), although you may still occasionally run into an older table that operates by manually turning the cranks.

**WATCH OUT!** Operating Room Table Weight Limits

It is imperative that you know the weight limit of the OR table you are using BEFORE placing the patient on it. Failure to use the proper table for large patients could result in severe injury to the patient or staff.

As with any piece of medical equipment, it is important to know how to use the OR table in the room to which you are assigned (Fig. 2–2). Make sure you know the manufacturer's instructions for table use. All personnel should receive instruction on the tables in use at their institution as part of their orientation as well as when any new table is purchased. Failure to be familiar with proper use of the table use could result in surgery delays, increased anesthesia time for the patient (while personnel try to figure out how to work the bed during a procedure), or injury to the patient or staff.

### Parts of an Operating Room Table

**Headpiece (Head Plate):** The headpiece is a removable padded section attached to the head of the bed (usually with metal rods or bars). This section can be adjusted up or down to aid in airway maintenance. The headpiece can be removed to allow for attachment of other headrests such as a Mayfield headrest (neurosurgery) or a horseshoe headrest. The headpiece also can be removed and placed at the bottom of the table for some gynecological procedures.

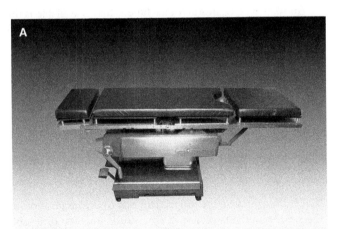

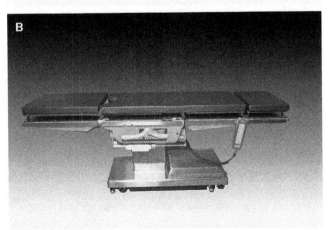

FIGURE 2–1 (A) Manual operating room (OR) table. (B) Electric OR table.

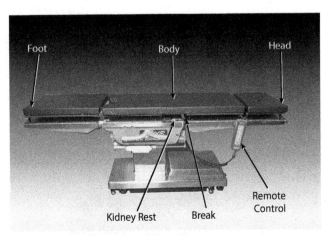

FIGURE 2–2 Operating room table parts.

**Body (Back Plate and Seat Plate):** The body of the table usually consists of two padded pieces with a "break" in between them. The break allows for each piece to be flexed or extended independently for patient positioning (e.g., Fowler's or sitting position). There is a metal bar in the break area that can be moved up and down. This bar is known as a *kidney rest* or *kidney break* and is used to elevate the flank area for better exposure during renal procedures.

**Footpiece (Foot Plate):** The footpiece or bottom of the bed is a padded removable section where the patient's lower legs and feet rest. The footpiece can be flexed or extended independently of the rest of the bed for patient positioning, or it can be moved out of the way during vaginal procedures.

## Operating Table Attachments

**Headrest Attachments:** The Mayfield attachment (Fig. 2–3) is used for some craniotomy procedures. The Mayfield generally is used to hold the horseshoe attachment or tong attachment (Fig. 2–4).

As its name implies, the horseshoe headrest is shaped like a horseshoe (Fig. 2–5). This headrest can be used to support

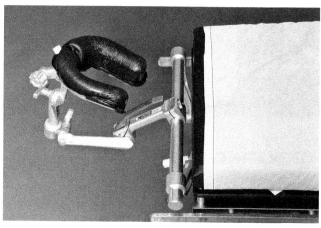

FIGURE 2–5 Horseshoe headrest.

the patient's forehead when he or she is in the prone position or the back of the head when he or she is supine. It is attached to the OR bed where the headpiece would normally be attached.

The three-pin system is designed to hold the head still during craniotomy procedures. It uses three pins or clamps (two on one side and one on the other) to stabilize the head. The system can accommodate the patient in any position: prone, supine, or Fowler's.

Another type of headrest attachment that is available is the narrow headrest, which allows greater access to the patient's head during ear, nose, and throat surgery; plastic surgery; ophthalmology procedures; and cranial surgeries.

Many of the newer headrests have articulating attachments to allow for more flexibility in head adjustment. Some headrests are available in pediatric sizes for use in children.

**Arm Boards:** Arm boards are attached to each side of the bed to support the patient's outstretched arms (Fig. 2–6). The boards are padded, but extra padding may be needed in the areas of the shoulder, elbow, wrist, or hand, depending on the patient. Make sure you have the proper arm boards before positioning the patient on the table; not all arm boards are interchangeable (i.e., fit more than one OR table).

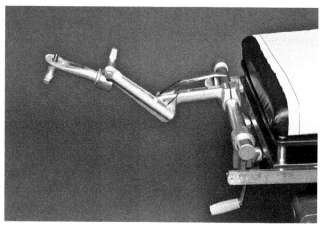

FIGURE 2–3 Mayfield attachment.

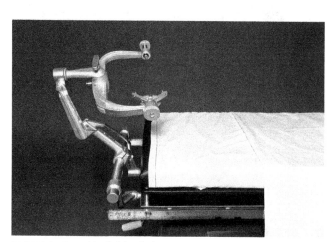

FIGURE 2–4 Mayfield with three-pin system.

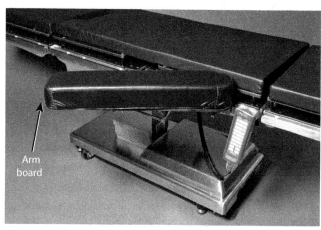

Arm board

FIGURE 2–6 Arm board.

**Shoulder Braces:** Padded shoulder braces can be attached to the head of the bed when the patient is placed in the Trendelenburg position (Fig. 2–7). They are used to prevent the patient from sliding upward, off the top of the bed. Care should be taken when using these braces; improper positioning of the braces could cause undue pressure to the brachial plexus, resulting in injury to the patient. Shoulder braces should be applied only when absolutely necessary.

**Toboggan:** Also known as a *sled* or *arm shield,* the toboggan is a Plexiglas, three-sided box used to brace the arm or leg at the patient's side, preventing the appendage from falling off the table (Fig. 2–8). The device is held in place by sliding it under the mattress.

> **WATCH OUT!** **Hyperextension of the Arms**
>
> A patient's arm should NEVER be extended (abducted) >90 degrees on an arm board. Extending a patient's arm >90 degrees could result in damage to the brachial plexus with resulting temporary or permanent nerve damage.

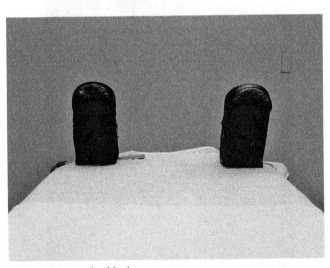

FIGURE 2–7 Shoulder braces.

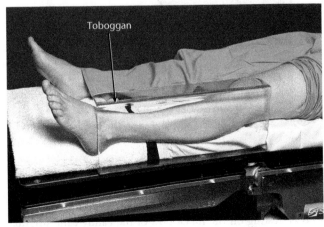

FIGURE 2–8 Toboggan.

**Allen Arm Support:** The Allen arm support (Fig. 2–9) can hold the hand and wrist in the prone, lateral, or seated position. The handrest is malleable to allow for flexibility in positioning. The arm rest is made of metal; therefore, padding (e.g., gel pad) must be applied before placing the patient's hand and wrist on it.

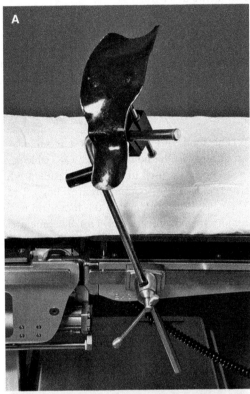

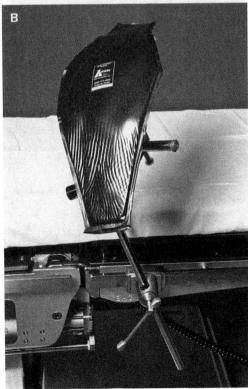

FIGURE 2–9 (A) Allen arm support. (B) Allen arm support with gel pad.

**Hand Table:** The hand table (Fig. 2–10) is a rectangular or hourglass-shaped folding table used to support the entire arm and hand during surgery. It attaches to the side of the OR table and can be moved easily for repositioning. It has one or two telescoping legs to support the distal end of the table. It is available in several sizes, ranging from 14 to 23 inches in width to 29 to 38 inches in length.

**Beach Chair:** Also known as a *captain's chair,* the beach chair attachment supports the patient in an upright siting position for shoulder surgery. The patient's head is strapped into a headrest and the nonoperative arm is strapped to the patient's waist. The device requires specially designed disposable padding (Fig. 2–11).

**Footboard:** The footboard (Fig. 2–12) is a rectangular metal board that attaches to the bottom of the OR table at a right angle. The footboard is used to prevent the patient who is in the reverse Trendelenburg position from sliding off the bottom of the table. Place padding on the footboard to prevent pressure injury to the patient's feet. This attachment can also be used as a "shelf" during vaginal procedures by attaching it at a right angle to the bed's footpiece, which is lowered all the way down.

## Stirrups

**Candy Cane Stirrups:** Also known as *sling stirrups,* candy cane stirrups (Fig. 2–13) support the foot and heel of the patient

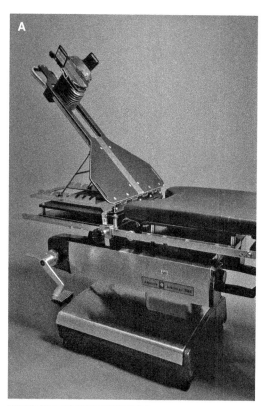

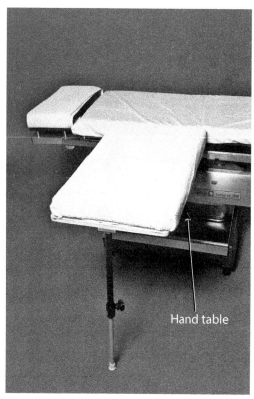

FIGURE 2–10 **Hand table.**

Hand table

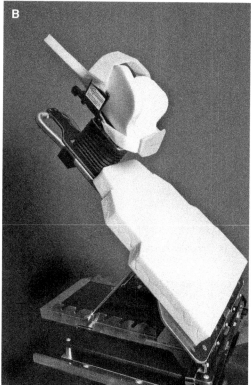

FIGURE 2–11 (A) Beach chair. (B) Padding for beach chair.

in the lithotomy position. These stirrups can be used for gynecological, urological, and laparoscopic procedures. Care must be taken to make sure the side of the patient's lower leg is NOT resting on the metal post of the candy cane stirrup.

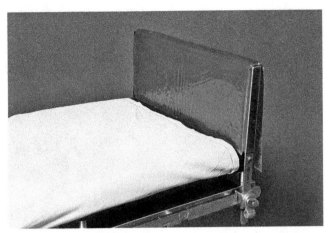

FIGURE 2-12 Footboard.

## Guidelines for Placing the Patient's Legs in Stirrups

- When placing the patient in stirrups, both legs must be lifted slowly, at the same time, by two people. Failure to do this could result in injury to the spine or hips.
- Removing the patient from stirrups requires two people to lower the legs slowly, at the same time, to prevent stress on the patient's lower back.
- If legs are lowered too quickly, hypotension could occur.
- Caution needs to be taken to make sure the hip flexion is not too severe because this can damage the femoral nerves.
- Patients with knee or hip replacements or those with limited range of motion should be positioned while awake in order to avoid damage or severe pain due to hyperextension of the knee or hip joints.

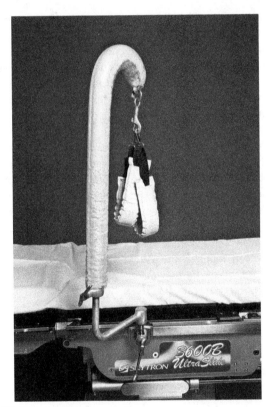

FIGURE 2-13 Candy cane stirrups.

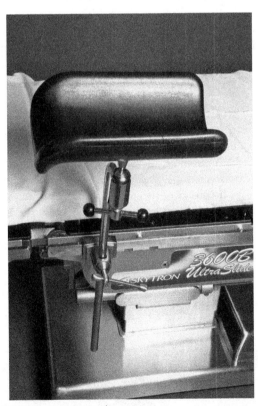

FIGURE 2-14 Knee-crutch stirrups.

Do not place the sling directly over the Achilles area because pressure could cause injury to the peroneal nerve.

**Knee-Crutch Stirrups:** These stirrups provide support under the knee and areas just above and below the knee (Fig. 2–14). They are generally used for short-duration knee arthroscopy or cystoscopy procedures. Care must be taken to properly pad and position the stirrups to prevent popliteal nerve damage.

**Boot Stirrups:** Rapidly becoming the stirrup of choice for many gynecological and rectal procedures, the boot stirrup provides support to the patient's foot and entire lower leg

(Fig. 2–15). This type of stirrup is completely adjustable both vertically and for abduction. The boot is padded, but care must be taken to properly place the patient's leg in the boot. Ensure the heel is all the way back into the boot to prevent nerve injury. There are several manufacturers of boot-type stirrups, so make sure you are familiar with the operation of the stirrups (how to raise, lower, and abduct them) used at your facility.

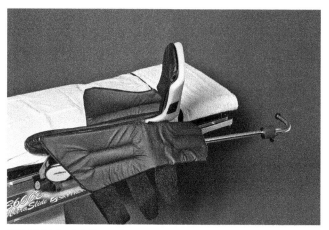

FIGURE 2–15  Boot stirrups.

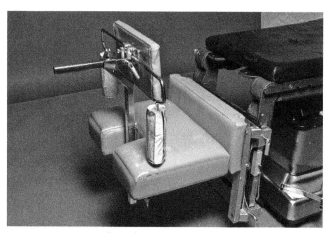

FIGURE 2–17  Andrews frame.

**Nissan Thigh Straps:** These are a thick, padded strap that fit around the top of the thigh and are attached to clamps on the side of the OR table. They are used, one on each thigh, when the patient is going to be placed in steep reverse Trendelenburg position (for example, the Nissan fundoplication procedure). They are available in regular or bariatric sizes. It is imperative you know the weight limit of the straps you are using and use the correct size for your patient.

## Frames for Lumbar Surgery

**Wilson Frame:** The Wilson frame (Fig. 2–16) supports a patient's torso in a flexed, prone position. This frame is used for surgeries of the lumbar spine, including laminectomy, diskectomy, and microdiscectomy as well as insertion of bladder control stimulators. It consists of two padded half circles mounted on a frame that is placed under the prone patient's torso. Using a crank system, the supports can be raised or lowered to achieve the desired amount of flexion. The supports also can be adjusted laterally to fit multiple patient body types.

**Andrews Frame:** The Andrews frame (Fig. 2–17) is used to support the patient in the knee-chest position for surgery on the lumbar spine. This frame is mounted on the bottom end of an OR table where the footpiece has been removed. The patient is anesthetized in a supine position and carefully rolled prone and into the knee-chest position on the frame. Ventilation is a major concern with the use of this frame—make sure the patient's chest has room to expand once the patient is positioned.

**Jackson Table:** The Jackson table (Fig. 2–18) is a frame with interchangeable accessories that allow it to be adapted for cervical, thoracic, and lumbar surgical procedures. The table has a flat surface for positioning the patient for cervical spine surgery. A Wilson frame can be mounted on the table for lumbar surgery along with a sling footpiece or flat footpiece. The table has a top that can be placed over the patient and secured to allow for "flipping" the patient 180 degrees.

## Miscellaneous Tables

**Orthopedic Surgery (Fracture) Table:** The orthopedic or fracture table (Fig. 2–19) is used for procedures such as hip nailing,

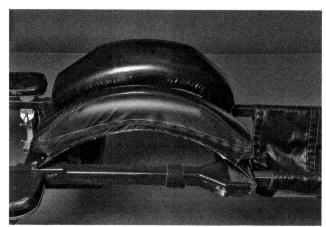

FIGURE 2–16  Wilson frame.

### Guidelines for Orthopedic Tables

- The orthopedic table can be configured in several ways. Make sure you know which configuration is needed for the procedure being performed.
- Make sure you know how to use the table and accessories BEFORE the procedure. If you are unsure, ask someone experienced with its use and consult the user manual.
- Make sure that the perineal post is well padded. The patient's perineal area should NOT rest directly against the post.
- Traction to the affected leg should be directed and applied by the surgeon. Make sure the foot is secure in the boot before applying the traction. Failure to do so could result in the foot slipping out, causing further damage from the fracture or damage to the skin of the foot.

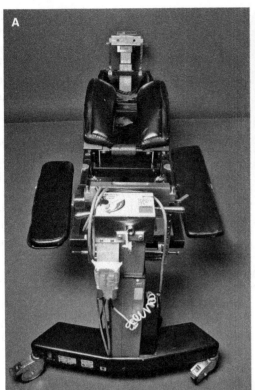

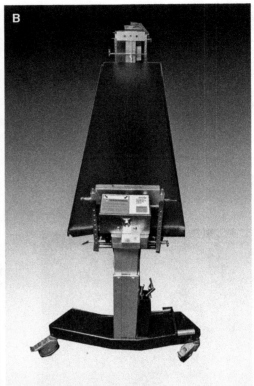

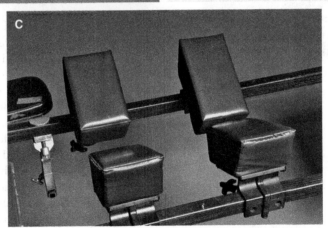

FIGURE 2-18 Three configurations for the Jackson table. (A) With Wilson frame. (B) With flat frame. (C) With padded bolsters.

femoral rodding or plating, tibial nailing, anterior hip arthroplasty, total knee replacement, and hip arthroscopy. The table has leg positioners that can be moved laterally to position the nonoperative leg out of the way and allow for C-arm access. Traction and rotation can be applied to either leg. The table can be fitted with different accessories that allow it to be configured for many types of procedures. All personnel working with this table must be familiar with the manufacturer's instructions and the institution's policy regarding the use of the table and its accessories.

**Top Sliding Table:** The tabletop slides toward the head or toward the foot, allowing for imaging access to any part of the body

(Fig. 2–20). These tables can be used for any surgical procedure in which C-arm or other imaging may be needed, such as some urology and major endovascular, orthopedic, or general surgeries. Similar to other OR tables, they can be rotated or flexed as needed.

## OPERATING ROOM FURNITURE

One of the first things that new personnel in an OR environment notice is that the furniture is different from furniture found in other patient care areas. The OR furniture is generally made of stainless steel (for ease of cleaning), has wheels to make it portable, and is designed to perform a specific purpose.

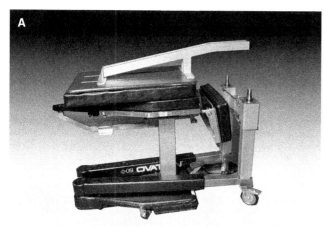

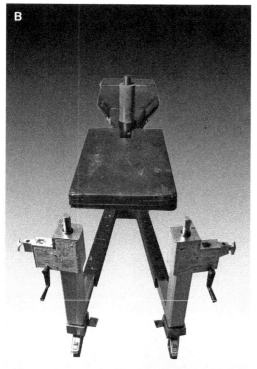

It is not decorative but plain and utilitarian. In this section, the most common pieces of furniture (except for the beds, which have their own section) are described.

All OR furniture should be wiped down thoroughly (all surfaces) with a hospital-grade disinfectant at the beginning of the day and between cases according to your institutional policy.

**Back Table:** The back table (also known as an *instrument table*) is a large one- or a two-tiered stainless steel table that, when covered with a sterile drape, is used to hold the sterile instruments and supplies (Fig. 2–21). The sterile large pack is opened on the back table to create a sterile field onto which the instruments, sutures, and other sterile supplies are opened and placed. If a large number of instruments or supplies are needed for the case, more than one back table may be used.

Back tables come in a variety of sizes and heights. The table may have one or two top shelves. The model with two top shelves is generally used for cases requiring a large amount of supplies and equipment, such as vascular, orthopedic, or neurosurgery. Both top shelves are covered with a sterile drape. Some back tables have a bottom shelf about 12 to 18 inches under the top shelf. On these models, the bottom shelf is not covered with a drape and is NOT considered sterile.

**Mayo Stand:** The Mayo stand is covered with a special sterile drape made specifically for that purpose and is used to set up instruments that need to be readily available for the case (Fig. 2–22). The instruments placed on the Mayo stand vary depending on the case but should be kept to a minimum to avoid disorganization and wasted time hunting for needed items. The space on top of the Mayo stand is limited; use it only for the items needed to start the case (e.g., scalpels and superficial retractors) and those that will be used repeatedly (e.g., common rings such as Kocher, Allis, and hemostats; Mayo and Metzenbaum scissors; smooth and tissue forceps). The rest of the instruments should be organized on the back table. Instruments can be removed and replaced with others (e.g., deeper retractors) as the surgery progresses.

FIGURE 2–19 (A) Fracture table closed. (B) Fracture table opened.

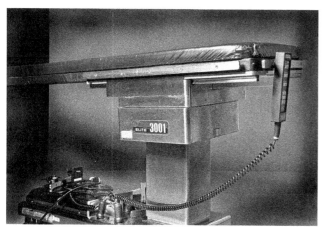

FIGURE 2–20 Top sliding table.

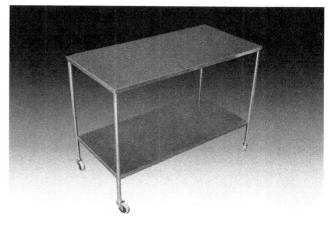

FIGURE 2–21 Back table.

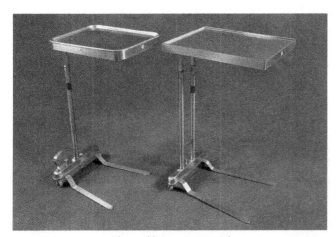

FIGURE 2-22 Regular and large Mayo stands.

Mayo stands come in a variety of styles. The height on most Mayo stands can be adjusted from 36 to 62 inches to allow them to be moved up to the field and over the patient. Height adjustment is made either by stepping on a foot button or pulling a hand lever, depending on the model. Standard Mayo stands have a tray surface area of 12 × 19 inches or 16 × 21 inches. Extra-large Mayo stands (used mostly in orthopedic or neurosurgical procedures) have a surface area of 20 × 25 inches. The extra-large stand requires an extra-large sterile Mayo cover.

**Utility Table:** The utility table (also called a *prep table*) is a small, stainless-steel table (Fig. 2–23) that can be used for a variety of things. When it is covered with a sterile drape, it can be used to hold the basins and other supplies used for skin prep or as a separate small sterile field (e.g., for a local anesthesia supply set-up or for a sigmoidoscopy set-up). Unsterile, it can be used to hold paperwork, specimen containers, scales (for weighing specimens), or other items.

Utility tables come in a variety of styles, some with drawers and some without. They are small, with a surface area of about 16 × 20 inches.

**Mobile Instrument Stand:** The mobile instrument stand (Fig. 2–24) is a small, single-post stand that can be covered with a sterile drape and used to hold instruments and supplies for a minor surgical or dental case. The surface area is 12 × 19 inches, and the height is adjustable from 31 to 50 inches. Unlike a Mayo stand, the mobile instrument stand is made to go beside the OR table, not over the patient's body or feet.

**Kick Bucket:** The kick bucket (Fig. 2–25) is a stainless-steel, 13-quart bucket set into a round, rolling stainless-steel frame. The bucket is commonly used to contain dirty sponges discarded from the field. The circulator (using proper standard precautions) may drape the sponges over the side of the bucket for ease of counting. Some institutions require that discarded sponges be placed in plastic-impervious sponge count bags for counting. Check your institution's policies and procedures.

**Ring Stand:** The ring stand (also known as a *basin stand*) is a round, stainless-steel ring mounted on a rolling stand (Fig. 2–26). The

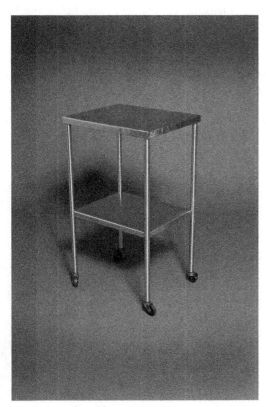

FIGURE 2-23 Utility table.

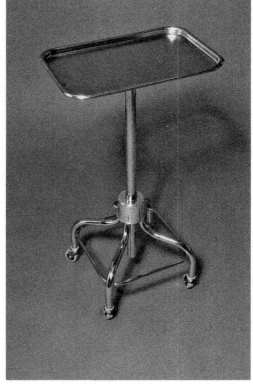

FIGURE 2-24 Mobile instrument stand.

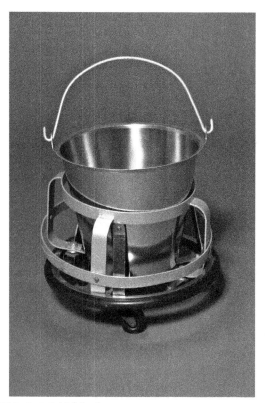

FIGURE 2-25 Kick bucket.

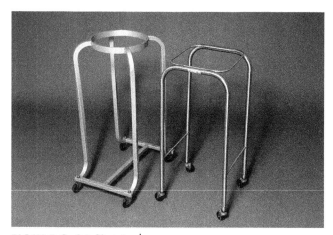

FIGURE 2-26 Ring stand.

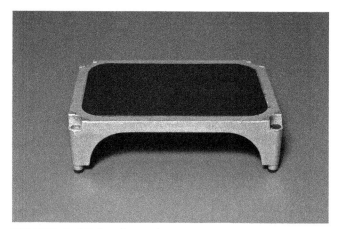

FIGURE 2-27 Standing stool.

members of the surgical team better visualization of the surgical field during a procedure. The important thing to check on a standing stool is that all four rubber feet are solid and intact; otherwise, the stool may wobble and pose a safety hazard.

Standing stools are 11¼ inches high and come in regular (350-lb weight limit) or bariatric (600-lb weight limit) styles.

**Sitting Stool:** The surgeon and staff use sitting stools when it is more advantageous to sit during the procedure rather than stand (e.g., hand surgeries, vaginal procedures). These stools adjust in height from 17 to 24 inches (Fig. 2–28). Depending on the model, they are adjusted by turning the seat, which is mounted on a large screw-type pole, or by using a pneumatic lever. The seats are padded for comfort. Check the weight capacity of the stools in your institution before use, because some have weight capacities as low as 250 lb.

**Specialty Surgery Stool:** Commonly used for ophthalmological; ear, nose, and throat; or microsurgery, the specialty surgery stool is more like a chair (Fig. 2–29). It has two armrests to support and help steady the surgeon's forearms. The armrests can be individually adjusted vertically and radially (outward or inward). The height of the stool can be adjusted from 19 to 28 inches using a foot control.

large (8.5 quart) sterile basin is open in this stand, with the wrapper opened outward to cover the top and side of the stand, creating a sterile field. The sterile basin can then be used as a place to organize drapes or gowns or to open other sterile items.

Ring stands are available as single or double models. The double model holds two basins side by side. The stands have open frames to allow easy access from any side and may or may not have a shelf underneath.

**Standing Stool:** The standing stool (also known as a *step stool*) comes in a variety of styles (Fig. 2–27). This stool gives

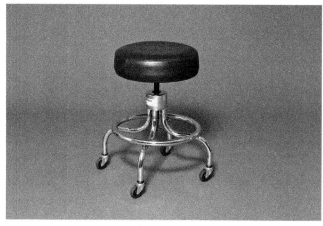

FIGURE 2-28 Sitting stool.

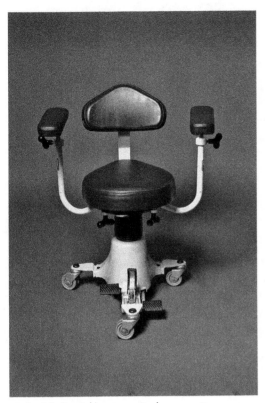

FIGURE 2-29 Specialty surgery stool.

**Surgical Spotlights:** Surgical spotlights come in a variety of sizes and configurations, but they are made for one purpose: to provide a concentrated beam of light into the surgical field that allows for better visualization (Fig. 2–30). The focus of the beam and beam location are controlled by sterile light handles that are inserted into the lights when the room is prepared for surgery.

Most ORs have two or three surgical spotlights located above the surgical bed. The lights are mounted on arms so they can be moved and adjusted.

Surgical spotlights should be turned on and checked—at the beginning of the day and between cases—for burned-out bulbs. Any bulbs that are burned out or dim should be changed before the start of the case. Spotlights should be wiped down with disinfectant at the beginning of the day and between cases, according to your institution's infection control policies.

**Intravenous Pole:** Intravenous (IV) poles come in a variety of styles, but they are all used to hang IV fluid, medication, or blood transfusion bags. The IV poles are mounted on a stand with wheels to allow for portability (Fig. 2–31). They generally have two or four rings at the top for hanging the solution bags. The height is adjustable; generally, pediatric IV poles adjust from 56 to 89 inches, and adult models adjust from 68 to 99 inches or 75 to 101 inches. Some IV poles come with a shelf to allow for pumps to be mounted onto them.

**Irrigation Tower:** An irrigation tower performs a function similar to an IV pole: it is made to hold bags of fluid. Unlike the IV pole, however, the height of each arm (the metal hook that holds the bag) of the irrigation tower can be adjusted separately, and it is designed for greater stability to hold larger amounts of fluids (Fig. 2–32). These towers are used when large amounts of irrigation fluid may be needed, such as during arthroscopic or cystoscopic procedures. The total capacity for fluid that can be hung on each tower varies by manufacturer; make sure you are familiar with the specific tower in your OR before use.

**In-Line Gas and Electric Columns:** ORs sometimes have the gas (e.g., nitrogen, oxygen, and nitrous oxide), suction, and

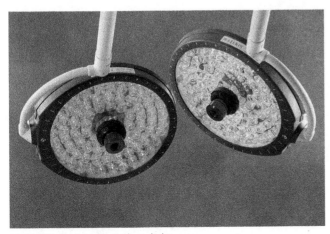

FIGURE 2-30 Surgical spotlights.

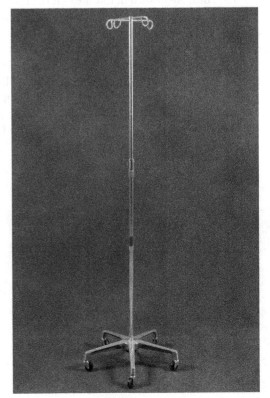

FIGURE 2-31 Intravenous pole.

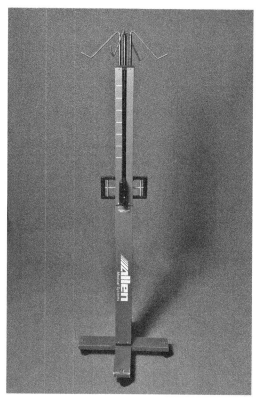

FIGURE 2–32 Irrigation tower.

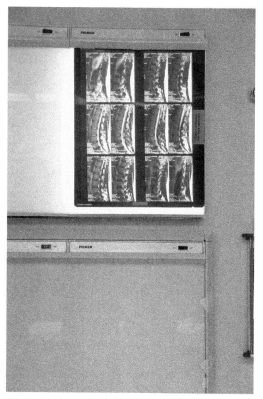

FIGURE 2–34 X-ray viewing box.

electrical outlets built into various types of ceiling-mounted columns (Fig. 2–33). The advantage to the columns is that the hoses and cords are housed in one area off the floor, lessening the number of cords running across the floor and thus decreasing potential tripping hazards.

**X-Ray Viewing Box:** Some ORs have one or more x-ray viewing boxes mounted on the wall (Fig. 2–34). These illuminated boxes allow patient films to be viewed during the procedure. The most common configurations are single panel (14 × 17 inches) or double panel (28 × 17 inches). The boxes

should be checked before the start of the case to ensure that they are functioning properly.

**Picture Archiving and Communication System:** The picture archiving and communication system (PACS) allows institutions to archive a patient's radiological studies and retrieve them on a computer system installed in a remote location (e.g., the OR or an off-site location) (Fig. 2–35). This system archives and retrieves not only regular x-ray films but also ultrasounds, magnetic resonance imaging scans, computed tomography scans, positron emission tomography scans, mammograms, and arteriograms.

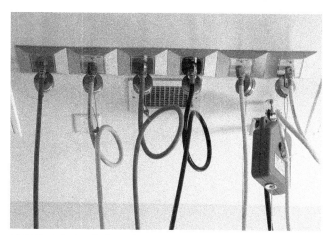

FIGURE 2–33 In-line column.

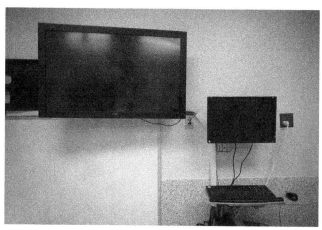

FIGURE 2–35 Picture archiving and communication system.

**X-Ray Cassette Holder:** There are many styles of x-ray cassette holders but those used in ORs are small and mounted on wheels so that they can be moved easily (Fig. 2–36). The height of the bars can be adjusted to accommodate several cassette sizes. These holders are used to keep the cassette in place when lateral x-rays are needed intraoperatively. The holders and cassette are not sterile; therefore, they must be draped (e.g., by using a sterile half drape) before they are moved close to the surgical field.

**Lead Door:** The lead door (also known as a *mobile barrier*) shields staff from radiation during the taking of intraoperative x-rays. The door is mounted on wheels to allow for portability, and it is rolled to a location away from the sterile field. Staff stand behind it while x-rays are being taken. The door has clear lead windows (Fig. 2–37) to allow staff to see the patient. Doors are available with 0.5 mm, 1.0 mm, or 1.5 mm of lead protection.

## ELECTROSURGICAL UNITS

The invention of electrosurgery helped to revolutionize the speed at which surgery was performed. Surgeons could now cut and cauterize tissue with the push of a button or a touch of the foot pedal instead of having to tie off each bleeding blood vessel individually. In modern surgical suites, some form of electrosurgery is used in most procedures. In this section, common types of electrosurgery (i.e., monopolar, bipolar, and argon beam) as well as parts of the electrosurgical unit (e.g.,

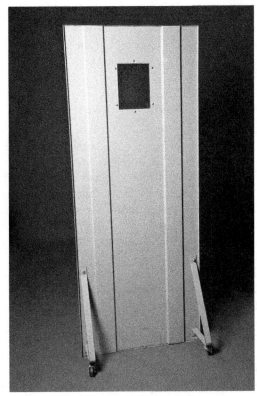

FIGURE 2–37 Lead door.

active and inactive electrodes, bipolar devices, argon beam wand and tips) are covered. Following this section are pages discussing electrosurgery safety, what to do if the patient sustains a burn, and simple troubleshooting.

### Control Panel for the Electrosurgical Generator

Several different models of electrosurgery generators are available. Figure 2–38 shows one common type with the plugs and controls labeled. This figure is intended as a guide to basic features of most generators; refer to the instruction manual

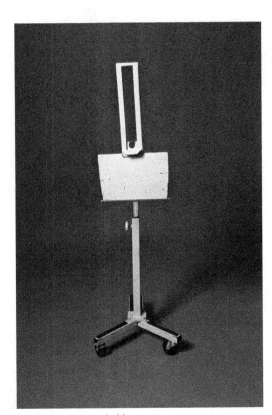

FIGURE 2–36 Cassette holder.

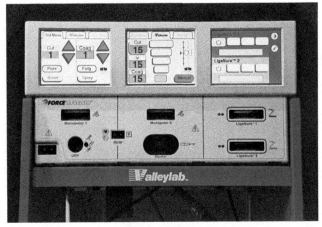

FIGURE 2–38 Control panel of an electrosurgery unit.

for specific information regarding the generators used in your institution.

Most electrosurgical units (ESUs; also referred to as *ESU generators*) are capable of producing two modes of current: monopolar and bipolar.

## Monopolar Electrosurgery

Monopolar is a commonly used form of electrosurgical current. In the monopolar mode, electrical current goes from the ESU generator to the handpiece (called the *pencil;* this is the *active electrode*), where it contacts the tissue. Once the tissue is cut or cauterized, the current travels through the patient's body until it gets to the *dispersive pad* (commonly called the grounding pad; this is the *inactive electrode*). The current exits through the grounding pad back to the generator and ground.

When using the monopolar current mode, it is essential that the patient have a properly placed grounding pad on the skin (Fig. 2–39). ESU generators will not work unless the grounding pad is plugged into the proper outlet. Many ESU generators will also sound an alarm (and not work) if the pad has come loose or is folded on itself. However, the staff person applying the dispersive pad is responsible for ensuring it is *properly* applied. An improperly or misplaced pad has the potential to cause burns to the patient's skin!

## Monopolar Handpieces and Tips

The *active electrode* is what the surgeon uses to cut or cauterize tissue. The most common form of active electrode is the pencil (see Figs. 2–40 and 2–41). A tip is inserted into the pencil. The type of tip depends on what surgery is being performed.

### Styles of Tips

Common tips (Fig. 2–42) for open procedures include spatula (flat blade), needle point (for working in small or delicate areas), ball tip, or loop (for resection in such procedures as a loop electrosurgical excision procedure [LEEP]). Long extension tips (most commonly spatula and needle point) for working on tissue deep within a body cavity are available.

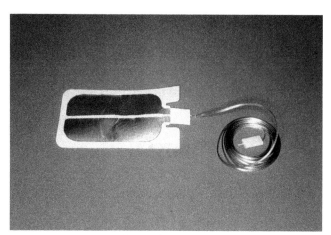

FIGURE 2-39 Grounding pad.

### Guidelines for Properly Placing a Dispersive (Grounding) Pad

- Before placement, inspect the pad for any tears, kinks in the cord, splits in the cord, or other damage. Remove the plastic protective backing and check the gel to ensure that it is sticky and fresh, not dried out. DO NOT use a damaged pad. If there is any doubt about the integrity of the pad; toss it out and get a new one!
- Make sure the site is clean and dry. Remove any lotions or creams as necessary.
- DO NOT apply on excessively hairy areas. If necessary, remove hair before pad application.
- Place over a large muscle mass with good vascularization. The upper thigh and outer thigh are two of the best areas.
- Uniform, smooth skin contact is essential. The pad should not be folded, bunched up, or torn. The pad should be placed AFTER final positioning of the patient to avoid damaging the pad or having the pad pull away from the skin.
- DO NOT apply over a bony prominence or over an area containing an artificial prosthesis (e.g., a total hip prosthesis). Excessive scar tissue at the site of the prosthesis can impede conduction.
- Apply the pad as close to the operative site as possible (e.g., for a patient undergoing an appendectomy, place the pad on the right thigh if possible).

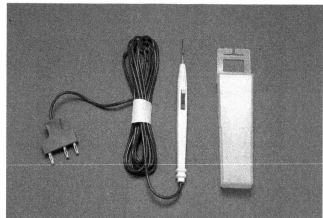

FIGURE 2-40 Pencil electrode.

Teflon-coated tips may be used when a great deal of cautery is anticipated (these tips are easier to keep free of tissue debris). Endoscopic procedures require special electrodes that are long and thin. There are a variety of endoscopic electrodes, including probes and graspers.

The pencil can be activated by pressing a button or stepping on the foot pedal. While the electrode is activated, the ESU makes an audible signal that alerts personnel that the tip is hot and therefore a potential hazard. These signals are intended for patient safety and should never be disabled or turned down so low as to make them inaudible.

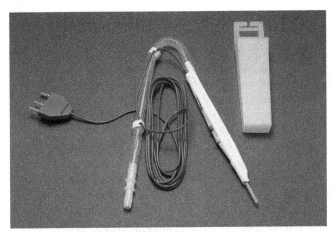

FIGURE 2-41 Suction electrode.

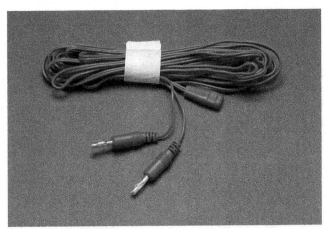

FIGURE 2-43 Bipolar cord.

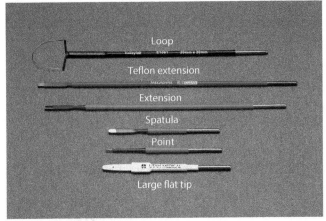

FIGURE 2-42 Loop, Teflon extension, extension tip, spatula, point, large flat tip.

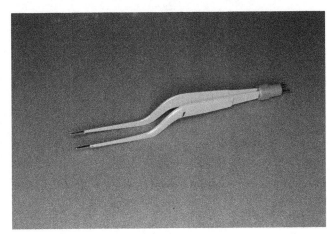

FIGURE 2-44 Bipolar forceps.

## Bipolar Electrosurgery

In bipolar electrosurgery, the current passes from one tine of the forceps to the other. The power is lower than what can be achieved with monopolar cautery and is used for cauterization during neurosurgery or on delicate tissue. The current does not pass through the patient, thus a dispersive (or grounding) pad is *not* needed.

*Note:* If the surgeon is going to be using *both* monopolar and bipolar current during the procedure, a dispersive electrode pad *must* be placed on the patient.

The special forceps used to deliver bipolar current are available in a wide variety of styles and plug into the ESU using a bipolar cord (Fig. 2–43). Many of the forceps resemble regular grasping forceps (Fig. 2–44) but with one important difference: these forceps have a plug on the end of the handle to plug them into the bipolar cord.

## Argon Beam Coagulation

Argon beam coagulation (also referred to as *ABC* or *argon plasma coagulation*) uses a combination of argon gas and monopolar electrosurgery to coagulate tissue. Within the machine (Fig. 2–45), the gas is ionized, making it electrically conductive.

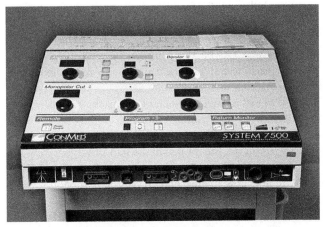

FIGURE 2-45 Argon beam machine.

This provides a more efficient pathway for the current to travel along to the tissue. The tip of the instrument (Fig. 2–46) does not need to touch the tissue; the beam of ionized gas coagulates bleeders within 2 to 10 mm of the tip. Argon beam coagulation produces less tissue damage, less smoke plume, and less charring than traditional electrosurgery methods.

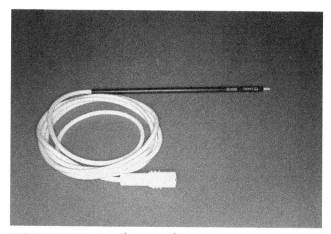

FIGURE 2-46 Argon beam wand.

On some argon beam machines, you can turn the gas tank off and use the machine as a monopolar device with a traditional pencil or as a bipolar device with ESU forceps. Be sure to refer to the manufacturer's instruction book to see if the unit in your institution can be used this way.

*Remember:* Argon beam coagulation allows the electrical current to travel through the patient's body; therefore, a dispersive electrode (grounding pad) *must* be used.

## Electrosurgical Safety

As with any electrical device, there are certain safety measures that should be followed when an ESU is in use.

- Know your machine. Only personnel knowledgeable about electrosurgical use and safety precautions should use the device. If you have questions, refer to the manufacturer's instructions.
- Check the unit for frayed cords or damaged plugs before use. If the electric cord is split, frayed, or otherwise compromised or the prongs on the plug are bent, damaged, or missing, DO NOT use the machine. Obtain a different machine and send the damaged one to biomedical engineering to be checked.
- Do not store liquids on top of the machine. Spills could occur and cause electrical shock or shortage.
- Make sure the electrosurgical dispersal pad is properly placed on the patient before the start of surgery. Plug the patient-dispersive pad into the machine (machines will not allow the machine to activate in monopolar mode unless the dispersive pad is plugged in).
- Fire safety precautions must be followed. These include:
  - Allow all prep solutions to dry completely before using the ESU.
  - Use a special endotracheal tube if electrosurgery will be performed near the airway.
  - Use flame-retardant drapes.
  - When not using the handpiece, place it back in the holder; DO NOT place it on dry drapes or towels.
  - Oxygen should be delivered at the lowest possible concentration.

- Water or saline must be available on the surgical field (usually on the back table).
- Portable fire extinguishers must be readily available (halon extinguishers are recommended).
- Nonflammable anesthetics must be used.
- During anorectal procedures, the rectum must be packed with a sterile, water-soaked sponge to prevent a methane gas fire.
- NEVER turn off or disable alarms. Do not turn the volume too low; personnel should be able to hear the "beeping alert sound" when the electrode is activated (hot).
- Use an instrument, such as a clamp, to change the electrode tip. DO NOT use your hands!
- Do not loop the cords around metal devices or instruments.
- Make sure all jewelry is removed from the patient before surgery. Metal jewelry can act as a conductor and cause alternate-site burns. If jewelry cannot be removed, check with your institution policy for necessary steps and documentation requirements.
- If the patient has a pacemaker or an implanted defibrillator, consult the cardiologist before surgery to find out whether or not the device needs to be shut off.
- DO NOT allow the patient to come in contact with metal surfaces on the OR bed.
- Suction smoke and plume during electrosurgery use (a smoke evacuation system is recommended instead of regular suctioning).

## What to Do If the Patient Sustains a Burn

If a patient is burned and the electrosurgical device might have been the cause (e.g., the patient's skin underneath the pad is burned), the incident falls under federal mandatory reporting laws. What does staff need to do?

- Notify the surgeon immediately that a burn has occurred and have him or her look at the area. The surgeon will need to talk to the patient about what happened and may need to order treatment (e.g., ointments or dressings) for the burn.
- Document the facts of how the skin looks in the patient's perioperative record. Document that the surgeon was notified and what was done to treat the burn area.
- Save ALL disposable parts of the electrosurgical unit used on that patient, including the grounding pad, electrosurgical pencil, and tips. Put these supplies in a bag and send them with the machine to biomedical engineering to be checked.
- The electrosurgical machine should NOT be used on any other patient until it has been checked and cleared by biomedical engineering.
- Notify your supervisor (who in turn needs to notify risk management). Fill out your institution's quality assurance paperwork (usually known as an *incidence* or *variance report*).

## Electrosurgical Unit Troubleshooting Tips

As with any device, troubleshooting starts with the seemingly obvious and simple:

| PROBLEM | WHAT TO LOOK AT |
|---|---|
| When the surgeon presses the button, the handpiece doesn't work. | ▪ Make sure the machine is turned on.<br>▪ Check to see that the machine is in "ready" mode, not "standby."<br>▪ Is the handpiece plugged into the proper place?<br>▪ Is the handpiece plugged in all the way (snuggly)?<br>▪ Is the grounding pad plugged into the machine?<br>▪ Is there a problem with the grounding pad (has it lifted off the skin, folded on itself, or torn)? |
| The grounding pad light is lit up. | ▪ Is the grounding pad plugged into the machine?<br>▪ Has the grounding pad begun to lift off the patient's skin?<br>▪ Is there a kink or tear in the grounding pad cord?<br>▪ Has the grounding pad torn or folded (especially if the grounding pad was applied before positioning)? |
| I turn the machine "on," but the power doesn't come on. | ▪ Is the machine plugged in?<br>▪ Is the cord kinked or frayed? If the cord is frayed or split, do not use this machine—get another one.<br>▪ Try another electrical outlet (sometimes there is a problem with power to one outlet).<br>▪ If the machine is plugged in and you've tried other outlets without any luck, get another machine and have biomedical engineering check out the problematic machine. |

▪ The supervisor and/or risk management department will report the incident to the proper federal reporting agency following your institution's policy.

## MEDICAL GASES

There are five common medical gases used in the OR: oxygen, nitrogen, nitrous oxide, carbon dioxide, and argon. Each gas has a specific purpose, and a mix-up could be *disastrous*.

The Food and Drug Administration (FDA) recommends that each medical gas be stored in a cylinder of a specific color to make identification easier and a mix-up less likely. DO NOT rely solely on the cylinder color; *read the label on the cylinder carefully!* The regulator for the cylinder is another safety feature. Regulators are gas specific and are not interchangeable; never modify a gas regulator from one type of gas to try to make it fit another.

This section contains photographs and descriptions of each gas as well as specific safety tips. At the end of this section, general safety tips for handling medical gases are presented.

### General Medical Gas Cylinder Safety

Medical gases are the only ones that have a regulated color system for the cylinders. Although it is *never* recommended that you rely on cylinder color alone (*read the label!*), here are the FDA cylinder color recommendations to help with identification:

- **Air:** yellow
- **Carbon dioxide:** gray
- **Argon:** teal
- **Nitrogen:** black
- **Nitrous oxide:** blue
- **Oxygen:** green

## General Guidelines for the Safe Handling of Medical Gas Cylinders

1. Read the label! Know what you are using before you use it. Never use an unmarked cylinder or one bearing a label that is unreadable.
2. Store cylinders away from flammable material. Do not use oily or greasy substances to clean the cylinders.
3. Store cylinders in an upright position and make sure they are secured at all times. Use handcarts to transport cylinders. Do not allow cylinders to hit against one another.
4. Store cylinders away from sources of heat or electricity.
5. Do not try to modify regulators from one type of gas to fit another type of gas cylinder. *Remember:* regulators are gas specific and NOT interchangeable!
6. Store all cylinders in a well-ventilated area.
7. Let the experts do any repairs that are necessary. Do not try to repair damaged cylinders, regulators, or gauges.
8. Never use a cylinder that is damaged or has a damaged pressure gauge or regulator.

**Name:** oxygen

**Alias:** $O_2$

**Medication Class:** essential gas

**Use:** provides supplemental oxygen to organs and tissue

**Features:** can be delivered via cannula, mask, Ambu bag, or ventilator

**Additional Information:** liter flow is dependent on the delivery device: a flow rate should be 1 to 3 L for a cannula, a flow rate of 8 to 10 L is best for a mask, and a flow rate of at least 15 L is needed for an Ambu bag or ventilator

- **Cylinder Color:** green
- **Safety Tips:** flammable: caution must be taken when using the ESU or laser in areas where oxygen concentration may be high (e.g., the face or neck or under drapes)

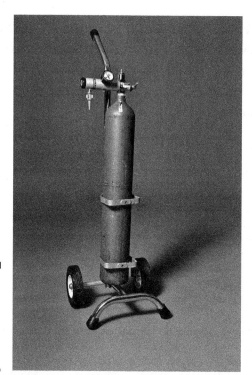

**Name:** nitrous oxide

**Alias:** none

**Medication Class:** inhalation anesthetic

**Use:** used in conjunction with other agents to provide balanced anesthesia; can be used in specific circumstances to create a pneumoperitoneum

**Features:** has little effect on heart rate or blood pressure; not potent enough to be used alone for general anesthesia

**Additional Information:** gas diffuses into closed spaces, thus making it contraindicated for some surgeries (e.g., tympanoplasty)

- **Cylinder Color:** blue
- **Safety Tips:** nonflammable but does support combustion; use ESU or laser with caution in areas where high concentrations are likely (e.g., face or neck)

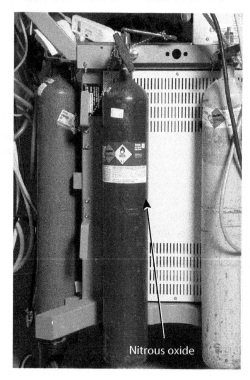

Nitrous oxide

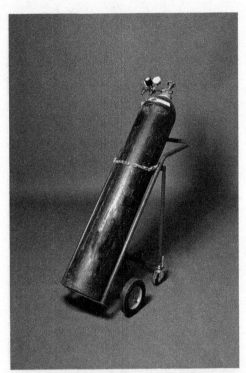

**Name:** nitrogen

**Alias:** none

**Use:** provides pneumatic power to equipment such as saws, drills, bone cement mixers, and irrigators

**Features:** nonflammable

**Additional Information:**

- **Cylinder Color:** black
- **Safety Tips:** make sure all connections to equipment are secure

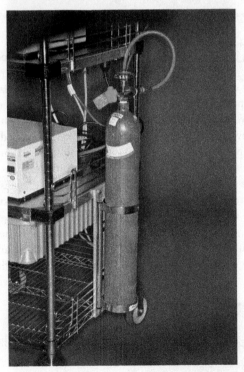

**Name:** carbon dioxide

**Alias:** $CO_2$

**Use:** insufflates the abdomen during laparoscopic surgery; used in cryosurgery

**Features:** odorless; does not support combustion; readily absorbed by the body

**Additional Information:** has the potential to cause hypercarbia leading to metabolic acidosis

- **Cylinder Color:** gray
- **Safety Tips:** monitor patient for signs of respiratory or cardiac problems (signs of acidosis due to break down of carbon dioxide into carbolic acid)

**Name:** argon

**Alias:** none

**Use:** argon beam coagulation

**Features:** colorless; odorless; nonflammable; when ionized by electricity the argon provides the current an efficient pathway on which to travel

**Additional Information:**

- **Cylinder Color:** teal
- **Safety Tips:** a grounding pad must be placed on the patient before using argon beam coagulation (electrical current is passing through the patient)

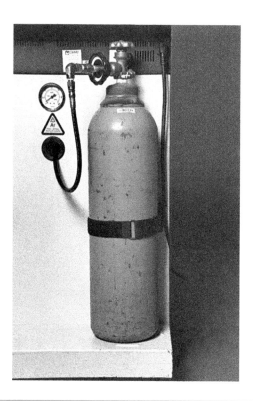

## PNEUMATIC TOURNIQUET

The pneumatic tourniquet is used to create a bloodless surgical area by limiting circulation to a patient's operative limb. This device is used for procedures involving the knee, lower leg, ankle, foot, distal humerus, elbow, forearm, wrist, and hand. Sometimes it is used in the administration of regional anesthesia.

The tourniquet cuff is an air bladder surrounded by a nylon cover (Fig. 2–47), similar to a blood pressure cuff. It is placed proximal to the surgical site. Cuffs are available in sizes ranging from 8 to 42 inches.

Before applying the tourniquet cuff, check the skin for breaks or lesions and then pad the area circumferentially with

Webril and stockinette (or whatever type of padding your institutional policy requires). The padding helps to prevent undo pinching or damage to the skin. Once the padding is applied and smoothed (it should not have wrinkles that could dig into the skin when the tourniquet is inflated), the tourniquet cuff is applied around the entire circumference of the limb and fastened snugly in place (Fig. 2–48A). It is hooked to the inflation machine tubing. The limb is then exsanguinated using an Esmarch or other type of elastic bandage **approved by institutional policy** (Fig. 2–48B). Once the limb has been exsanguinated, the cuff can be inflated.

The surgeon is the one who decides at what point the cuff should be inflated and deflated. The circulating nurse must note the time of inflation and deflation in his or her documentation. The tourniquet is inflated using a machine that

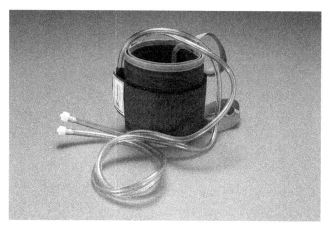

FIGURE 2-47 Tourniquet cuff.

### Guidelines for Inflation Pressures

- Keep the inflation pressure to a minimum, based on patient need rather than standardized pressures. The limb occlusion pressure should be measured using a device such as a Doppler. A safety margin should be added to it, according to the manufacturer's instructions.
- Inflation pressures may need to be increased for patients with larger limb circumferences.
- Inflation pressure recommendations may vary by device. Make sure you know the manufacturer's recommendations for the device used in your institution.

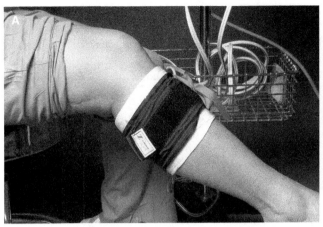
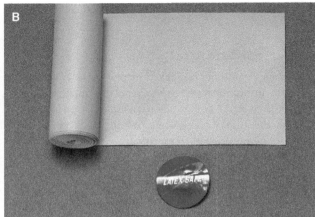

FIGURE 2-48 (A) Padded tourniquet applied to leg. (B) Esmarch bandage.

pumps compressed gas into the cuff. Generally, the surgeon will tell the circulator at what inflation pressure he or she wants the tourniquet set, based on patient systolic blood pressure, but there are some general safety guidelines for inflation pressures.

There are several pneumatic tourniquets available, each having a slightly different control panel. Although they may look different, each machine's control panel (Fig. 2–49) has similar functions. Most machines can have two separate cuffs connected to them simultaneously, allowing for placement of

the cuffs on two extremities (e.g., bilateral knee replacements) at the beginning of the procedure rather than trying to remove the cuff from one extremity and apply it to another in the middle of a procedure. Each cuff is attached to a separate set of tubing and controlled by a separate set of controls. Only one cuff is inflated at a time. The timer is reset when the first cuff is deflated and the second one inflated.

The control panel includes these buttons: power on/off switch, inflate and deflate buttons for each cuff, and buttons to increase and decrease cuff pressure. Located on the front

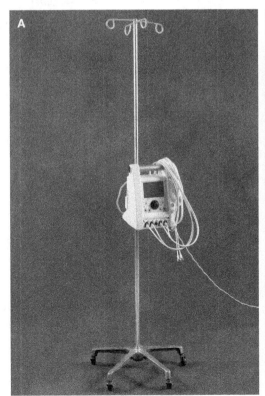
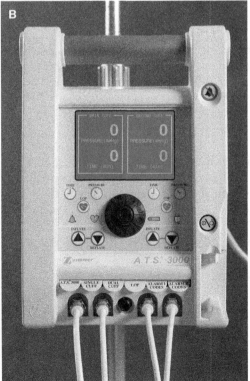

FIGURE 2-49 (A) Tourniquet machine. (B) Control panel.

of the machine is a display of inflation time and cuff inflation pressure.

## Tourniquet Safety

- Tourniquets should be applied by personnel approved by the institutional policy. Personnel may include surgeons, registered nurses, physician assistants, or, in some cases, the surgical technologist. Be sure to check your policy before applying a tourniquet to a patient.
- Only personnel who are familiar with the use of the device should be using it. If you are unsure of how to use the device, read the manufacturer's instructions and seek help from experienced personnel.
- All staff who will be using the device need to demonstrate ongoing competency in its use.
- Policies and procedures must be in place regarding device use.
- The limb where the tourniquet cuff will be placed must be assessed by the circulator before cuff application and after cuff removal at the end of the procedure. Both assessments must be documented in the patient record.
- Document the time from inflation of the cuff to deflation of the cuff (known as "tourniquet time") in the patient record.
- Make efforts to ensure prep solutions do not seep underneath the tourniquet or into the padding. Fluid pooling under the tourniquet could cause tissue damage such as burns.
- If the tourniquet appears to be malfunctioning, use another one and have biomedical engineering check the malfunctioning device. Repairs should be done by qualified personnel only.
- As with any electrical device, check all cords for fraying, cracks, or exposed wire before use. If any of these things are found, DO NOT use the device.
- Before use, check tubing that connects the cuff to the machine for cracks or holes. Check connections to make sure there are no leaks.
- Most cuffs are designed for single patient use and are discarded after the procedure. Machines and tubing need to be decontaminated according to the manufacturer's instructions and institutional policy.
- Do not disable or make inaudible the time or pressure alarms. They are there for patient safety and need to remain audible to personnel.

## AUTOTRANSFUSION

Autotransfusion is the reinfusion of the patient's own blood or blood products. Autotransfusion is sometimes preferable to a donor transfusion because it eliminates the danger of blood incompatibility and possible disease transmission. In some cases, patients who refuse a blood transfusion from an outside source may be willing to accept an autotransfusion. These products may be donated before surgery, or blood may be collected intraoperatively or postoperatively and then reinfused.

There are times when you should not collect the patient's blood and reinfuse it:

- If the patient has a known infection (localized or systemic)
- If the blood has been exposed to antibiotics (including antibiotic irrigating solutions) or collagen hemostatic agents; this can cause blood to coagulate in the machine
- If the blood has mixed with amniotic fluid or gastric or bowel contents

Several types of devices can collect blood, process it, and prepare it for reinfusion back into the patient. This section

## Tourniquet Troubleshooting Tips

| PROBLEM | WHAT TO LOOK AT |
|---|---|
| The surgical field suddenly starts to fill with blood | ■ Has the cuff come loose or off?<br>■ Is the tubing still connected to both connections?<br>■ Are the tubing connections tight?<br>■ Are the connections still attached to the cuff? (Did one of the connections rip out of the cuff?) |
| The cuff doesn't inflate | ■ Is the pressure reading still where you set it?<br>■ Is the machine on?<br>■ Is the cuff securely connected to the tubing?<br>■ Are you using the inflation control for the correct cuff? (Most machines allow you to connect two tourniquets, but each is connected to separate tubing and controlled by separate controls.)<br>■ Is there a hole or leak in the cuff? |
| The machine isn't working | ■ Is the power switch on?<br>■ Is it plugged in? (If there is battery backup, is the battery dead?)<br>■ If it is plugged in and switched on and it still doesn't work, get another machine and have this one evaluated. |

covers the most common intraoperative and postoperative blood collection and reinfusion devices.

## Cell Saver or Cell Salvager

The cell saver or cell salvager allows the blood to be suctioned directly from the surgical field into the machine (Fig. 2–50). It can also suction bloody saline from a basin in which bloody sponges were immersed in saline. The machine filters and anticoagulates the blood and fluid, readying it for IV reinfusion back to the patient. This process causes little or no harm to the red blood cells.

The cell saver is capable of processing large quantities of blood and irrigation fluid and is used when a large blood loss is possible, such as a ruptured spleen or large blood vessel, major spinal surgery, major orthopedic procedures, or multiple traumas with suspected major bleeding.

One major disadvantage to the cell saver device is that it may require a dedicated operator to run it. Check your institution's policy regarding who can operate a cell saver.

## OrthoPAT Blood Salvaging Device

This blood salvaging device is designed for use during orthopedic procedures in which blood loss may be sufficient to require transfusion (e.g., total hip replacement). The blood is suctioned from the surgical field into the machine, where it is cleansed, anticoagulated, and collected in a bag for IV reinfusion.

The OrthoPat (Fig. 2–51) can be used postoperatively to collect and prepare blood for reinfusion. Instead of suctioning blood from the surgical field, the OrthoPat device is attached to the drain. The blood is drained from the surgical wound into the machine and cleansed and prepared for reinfusion.

This device is capable of processing smaller amounts of blood and fluid than a cell saver and is designed for use in orthopedic procedures in which blood loss is intermittent. It is *not* designed to be used for major blood loss such as with a ruptured spleen or bleeding aorta. One major advantage is that the machine is fully automated and can be monitored by the circulating personnel. It does not require a dedicated operator.

## Autotransfusion Drains

The simplest of autotransfusion devices are the postoperative collection drains (Fig. 2–52). These devices are closed collection systems that use a three-spring evacuator (similar to a Hemovac drain) or controlled wall suction to suction blood from the surgical wound postoperatively and collect it for possible reinfusion. Please see the "Autotransfusion Drains" section in Chapter 4 for information on various types and their usage.

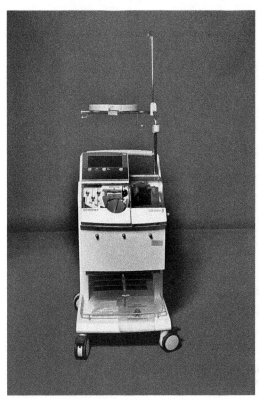

**FIGURE 2–50** Cell saver machine.

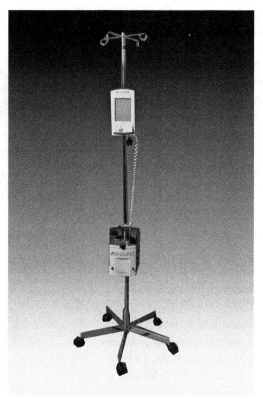

**FIGURE 2–51** OrthoPAT machine.

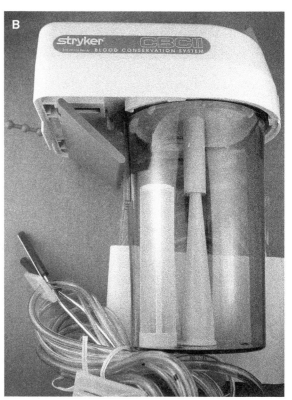

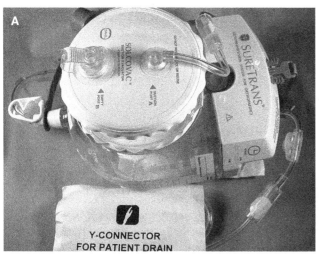

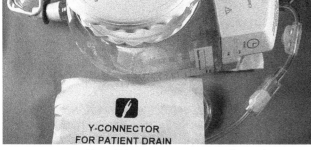

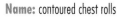

FIGURE 2-52 (A and B) Postoperative autotransfusion drains.

# PATIENT POSITIONING EQUIPMENT

**Name:** gel pad

**Alias:** none

**Use:** intraoperatively pads pressure points (e.g., heels, ankles, knees, elbows, hands)

**Features:** contains a gel substance that supports the area without placing pressure on it

**Additional Information:** available in many sizes, shapes, and levels of firmness

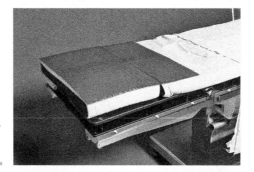

**Name:** contoured chest rolls

**Alias:** none

**Use:** lift the chest off the stretcher during prone positioning to allow for chest expansion during respiration

**Features:** contains a gel substance for softness

**Additional Information:** available in many sizes and levels of firmness; should be placed so that it extends from the top of the chest to the waist

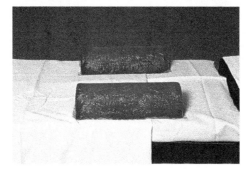

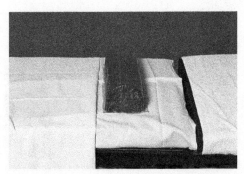

**Name:** axillary roll
**Alias:** none
**Use:** helps avoid pressure on the axillary nerves and blood vessels during lateral positioning
**Features:** padded gel material to provide padding and protection
**Additional Information:** available in several sizes and shapes

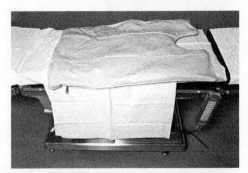

**Name:** bean bag positioner
**Alias:** none
**Use:** stabilizes the torso in lateral positioning
**Features:** air is taken out of the bean bag using suction to firm the bag and hold the patient in place
**Additional Information:** air is suctioned out after the patient is positioned; some bean bags have optional gel inserts for added protection

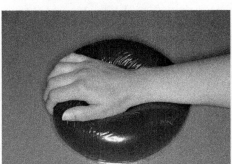
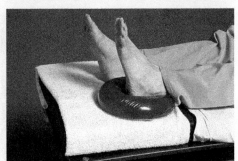

**Name:** closed head ring
**Alias:** none
**Use:** supporting the patient's wrist and hand, heel, or head in supine position
**Features:** gel padding for support and comfort
**Additional Information:** available in several sizes

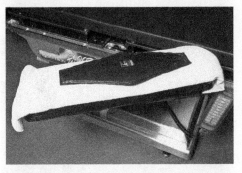

**Name:** elbow gel pad
**Alias:** none
**Use:** intraoperatively pads elbows
**Features:** has gel inside for padding; Velcro strap allows for secure fastening around the arm
**Additional Information:** available in several styles and sizes; can be strapped around the elbow or laid out straight with the elbow resting on the widest area

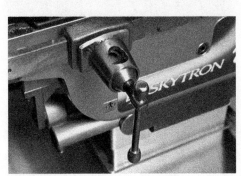

**Name:** stirrup holders
**Alias:** none
**Use:** attach stirrups or other positioning devices to the surgical bed
**Features:** attach onto OR table rails
**Additional Information:** comes in many sizes and styles

**Name:** lateral hip post

**Alias:** none

**Use:** supports the lateral aspect of the thigh during orthopedic surgery

**Features:** padded support area, post is solid; to adjust height, slide up or down in the stirrup holder

**Additional Information:** positioned using stirrup holder attached to the OR bed rail

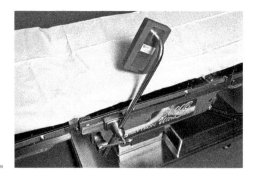

**Name:** Shea headrest

**Alias:** none

**Use:** positions the head during supine or lateral positioning

**Features:** made of foam to cushion head

**Additional Information:** available in adult and pediatric sizes

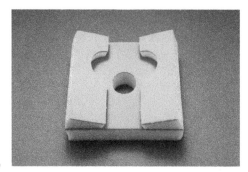

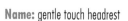

**Name:** gentle touch headrest

**Alias:** none

**Use:** supports the head and airway while the patient is in the prone position

**Features:** soft padding for face (white side is placed toward patient's face); cut-out area is for positioning of the endotracheal tube

**Additional Information:** comes vacuum sealed; needs to be taken out of the package and allowed to "puff up" before use

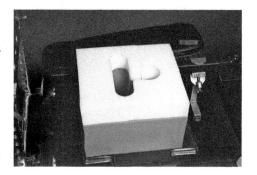

**Name:** prone view positioner

**Alias:** none

**Use:** supports head and airway while the patient is in the prone position

**Features:** mirrored bottom allows for viewing of patient airway; foam padding is placed inside the rigid support

**Additional Information:** use only the prone view padding with the prone view positioner; padding is single patient use; rigid support is disinfected between patients

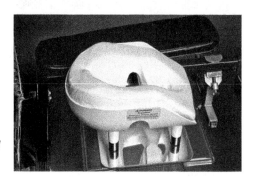

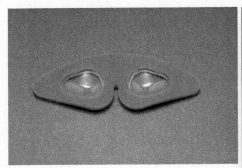

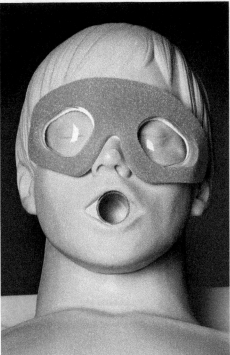

**Name:** Opti-Gard eye protector

**Alias:** none

**Use:** protects patient's eyes while patient is in the prone position

**Features:** padding on the borders of the glasses with rigid plastic eye shields keeps the eyes from being compressed while the patient is prone

**Additional Information:** none

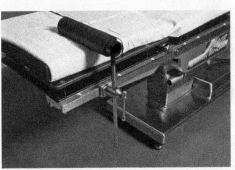

**Name:** total knee stabilizer

**Alias:** none

**Use:** supports the foot while the leg is flexed (e.g., during total knee arthroplasty)

**Features:** padded to protect the sole of the foot

**Additional Information:** available in several styles; foot pad is replaceable

**Name:** pelvic positioner

**Alias:** none

**Use:** supports and holds the pelvic area in place during lateral positioning (e.g., during hip surgery)

**Features:** padded; attached to the OR table using stirrup holders

**Additional Information:** available in several styles

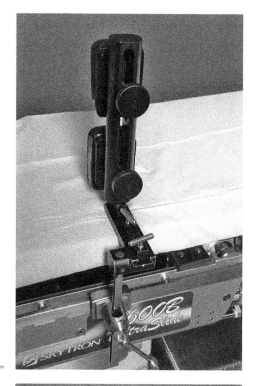

**Name:** safety belt

**Alias:** safety strap; restraint strap

**Use:** helps to keep the patient's legs secured in place during surgery

**Features:** some have Velcro straps for fastening whereas others have buckles; available in various lengths

**Additional Information:** the belt should be placed approximately 2 inches above the patient's knees; the strap should be snug but not tight (you should be able to slip two fingers under the belt); bariatric-sized straps are available

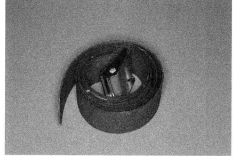

**Name:** hand positioner

**Alias:** Allen Hand positioner

**Use:** spreads out fingers for surgery on the palm

**Features:** can be adjusted to hold one or all fingers; padded with foam to cushion the hand

**Additional Information:** single patient use

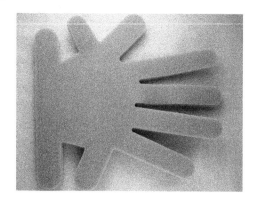

# MISCELLANEOUS EQUIPMENT

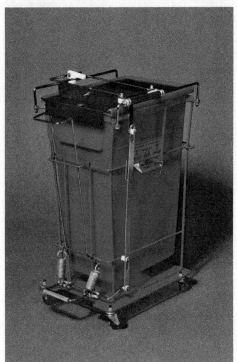

**Name:** sharps container

**Alias:** none

**Use:** safe disposal of all contaminated sharps (e.g., needles, blades, trocars)

**Features:** puncture proof; marked with biohazardous waste symbol

**Additional Information:** available in a variety of sizes

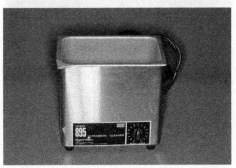

**Name:** ultrasonic cleaner

**Alias:** none

**Use:** cleans debris from delicate instruments (e.g., eye instruments); cleans debris from hard-to-reach places on instruments (e.g., box locks, serrations)

**Features:** *cavitation* is used to remove the debris; in other words, high-frequency sound waves are converted to vibrations, which create bubbles and cause the bubbles to *implode* (collapse inward); the implosion of the bubbles creates a vacuum that pulls debris from the instruments

**Additional Information:** instruments made of dissimilar metals should not be placed in the ultrasonic cleaner together; gross debris must be removed from instruments before placing them in the ultrasonic cleaner; various models are available; models can contain one to three chambers

**Name:** sequential compression device

**Alias:** SCD

**Use:** helps to prevent venous stasis and decrease the chance of thrombus formation postoperatively

**Features:** stockings massage the legs in an upward pattern to help prevent pooling of blood in the lower extremities

**Additional Information:** stockings are available in small, medium, large, and extra-large sizes

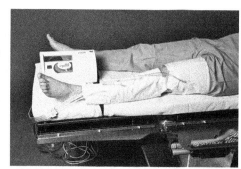

**Name:** head light

**Alias:** head lamp

**Use:** provides a concentrated area of light on the wound site for visualization by the surgeon during a procedure

**Features:** adjustable headpiece allows for snug fit to the surgeon's head; beam can be adjusted to the area the surgeon is viewing

**Additional Information:** available in many styles and sizes

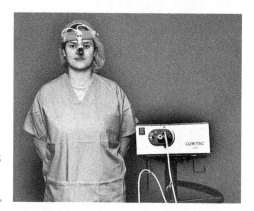

**Name:** sponge collection bag

**Alias:** none

**Use:** separates used sponges for ease of count

**Features:** each holder has 5 large or 10 small individual compartments; see-through front allows for ease of visualization of sponges

**Additional Information:** for ease and efficiency of counting, each type of sponge should be placed in a separate holder; do not "mix" different types (e.g., lap pads and Ray-Tecs) in the same holder

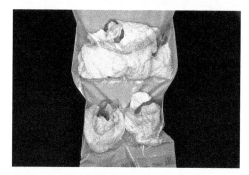

**Name:** smoke evacuation system

**Alias:** none

**Use:** suctions and filters surgical plume

**Features:** system contains HEPA filters and absorbers to trap surgical plume

**Additional Information:** nozzle tip must be as close to the surgical site as possible in order to be effective; filters, wands, and tubing must be changed between patients; filters, tubing, and wands are considered biohazardous waste and must be disposed of properly

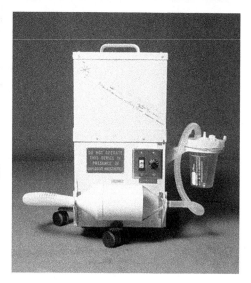

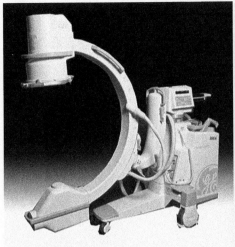

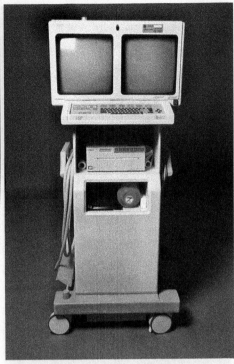

**Name:** C-arm

**Alias:** image intensifier

**Use:** intraoperative fluoroscopy

**Features:** image is immediately available to view; C-arm can be manipulated to give multiple views of the operative site

**Additional Information:** personnel need to wear lead aprons or stand behind a lead shield when C-arm is in use; C-arm is draped with a sterile C-arm drape

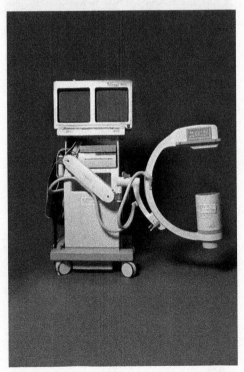

**Name:** mini C-arm

**Alias:** image intensifier

**Use:** intraoperative fluoroscopy; used primarily for imaging fingers, hands, wrists, or knees

**Features:** smaller and more easily maneuvered than conventional C-arms; exposes patients and staff to less radiation

**Additional Information:** lead apron should be worn when operating the machine (lighter mini C-arm lead aprons are available in some institutions); mini C-arm is draped with sterile mini C-arm cover; machine can be operated by the surgeon using a foot pedal

**Name:** fire extinguisher

**Alias:** none

**Use:** extinguishes small fires

**Features:** pin must be pulled to operate extinguisher; there are several models available, each one specific to certain types of fire; make sure you use the correct extinguisher for the type of material that has ignited

**Additional Information:** most ORs are equipped with multipurpose (ABC) extinguishers that can be used on most materials; only use the extinguisher if the fire is small and you have been properly trained in extinguisher use

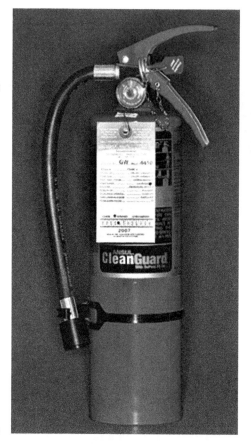

**Name:** vascular Doppler

**Alias:** SonoTrax

**Use:** assesses blood flow through a blood vessel before, during, and after surgery

**Features:** sterile probe cover should be available if intraoperative use is expected

**Additional Information:** available in many models and styles; pictured is one example

(Edan Diagnostics, Inc.)

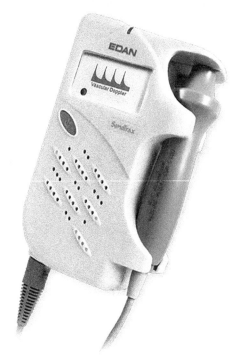

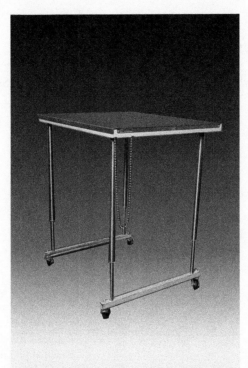

**Name:** Mayfield instrument table

**Alias:** overhead table

**Use:** holds instruments and supplies during craniotomy or spine procedures

**Features:** provides a large work area for the scrub; person (33.5- × 42-inch surface)

**Additional Information:** draped with an overhead table drape; can be draped continuously with the patient to produce a single large sterile field

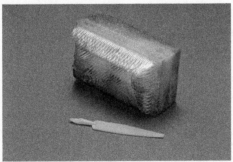

**Name:** surgical scrub brush

**Alias:** none

**Use:** performing the surgical scrub before entering the surgical suite

**Features:** soft foam side for performing skin scrub; bristle side for performing fingernail scrub

**Additional Information:** available with hexachlorophene or povidone-iodine (Betadine) soap impregnated in the brush; single use only

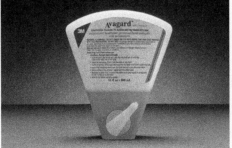

**Name:** waterless surgical scrub

**Alias:** several brand names: Avagard, Triseptin, Purell Surgical Scrub

**Use:** performing the surgical scrub before entering the surgical suite

**Features:** does not require the use of water; nonabrasive to the skin; has built-in emollient to control drying out of the skin

**Additional Information:** follow manufacturer's instructions for use; use only the amount the manufacturer recommends and the procedure suggests; procedures vary for each type of scrub

**Surgical Session Review**

1) A Mayfield attachment is most likely going to be used for which type of surgery?
   a. Total knee
   b. Craniotomy
   c. Total hip
   d. Endoscopic AAA repair

2) The PACS system is used to archive which type of studies?
   a. Radiological
   b. Laboratory values
   c. EEG results
   d. ECG tracings

3) Nissan thigh straps are used when the patient is being placed in what position?
   a. Lithotomy
   b. Prone
   c. Trendelenburg
   d. Steep reverse Trendelenburg

4) During which of the following surgeries might a cell saver be used?
   a. Shoulder arthroscopy
   b. Bowel resection
   c. Splenectomy for a ruptured spleen
   d. Strangulated hernia repair

5) The case is completed, and you are tearing down the smoke evacuation system. Which of the following is NOT considered hazardous waste?
   a. Machine control knobs
   b. Wand
   c. Filter
   d. Tubing

6) Which of the following is TRUE about grounding pad placement?
   a. Place over a bony prominence
   b. Place before the patient is positioned
   c. Check the pad for tears or kinks before placement
   d. If the pad is too large, fold it in half

7) Which of the following might be used to position a patient who is undergoing surgery on the lower back?
   a. Jackson table
   b. Wilson frame
   c. Andrews frame
   d. Any of the above

8) A horseshoe or Shea may be used to position the patient's _____.
   a. Head
   b. Arm
   c. Foot
   d. Shoulders

9) Arms should NEVER be extended more than _____ degrees on an arm board.
   a. 45
   b. 65
   c. 90
   d. 120

10) Hyperextension of the arm can cause damage to the:
    a. Peroneal nerve
    b. Popliteal nerve
    c. Brachial plexus
    d. Chordae tendineae

11) All of the following are types of stirrups *except:*
    a. Candy cane
    b. Boot
    c. Knee release
    d. Knee crutch

12) _____ is a gas that can be used to power equipment such as saws or drills.
    a. Oxygen
    b. Carbon dioxide
    c. Nitrogen
    d. Argon

13) Which of the following types of electrosurgery unit *does not* require the use of a grounding pad?
    a. Monopolar
    b. Argon beam
    c. Bipolar
    d. All of the above require a grounding pad

14) Fire safety rules during the use of electrosurgery include:
    a. Allow all prep solutions to dry completely
    b. Water or saline must be available on the surgical field
    c. When not in use, the handpiece should be placed back in a holder
    d. All of the above

15) In reference to electrosurgery units, ABC stands for:
   a. Aluminum beam coagulation
   b. Argon beam coagulation
   c. Argon beam cautery
   d. Aluminum beam cautery

16) Which of the following cases might you anticipate needing a back table with two top shelves?
   a. Appendectomy
   b. Inguinal hernia repair
   c. Bunionectomy
   d. Open multilevel spinal rodding

17) Ultrasonic cleaners use _____ to remove debris from instruments.
   a. Cavitation
   b. Steam
   c. Ethylene oxide
   d. Cidex

18) _____ is an anesthetic gas.
   a. Oxygen
   b. Nitrogen
   c. Nitrous oxide
   d. Argon

19) An Optigard protector is used when the patient is prone to protect his or her _____.
   a. Fingers
   b. Hands
   c. Toes
   d. Eyes

20) A Doppler is used to assess _____ flow.
   a. Urine
   b. Coronary artery
   c. Blood
   d. Brain wave

# 3

# General Surgical Supplies and Splints

## BASINS

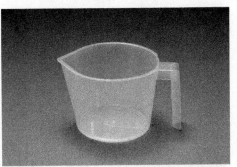

**Name:** graduate

**Alias:** graduated pitcher

**Use:** holds and measures irrigation fluids

**Features:** marked in cubic centimeters (cc) to allow fluid measurement; most common size is 1,000 cc

**Additional Information:** available in metal or plastic versions; all fluids, solutions, and medications on the sterile field must be labeled

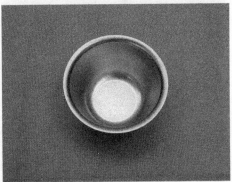

**Name:** alcohol cup

**Alias:** paint cup

**Use:** holds prep solution or medication

**Features:** able to fit in one hand so that it can be held by the person painting the skin (prep)

**Additional Information:** all fluids, solutions, and medications on the sterile field must be labeled

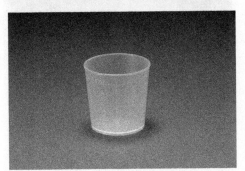

**Name:** medication cup

**Alias:** none

**Use:** holds and measures medications and solutions

**Features:** marked in cubic centimeters (cc) to allow for ease of measurement

**Additional Information:** available in plastic or metal versions; most common size holds 2 oz (60 cc); all fluids, solutions, and medications on the sterile field must be labeled

**Name:** round bowl

**Alias:** none

**Use:** stores solutions or medication on the back table; contains the specimen before it is passed off to the circulator

**Features:** available in many sizes to accommodate various uses

**Additional Information:** available in stainless steel or plastic disposal styles

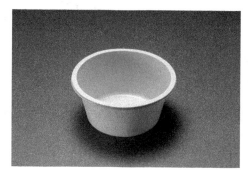

**Name:** wash bowl

**Alias:** extra-large basin

**Use:** soaks instruments intraoperatively; contains large specimens before passing them to the circulator; in some institutions, wash bowls are used to open small items into when first opening the supplies

**Features:** large capacity

**Additional Information:** available in stainless steel or plastic disposable styles

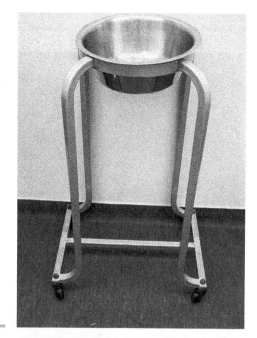

**Name:** soaking basin

**Alias:** none

**Use:** soaks instruments intraoperatively

**Features:** large capacity; rectangular shape allows for soaking of long instruments (e.g., femoral reamers)

**Additional Information:** available in shallow or deep styles

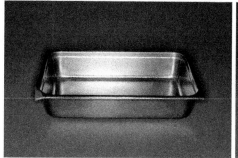
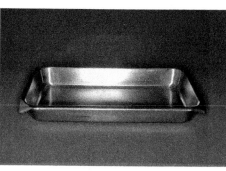

**Name:** kidney basin

**Alias:** emesis basin

**Use:** storage of specimens before basing them off the field; may be used as a "neutral zone" to pass sharps or instruments; may be used to contain vomit if patient is sick

**Features:** kidney shape allows for ease of fit under the patient's chin if they are vomiting

**Additional Information:** made of stainless steel or disposable plastic

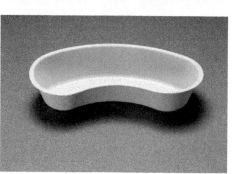

## EQUIPMENT DRAPES

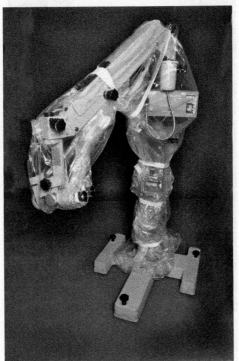

**Name:** microscope drape

**Alias:** none

**Use:** drapes the microscope for use in the surgical field

**Features:** tape closures ensure custom fit around oculars

**Additional Information:** available to fit several models of microscope

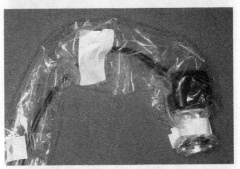

**Name:** camera drape

**Alias:** camera/laser arm drape

**Use:** drapes a nonsterile camera or a laser arm for use in the surgical field

**Features:** clear plastic so that equipment can be seen easily; telescopically folded for ease of application

**Additional Information:** 96 inches long; end width available in 5 or 7 inches

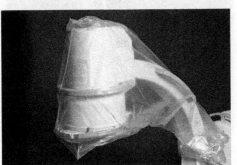

**Name:** C-arm drape

**Alias:** x-ray image intensifier drape

**Use:** drapes C-arm for use in the sterile field

**Features:** one-piece coverage; adhesive strips or patches help to customize fit to machine

**Additional Information:** available in sizes to fit regular C-arm or mini C-arm models

**Name:** banded bag

**Alias:** bonnet

**Use:** covers equipment for use in the sterile field; some surgeons use it to cover the end of the C-arm

**Features:** clear plastic to allow for equipment visualization; nonlatex elastic opening

**Additional Information:** available with 17-, 23-, 35-, or 45-inch opening

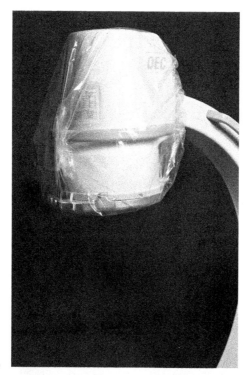

**Name:** half drape

**Alias:** medium drape

**Use:** general-purpose drape (e.g., can be used to drape arm boards and x-ray cassettes and cover small utility table)

**Features:** comes one to a package; can be folded to fit the area needed; has no adhesive; may need to use towel clamp to hold it in place

**Additional Information:** 60 × 44 inches

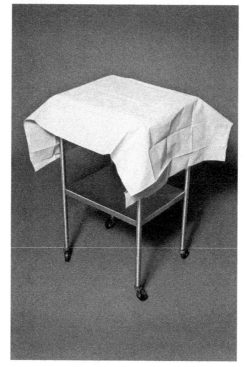

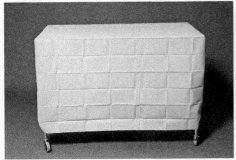

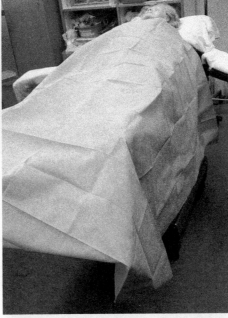

**Name:** large drape

**Alias:** three-quarters drape

**Use:** used as general-purpose drape to cover large areas

**Features:** comes one to a package; no adhesive

**Additional Information:** 60 × 76 inches

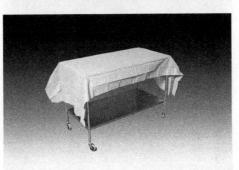

**Name:** back table cover

**Alias:** none

**Use:** drapes instrument table (back tables)

**Features:** reinforced for extra tear resistance; impervious backing to prevent fluid strike-through

**Additional Information:** 44 × 90 inches

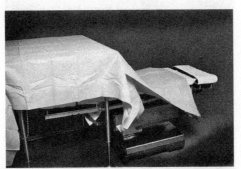

**Name:** overhead table cover

**Alias:** none

**Use:** drapes Mayfield (overhead) table

**Features:** sterile skirt around drape extends the sterile field to the top surface of the draped patient

**Additional Information:** available in regular or extra-large sizes

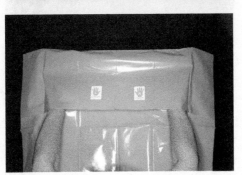

**Name:** Mayo stand cover

**Alias:** none

**Use:** drapes standard size Mayo stand

**Features:** reinforced to help prevent tears; impervious backing helps prevent strike-through contamination

**Additional Information:** 23 × 54 inches

**Name:** extra-large Mayo stand cover

**Alias:** none

**Use:** drapes large Mayo stands

**Features:** reinforced to help prevent tears; impervious backing helps prevent strike-through contamination

**Additional Information:** 30 × 57 inches; large Mayo stands are often used in orthopedic, neurosurgery, or spine cases

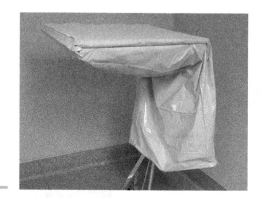

**Name:** woven sheet

**Alias:** cloth sheet

**Use:** generally covers a back table cover to give extra reinforcement; can be used as a sterile drape for the patient (e.g., could be put on a stretcher where a burn patient is going to be placed or used to cover a burn patient)

**Features:** washable and sterilizable

**Additional Information:** not impervious to fluids

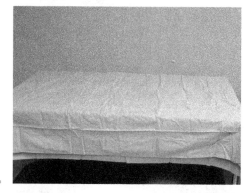

**Name:** controller drape

**Alias:** none

**Use:** drapes equipment remote controls

**Features:** drape is opened like a plastic bag and the nonsterile remote is dropped inside

**Additional Information:** none

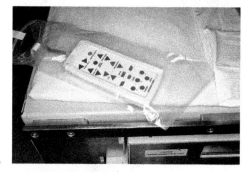

**Name:** x-ray cassette drape

**Alias:** none

**Use:** covers an x-ray cassette that needs to be placed in the sterile field

**Features:** deep cuff to protect the hands of scrub personnel

**Additional Information:** available in several sizes, ranging from 14 × 19 inches to 24 × 40 inches; clear plastic so that cassette can be seen easily for placement

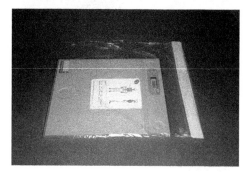

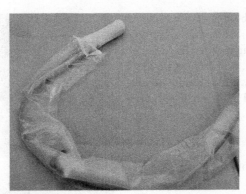

**Name:** ultrasound probe drape

**Alias:** none

**Use:** drapes probes for use in the sterile field

**Features:** available with several tips to accommodate different styles of probes (e.g., straight tip, angled tip, T-tip, and burr hole tip)

**Additional Information:** 5 × 96 inches; telescopically folded for ease of application

## SKIN PREPPING SOLUTIONS

The most common cause of surgical site infection is the first-line resident and transient (normal) flora found on the skin of the patient or surgical team members. In order to decrease the number of bacteria found on the patient's skin to an absolute minimum, the skin is prepped at the surgical site before the patient is draped. The prep removes oil and dirt that can harbor harmful bacteria and minimizes the normal bacteria on the skin.

Several types of prepping solutions are available to prepare the patient's skin before surgery. The solution used depends on the area to be prepped and the patient's allergy history. Only solutions approved for use on the skin are used as prep agents. Use of any other type of agents (e.g., disinfectants or chemical sterilants) could result in severe damage to the patient's skin. Covered in this section are the four most commonly used prepping solutions: alcohol, iodophors (povidone-iodine), DuraPrep, and chlorhexidine gluconate.

### Alcohol

The most common alcohol solutions used for skin preparation are those containing 70% isopropyl alcohol. At this concentration, the solution is 95% effective against both gram-positive and gram-negative bacteria; however, it is not completely effective against their spores. Alcohol works to kill bacteria by drying out the cell proteins. It is this drying characteristic that makes alcohol *not* appropriate for use on mucous membranes, in open wounds, or in eyes.

Isopropyl alcohol is colorless, although some manufacturers add a blue color to make it easier to distinguish from saline or other clear medications and solutions. It has a strong odor and is highly flammable. This flammability makes it imperative that the skin be given *adequate time to dry* before applying drapes; *all* traces of the alcohol must be gone. If alcohol is still present on the skin or drapes when laser or electrocautery is used, a fire could result.

Isopropyl alcohol in a 70% solution is available on swabs, on pads, in bottles, or in spray bottles. The most common container seen in the OR for skin prep is the 16-oz bottle

(Fig. 3–1). Isopropyl alcohol is also available in a 99% solution (bottle and spray bottle), although this is not as commonly used.

### Iodophors

Iodophors are a combination of iodine and povidone, which helps to make the iodine less irritating to tissue. The common concentration of povidone-iodine solution used for surgical skin prep is 10%. This type of solution is often referred to by the brand name Betadine.

In addition to the solution (sometimes referred to in the OR as *paint*), iodophors are mixed with detergents to make a 7.5% "scrub" solution. The scrub solution can be used by personnel to scrub their hands and arms before entering the sterile field or can be used to wash the patient's skin before applying the paint solution. Unlike the solution (or paint), iodophor scrub is *not* meant to be left on the skin and must be rinsed off. Scrub solutions should *not* be used around the eyes or on mucous membranes, although the paint solution can be used in these areas.

Iodophors are effective against gram-positive bacteria, but they are not as effective against gram-negative bacteria, viruses, and fungi. They do provide some residual antimicrobial effect.

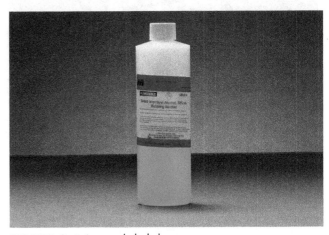

**FIGURE 3–1** Isopropyl alcohol.

Iodophor solution is available in bottles, on swab sticks, on pads, and in spray bottles (Fig. 3–2). The scrub solution is available in bottles and on surgical scrub brushes. **Because of the iodine content in this product, it *should not* be used on patients with an iodine allergy. This should not be placed in a warmer and then used on a patient due to the chance of thermal burns.**

## DuraPrep

DuraPrep is the 3M brand name for a popular prepping solution that combines 70% isopropyl alcohol and iodophor solution. The combination of the solutions combines the fast bacterial killing action of alcohol with the residual effect of the iodophor (kills bacteria up to 12 hours). It contains alcohol; therefore, it is flammable and must be allowed to dry completely (about 3 minutes) before applying drapes.

DuraPrep is packaged in a self-contained sponge applicator for ease of prep (Fig. 3–3). The applicator is available in two sizes: 6 mL (for small areas) and 26 mL (for larger areas).

Once applied, DuraPrep forms an antimicrobial film that can be difficult to remove. DuraPrep can be removed from the skin postoperatively using DuraPrep Remover.

## Chlorhexidine Gluconate

Chlorhexidine gluconate (also known as CHG) is used in a 2% or 4% solution for surgical skin prep or as a surgical hand scrub (Fig. 3–4). Upon application, it has a broad-spectrum antimicrobial effect and has a residual effect of up to 5 to 6 hours. One of the more common brand names for this solution is Hibiclens.

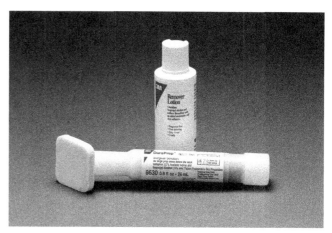

FIGURE 3–3 DuraPrep applicator and removing lotion.

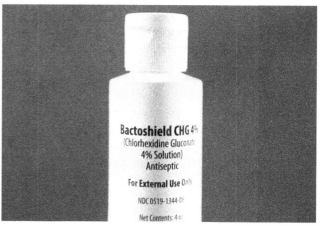

FIGURE 3–4 Chlorhexidine gluconate.

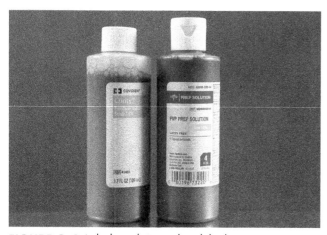

FIGURE 3–2 Iodophor solution and scrub bottles.

For surgical skin preparation, the manufacturer suggests chlorhexidine gluconate solution be swabbed onto the skin for 2 minutes. The area is then dried with a sterile towel, and the solution is reapplied and swabbed for 2 more minutes. The area is then dried again with a sterile towel. (Skin preparation procedures vary among institutions; check your institution's policy or procedure.) This solution is available in bottles of varying sizes and on surgical scrub brushes.

WARNING: Chlorhexidine gluconate has been associated with hearing loss when introduced into the middle ear; therefore, it should *never be used* for preparations around the ear. It also *should not* be used for preparation of the eye, of the mouth, or on large open wounds.

## PATIENT DRAPES

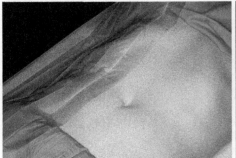

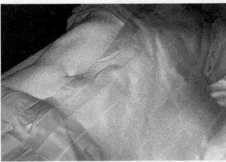

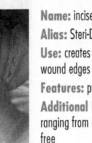

**Name:** incise drape

**Alias:** Steri-Drape

**Use:** creates a sterile operative area up to the wound edges

**Features:** provides a barrier to skin bacteria

**Additional Information:** available in many sizes ranging from 4 × 8 inches to 23 × 33 inches; latex free

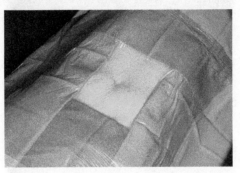

**Name:** antimicrobial incise drape

**Alias:** Ioban

**Use:** provides a sterile surface up to the wound edges; provides continuous antimicrobial activity intraoperatively

**Features:** stretches and contours to accommodate surgical site manipulation

**Additional Information:** available in several sizes ranging from 4 × 8 inches to 23 × 33 inches; latex free; cannot be used on patients with iodine sensitivity or allergy

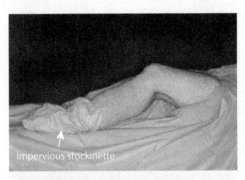

Impervious stockinette

**Name:** impervious stockinette

**Alias:** none

**Use:** drapes extremity

**Features:** fluid-proof barrier helps to reduce the chance of microbial migration

**Additional Information:** available in 8-, 10-, or 12-inch widths; some available with straps to help ease over the extremity

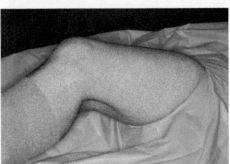

**Name:** impervious split drape

**Alias:** none

**Use:** drapes the top of an extremity (e.g., drapes the top of the thigh/buttock for hip surgery)

**Features:** split makes it easy to wrap around the extremity; fluid proof

**Additional Information:** 60 × 70 inches; large size is 60 × 81 inches; available with or without a built-in pouch

**Name:** extremity drape
**Alias:** none
**Use:** drapes an arm or leg
**Features:** 2.5-inch stretchable circular fenestration
**Additional Information:** 90 × 124 inches

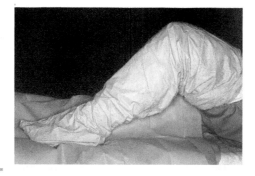

**Name:** bilateral limb drape
**Alias:** bilateral extremity drape
**Use:** drapes both legs at the same time (e.g., draping for bilateral knee arthroplasties)
**Features:** two 2.5-inch stretchable circular fenestrations
**Additional Information:** 76 × 120 inches

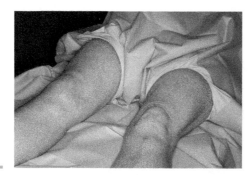

**Name:** beach chair shoulder drape
**Alias:** none
**Use:** drapes out the shoulder for open shoulder procedures
**Features:** available with or without a fluid pouch
**Additional Information:** 172 × 100 inches

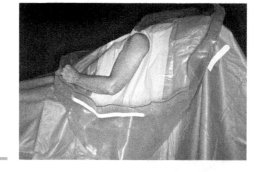

**Name:** laparotomy drape
**Alias:** none
**Use:** draping the abdomen for general or gynecological surgery
**Features:** 4 × 12-inch fenestration; attached arm board covers; attached tube holders
**Additional Information:** available in several adult and pediatric sizes; fenestration can be vertical (for midline incisions) or horizontal

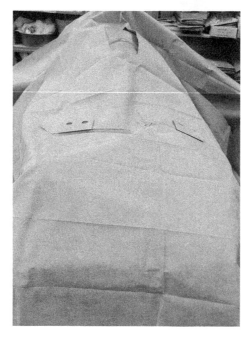

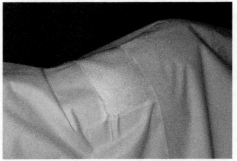

**Name:** laparoscopic cholecystectomy drape

**Alias:** lap chole drape, laparoscopic drape

**Use:** drapes the abdomen for laparoscopic cholecystectomy, splenectomy, etc.

**Features:** 12 × 13.5-inch laterally offset fenestration

**Additional Information:** 104 × 120 inches; available with or without instrument pouch

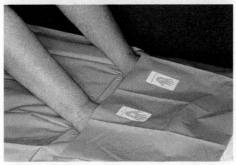

**Name:** cesarean section drape

**Alias:** C-section drape

**Use:** drapes the abdomen for a cesarean section

**Features:** fenestrated incise area with large 360-degree fluid collection pouch

**Additional Information:** 100 × 72 × 120 inches

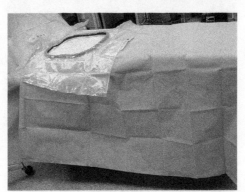

**Name:** under buttocks drape

**Alias:** none

**Use:** drape placed under the buttocks for gynecological procedures

**Features:** fluid proof; has pockets into which the scrub person can place his or her hands to protect them from contamination while sliding the drape under the patient's buttocks

**Additional Information:** available in small, medium, and large sizes

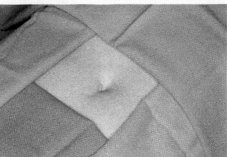

**Name:** utility drape

**Alias:** towel drape

**Use:** squares off the incision area

**Features:** built-in adhesive strip holds the drape in place

**Additional Information:** 15 × 26 inches; comes in a package of two; some surgeons use these in place of linen towels

**Name:** U-bar drape
**Alias:** bar drape
**Use:** usually used to drape chest or abdomen
**Features:** drape with a U cut out; 4 × 40-inch split (chest drape has 12 × 30-inch split)
**Additional Information:** 76 × 120 inches

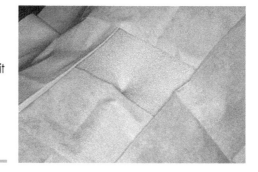

**Name:** incise utility towel
**Alias:** none
**Use:** drapes the surgical field (used like woven towel or utility drape)
**Features:** adhesive strip holds it in place; clear, which allows visualization around the wound area
**Additional Information:** none

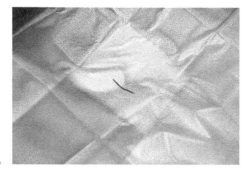

**Name:** woven towel
**Alias:** woven towel, cloth towel
**Use:** drapes the surgical site; covers Mayo stand or portions of the back table; can be rolled to make a place to hold instruments
**Features:** washable and sterilizable; generally packaged four or eight to a pack; if used to drape the surgical site either towel clips or incise/loban drapes can be used to hold them in place
**Additional Information:** Be cautious when using sharps so as not to slice the drape; it is *not* impervious to fluids; not radiopaque—should not be used inside body cavities

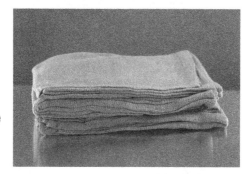

**Name:** leggings
**Alias:** none
**Use:** drape the feet and legs of patients who are in stirrups
**Features:** some drapes have clear tops so that feet and legs can be seen; drapes are marked "right" and "left"
**Additional Information:** come as a pair; have cuff to protect scrub person's hands while applying the drape

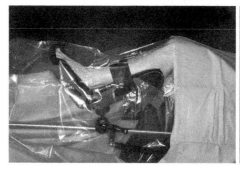
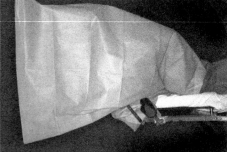

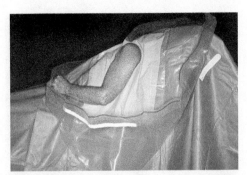

**Name:** arthroscopy drape
**Alias:** none
**Use:** drapes extremity for arthroscopic surgery
**Features:** 2.5-inch stretchable circular fenestration; fluid collection pouch with suction port
**Additional Information:** 90 × 124 inches

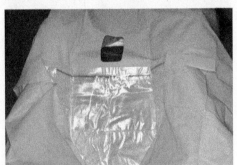

**Name:** cystoscopy drape
**Alias:** none
**Use:** drapes perineal area and abdomen for cystoscopic procedures
**Features:** T shape allows coverage of legs and abdomen with narrow part draping the perineum; 3 × 6-inch fenestration allows access to the perineal area
**Additional Information:** available in two sizes

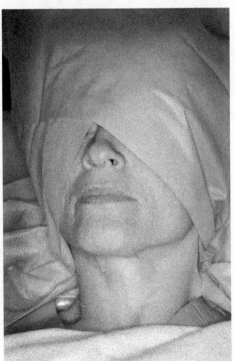

**Name:** head drape
**Alias:** turban drape
**Use:** drapes the head and covers the hair for eye, ear, nose, and throat (EENT) surgery
**Features:** has built-in turban to cover the patient's hair and keep it out of the operative field
**Additional Information:** available in two sizes (36 × 24 inches and 33 × 20 inches)

**Name:** craniotomy drape

**Alias:** none

**Use:** drapes the patient's head and body during a craniotomy

**Features:** oval fenestration; clear panels to allow anesthesia to visualize the patient

**Additional Information:** 122 × 74 × 134 inches

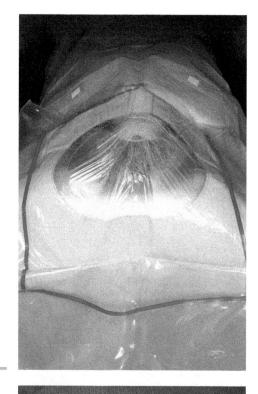

**Name:** EENT drape

**Alias:** none

**Use:** drapes the patient's head and body for EENT procedures

**Features:** available in two styles: one with a 3 × 28-inch split and one with a 2 × 2.5-inch fenestration

**Additional Information:** split drape is 76 × 124 inches; fenestrated drape is 76 × 90 inches

**Name:** ophthalmic drape

**Alias:** eye drape

**Use:** drapes the patient's eye, head, and upper body during ophthalmic procedures

**Features:** 3 × 2-inch oval fenestration; fluid collection pouch

**Additional Information:** 52 × 56 inches

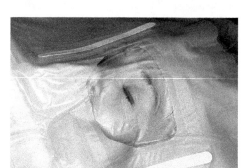

**Name:** breast/chest drape

**Alias:** none

**Use:** drapes patient for breast or thoracic procedures

**Features:** 13 × 14-inch fenestration; arm board covers; instrument pad

**Additional Information:** 100 × 72 × 124 inches

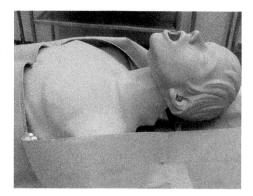

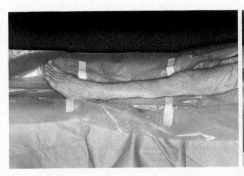

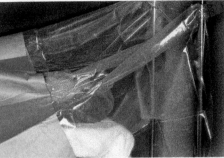

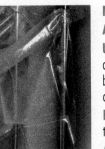

**Name:** CV drape

**Alias:** cardiovascular drape

**Use:** drapes the body, leaving the leg exposed for cardiovascular surgery (e.g., for femoral-popliteal bypass surgery or for harvesting of leg vein for cardiac bypasses)

**Features:** split all the way down, allowing one leg to be completely exposed; tubing pockets

**Additional Information:** 116 × 88 × 140 inches; 92-inch-long split

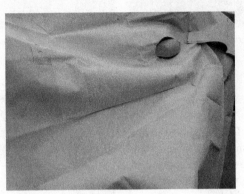

**Name:** split body drape

**Alias:** none

**Use:** used as general-purpose split body drape for orthopedic surgery

**Features:** 27-inch split

**Additional Information:** 88 × 116 inches

# SURGICAL SPONGES

Surgical sponges come in a variety of shapes and sizes, each with its own specific purpose. The most common use for surgical sponges is to absorb blood and fluid. They also can be used as padding to protect tissue from retractor blades, to wipe debris from instruments, or to perform blunt tissue dissection.

Sponges intended for use inside of the body cavity share several characteristics:

- Lint free
- Soft, to avoid damaging tissue
- Radiopaque strip sewn into them (to make them visible on radiography if left inside a wound)

Depending on your institution, various sponges are referred to by names other than what are listed in this section. I have chosen to go with the commonly accepted names for the various sponges.

## General Sponge-Handling Tips

- Sponges are contaminated with blood or body fluids. Use standard precautions.
- Gloves must be worn when handling sponges. Never use your bare hands.
- Sponges should be tossed off the field into a proper receptacle (e.g., kick bucket or basin), not onto the floor or into the trash.

- When setting up your table preoperatively, like sponges should be kept together and separate from other types (e.g., all laparotomy sponges in one area of the table, all Ray-Tec sponges in another area) to avoid confusion and to make counting more efficient.
- Soiled sponges should be separated, keeping all like sponges together. If using a clear sponge-counting bag, do not mix different sponges in the same bag; use a separate sponge bag for each type of sponge.
- Keep small sponges, such as cherries or dissectors, attached to a clamp or in the holder. Do not leave them loose on your table or Mayo stand. These sponges are very small and could easily be lost (or fall inside the wound).
- To avoid damaging tissue, moisten sponges that are being used inside the chest, abdomen, or pelvis with saline before use.
- Once the initial count has been done, never remove a sponge from the operating room (OR).
- When counting sponges, separate each sponge to avoid missing a sponge or miscounting. Each type of sponge should be counted separately.

## Ray-Tec

The Ray-Tec sponge is a 4 × 4-inch sponge with a radiopaque strip sewn into it. It is made of loosely woven gauze, which gives it a rough surface (Fig. 3–5). These sponges are used when the incision is small. Loose Ray-Tecs are generally not allowed on the field during a laparotomy because they could

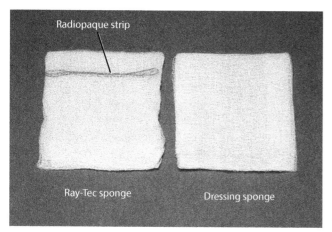

FIGURE 3-5 Ray-Tec sponge with radiopaque strip and plain dressing sponge.

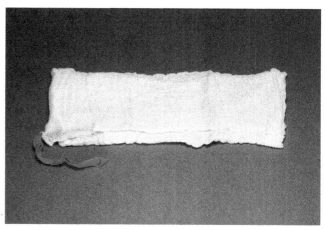

FIGURE 3-6 Laparotomy sponge. Notice placement of the blue radiopaque strip.

easily be lost in the abdominopelvic cavity. Instead, a large laparotomy sponge is used.

Wrapped around the fingers, Ray-Tecs can be used for blunt tissue dissection. They can be mounted on a sponge stick and used to absorb fluid or dissect tissue inside the abdominal cavity. Moistened with saline or sterile water, they are often used to keep surgical instruments free of debris.

Caution must be taken NOT to mix up Ray-Tecs with 4 × 4-inch gauze dressing sponges because they look very similar. The important difference is that dressing sponges DO NOT have the radiopaque strip sewn into them and therefore could easily be lost in the wound. Depending on the institution, dressing sponges are either kept in an area separate from the Ray-Tec sponges during the procedure or they are not introduced onto the sterile field until the wound is closed.

Ray-Tec sponges come in a package of 10. Ray-Tecs should be separated and counted individually (not in groups of two or three) to ensure an accurate count.

## Laparotomy Sponges and Tape

Laparotomy sponges, known as *laps,* are used when large incisions of the thoracic or abdominopelvic cavity are involved, during vascular surgery involving large blood vessels, or during major orthopedic cases (Fig. 3–6). These sponges are most commonly used for the absorption of large amounts of blood or body fluid. Moistened with saline, they can be used as padding between body tissue and retractors to decrease the chance of tissue injury. Laparotomy pads also may be used to wipe debris from instruments.

Laparotomy sponges measure 12 × 12 inches or 18 × 18 inches. They are made of surgical cotton and have a radiopaque strip sewn onto them. They come in packages of five. When counting laparotomy sponges, separate and count each one individually.

Laparotomy tape is a long, thin laparotomy sponge. Made of surgical cotton, it measures 4 × 18 inches and has a radiopaque strip sewn onto it (Fig. 3–7). These sponges are used to absorb blood or body fluid from a narrow, deep

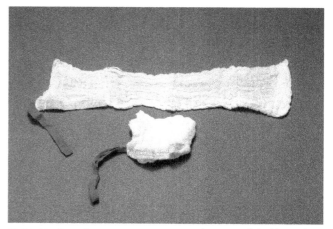

FIGURE 3-7 Laparotomy tape. Notice placement of the blue radiopaque strip.

incision (e.g., lumbar spinal surgery). Laparotomy tapes come in packages of five.

## Tonsil (Round) Sponges

Tonsil sponges are round pieces of cotton covered with gauze that have a string attached for easy retrieval from the throat. They have a radiopaque strip sewn into them (Fig. 3–8). Typically these sponges are mounted on a clamp (e.g., Pean) and placed in the throat to control bleeding in the tonsil bed. They can be used plain, or they can have a hemostatic agent applied to them. When you remove the sponges from the throat, it is important to make sure that you have *both* the sponge and the string because a string could get cut during the procedure. Tonsil sponges come in packages of five.

## Peanut Sponges

Peanut sponges, also known as *dissectors* or *pushers,* are small oval pieces of cotton wrapped in gauze. A radiopaque strip is sewn into the material (Fig. 3–9). These sponges can be used to absorb small amounts of blood or fluid but are used

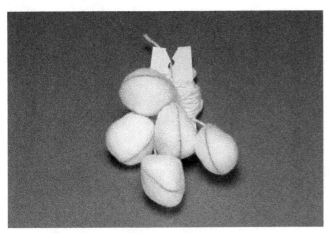

FIGURE 3-8 Tonsil sponges.

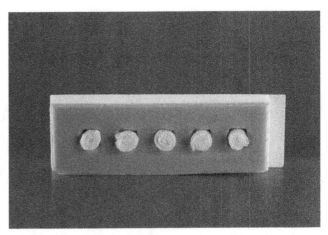

FIGURE 3-10 Kittner sponges.

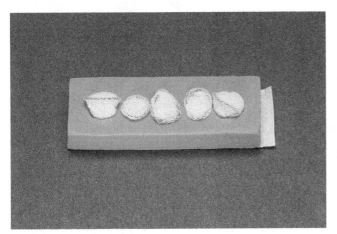

FIGURE 3-9 Peanut sponges.

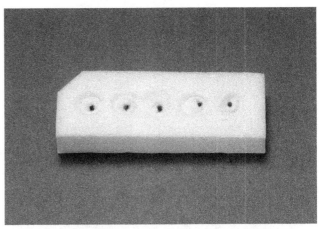

FIGURE 3-11 Beehive sponges.

more commonly for blunt tissue dissection. Peanuts are always mounted on a clamp (e.g., Pean) for use. They should never be loose on the field, table, or Mayo stand; they easily could be lost into the wound because of their small size. Peanuts come five to a package.

## Kittner Sponges

A Kittner sponge is a small, tightly wound roll of cotton tape containing a radiopaque strip (Fig. 3–10). Kittner sponges are used for blunt dissection. Kittners are always mounted on a clamp (e.g., Pean) for use. They should never be loose on the field, table, or Mayo stand; they easily could be lost into the wound because of their small size. Kittners come five to a package.

## Hard Dissectors

Hard dissectors or "beehive" sponges are small, round balls of tightly wrapped cotton with a radiopaque center. They may look similar to a peanut but are more tightly wrapped and stiffer (Fig. 3–11). These sponges are used for blunt tissue dissection. Beehive sponges are always mounted on a clamp (e.g., Pean) for use. They should never be allowed to be loose on

the field, table, or Mayo stand due to their small size; they easily could be lost in the wound. Beehive sponges come five to a package.

## Cherry Sponges

The largest of the dissectors, Cherry sponges are used for blunt dissection of large areas of tissue (Fig. 3–12). Cherry sponges are always mounted on a clamp (e.g., Pean) for use. They should never be loose on the field, table, or Mayo stand; they easily could be lost into the wound because of their small size. Cherry sponges come five to a package.

## Cylindrical Sponges

These sponges are cylinder-shaped tubes of cotton material, with an x-ray detectable marker (Fig. 3–13). An attached string makes them easy to remove when finished. They are designed for use in tonsil, adenoid, and nasal surgery. They come in regular or small sizes in packages of five.

## Neurosurgical Sponges

A neurosurgical sponge, also known as a *patty* or *cottonoid,* is a flat, square, or rectangular sponge made of cotton or synthetic

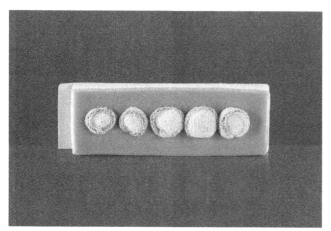

FIGURE 3-12 Cherry sponges.

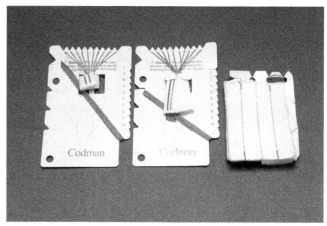

FIGURE 3-14 Neurosurgical sponges.

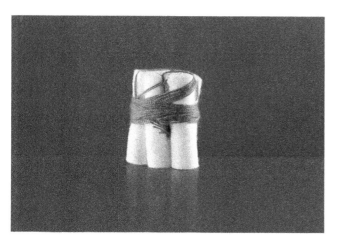

FIGURE 3-13 Cylindrical sponges.

tray called a *patty tray*. When passed to the surgeon, the sponges are mounted on a pair of smooth-jawed forceps (e.g., bayonet forceps). When receiving the sponge back from the surgeon, make sure you have *both* the sponge and the string; a string could get cut during the procedure. Neurosurgical sponges come in packages of 10.

### Eye Sponges

Eye sponges, also known as *spears* or *Weck Cel sponges,* are small, flat, triangular pieces of cellulose, each mounted on a small, thin piece of plastic (Fig. 3–15). These sponges are used to absorb small amounts of blood and fluid during eye procedures or some microsurgeries. They do not have a radiopaque strip because they are not used inside a body cavity. Eye sponges come in packages of 10.

material with a radiopaque strip down the center (Fig. 3–14). The sponge has a string attached for easy retrieval. These sponges come in a variety of sizes, ranging from ⅛ to 1 inch wide and ⅛ to 6 inches long.

Neurosurgical sponges are used for hemostasis during neurosurgery, but they also can be used during vascular or ear and nose procedures. They are moistened with either saline or thrombin before being placed on the tissue. Larger rectangular sponges can be moistened with a topical anesthetic (e.g., liquid cocaine) and inserted into the nose before nasal procedures. These sponges can be placed over an area to be suctioned and a small suction placed on top of them instead of directly on the tissue, thus protecting the tissue from damage.

To keep the sponges sorted and easily accessible, they are moistened with saline and mounted on a flat metal or plastic

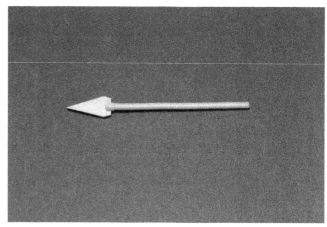

FIGURE 3-15 Eye sponge.

# HEMOSTATICS

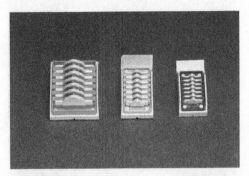

**Name:** hemoclips

**Alias:** clips, metal ligation system

**Use:** clip vessels or ducts

**Features:** available in sizes small, medium, medium-large, and large

**Additional Information:** clips may be metal or plastic; color of cartridge corresponds to the handle color of the applier; cartridges may be included as part of the count (not the individual clips)

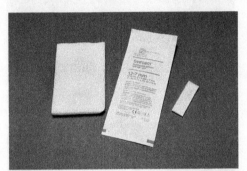

**Name:** absorbable gelatin sponge

**Alias:** Gelfoam, Surgifoam

**Use:** hemostatic

**Features:** dry; applied topically; absorbable

**Additional Information:** available in a variety of sizes; can be cut up for use in small areas

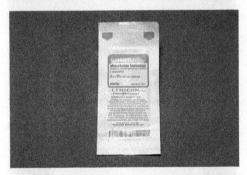

**Name:** oxidized cellulose

**Alias:** Surgicel, Oxycel, Gelita-Cel

**Use:** hemostatic

**Features:** absorbable; sheet can be cut to size needed; flexible

**Additional Information:** handle with dry forceps; comes in a variety of sheet sizes

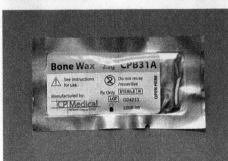

**Name:** bone wax

**Alias:** none

**Use:** stopping bleeding on the bone surface

**Features:** pliable; can be molded to size and shape needed

**Additional Information:** can be applied by hand or with an instrument; store away from heat

**Name:** microfibrillar collagen

**Alias:** Avitene, INSTAT MCH

**Use:** hemostatic

**Features:** absorbable; can be broken up into small pieces if necessary; conforms and adheres to irregular surfaces

**Additional Information:** should be handled with dry forceps; available in several sizes

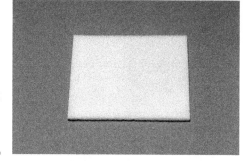

**Name:** collagen sponge

**Alias:** Collastat, Helistat

**Use:** hemostatic

**Features:** absorbable; comes as a sheet; sponge can be cut to desired size

**Additional Information:** handle with dry forceps; available in several sizes

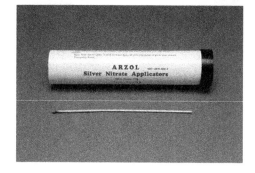

**Name:** Gelfoam sterile powder

**Alias:** none

**Use:** hemostatic

**Features:** mixed with sterile saline or thrombin and then applied

**Additional Information:** after mixing, it can be shaped and applied to the desired surface

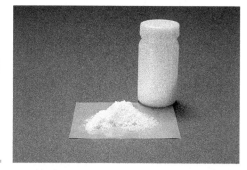

**Name:** silver nitrate sticks

**Alias:** none

**Use:** hemostatic

**Features:** when moistened (e.g., by blood from a bleeding vessel), the silver nitrate is activated and cauterizes the area

**Additional Information:** come in a canister to protect them from moisture; for use on small areas

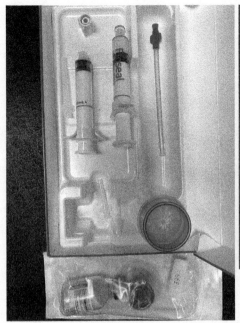

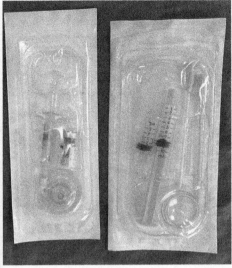

**Name:** hemostatic matrix

**Alias:** Floseal, Surgiflo

**Use:** adjunct to hemostasis when ligature or other conventional methods don't work or are impractical

**Features:** a mixture of hemostatic granules and human thrombin; applied directly to the bleeding area

**Additional Information:** CANNOT be injected directly into the circulatory system; applicator is needleless

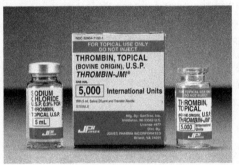

**Name:** thrombin, topical

**Alias:** none

**Use:** topical hemostasis; apply only to the surface of bleeding area; often Gelfoam (Surgifoam) is soaked in it and applied to bleeding

**Features:** comes as a powder; must be mixed with enclosed container of normal saline

**Additional Information:** available in 5,000 U or 20,000 U vials or 20,000 U spray kit; must ONLY be used topically; CANNOT be injected

# SYRINGES

Syringes are commonly used in the OR. Anesthesia care providers use them to measure and administer medications. Scrubbed personnel use syringes to measure medications, measure and dispense irrigating solutions, withdraw fluid from body cavities, and obtain liquid specimens to send for diagnosis. Circulators use syringes to measure and dispense medication to the field or administer medication to the patient. This section covers the two major categories of syringes—those that you can place a needle onto and those that are used for irrigation.

Syringes that have a tip where a needle (or needleless delivery system) can be placed come in many sizes and styles. Syringes are marked in milliliters (mL) or cubic centimeters (cc) for easy measurement. Milliliters and cubic centimeters are equivalent (1 mL = 1 cc). The most commonly used sizes are 1 mL, 3 mL, 5 mL, 10 mL, 12 mL, 20 mL, 30 mL, and 60 mL. Which size you use depends on what you are using it for—a 1-mL syringe would be used to measure out small amounts of medication (e.g., pediatric dosages), whereas a

60-mL syringe might be used to withdraw large amounts of fluid from a patient's joint.

Despite the size differences among syringes, they all have the same basic components (Fig. 3–16):

- Barrel
- Plunger
- Tip
- Measurement markings

Medication, solutions, and fluids are drawn up into the syringe by holding the barrel and pulling back on the plunger until you have the desired amount in the barrel of the syringe.

To inject medication or solution, you hold the top of the barrel in your fingers and push down on the top of the plunger slowly and steadily until you have injected the desired amount.

## Syringe Tips

There are two different types of syringe tips: Luer-Lok and plain (catheter tip; Luer-slip).

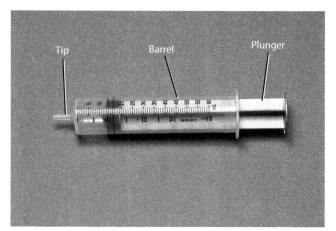

FIGURE 3–16 Parts of a syringe.

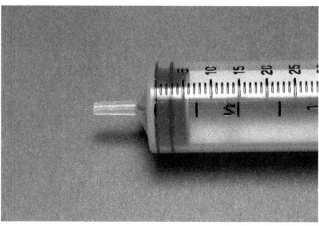

FIGURE 3–18 Plain catheter tip.

As the name implies, the Luer-Lok tip (Fig. 3–17) has threads, like a metal screw, to lock a needle in place. You place the hub of the needle onto the tip and, with a twisting motion, lock it in place. You must twist the needle onto the tip in order to secure it. This is the most commonly used type of syringe.

The plain-tip syringe, also known as a catheter or Luer-slip tip, does not have threads to lock the needle in place (Fig. 3–18). The hub of the needle or end of a catheter is pushed onto the end of the tip.

## Types of Syringes

Commonly used syringes are made of either plastic or glass. Plastic is by far the most common material used, but glass syringes are still used for certain tasks (e.g., some anesthesia providers prefer glass syringes when inserting an epidural, and some medication strengths could be affected by plastic) (Fig. 3–19).

One type of syringe has finger rings on the top of the barrel and plunger. These rings allow the user to insert fingers for better control of the rate of medication administration or force

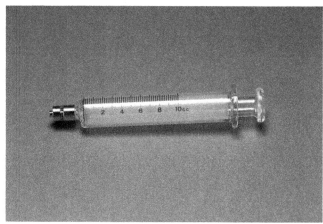

FIGURE 3–19 Glass syringe.

of irrigation. These are known as *three-ring, high-pressure,* or *control syringes* (Fig. 3–20).

## Irrigating Syringes

In the OR, there are three common types of irrigating syringes: the Asepto, the bulb, and the Toomey. These syringes

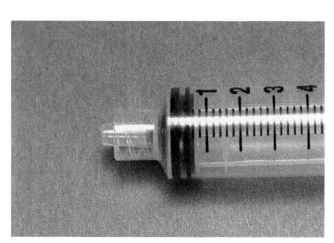

FIGURE 3–17 Luer-Lok tip.

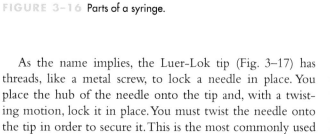

**WATCH OUT!** Tuberculin and Insulin Syringes

Tuberculin syringes and insulin syringes are both small syringes, but that is where the similarity ends. An insulin syringe should NEVER BE USED FOR ANYTHING OTHER THAN MEASURING AND ADMINISTERING INSULIN! The insulin syringe (Fig. 3–21) is marked in *units of insulin,* not milliliters (cubic centimeters) of volume. If you were to measure fluid or medication (other than insulin) in an insulin syringe, the measurement would be inaccurate and thus potentially dangerous. Only small dosages of medication should be drawn up using the tuberculin syringe (Fig. 3–21).

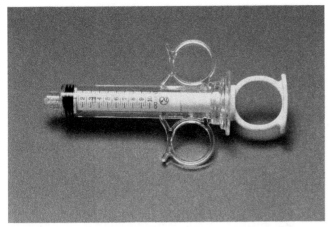

FIGURE 3-20 Three-ring, high-pressure, or control syringe.

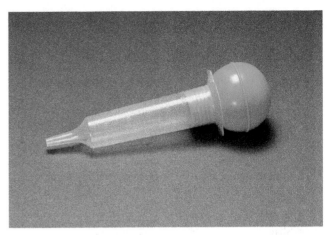

FIGURE 3-22 Asepto syringe.

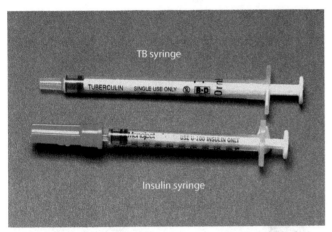

TB syringe

Insulin syringe

FIGURE 3-21 Tuberculin (TB) syringe: 1-mL capacity; marked in 0.1-mL increments (larger lines). Insulin syringe: marked in units of insulin (not mL).

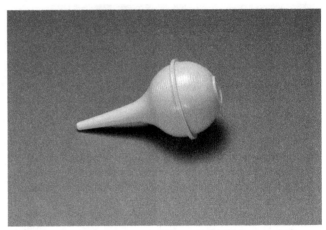

FIGURE 3-23 Bulb syringe.

a regular syringe, the tip is designed to irrigate or instill fluids only; a needle cannot be placed on it (Fig. 3–24).

## Hypodermic Needles

Hypodermic needles placed on syringe tips allow medication to be drawn up into the syringe, injection of fluid or

are used to draw up and dispense irrigating solutions and do not have a needle placed on them.

**Asepto Syringe:** The Asepto syringe is the most common irrigating syringe found on the surgical field. It has a capacity of 120 mL. The syringe has a bulb and barrel construction (Fig. 3–22).

**Bulb Syringe (Ear Syringe):** Most commonly thought of as a mechanism to remove fluid or mucus from an infant's nose or mouth, the bulb syringe can also be used for irrigation. In contrast to the Asepto, its construction is a bulb only (no barrel) (Fig. 3–23). The bulb syringe is used to irrigate small incisions or delicate structures such as the brain or ears.

**Toomey Syringe:** The Toomey syringe is used to irrigate or instill fluids into tubes or catheters. The plain style tip is long and tapered to fit inside the lumen of a catheter or tube. The Toomey has a capacity of 60 to 70 mL. The construction is the same as a regular syringe with a barrel and plunger but, unlike

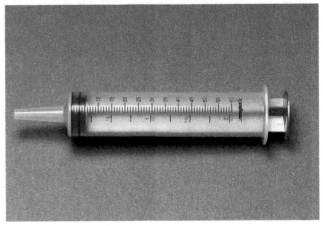

FIGURE 3-24 Toomey syringe.

medication into body tissue, and withdrawal of body fluid from tissues or joints. Small (fine) hypodermic needles may be used to remove small bits of tissue from biopsy needles.

Hypodermic needles are sized according to a numbering system. The important thing to remember is *the larger the number, the smaller the diameter of the needle.* The largest hypodermic needle is the #7, and the smallest needle is the #33 (Fig. 3–25). Hypodermic needles range in length from ⅜ to 4 inches.

Regardless of the size or length of the hypodermic needle, they all have the same basic components (Fig. 3–26):

- Hub
- Bevel
- Shaft

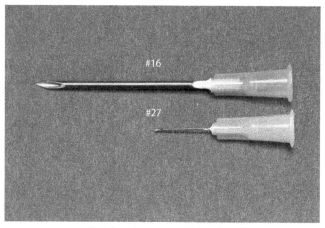

FIGURE 3–25 Tip of a 16-gauge needle and tip of a 27-gauge needle.

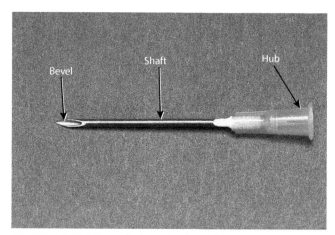

FIGURE 3–26 Parts of a hypodermic needle.

## WATCH OUT! Needle Safety

As with any sharp, hypodermic needles must be handled and disposed of with caution to avoid an inadvertent needlestick to yourself or other team member. Here are a few rules to follow to help promote safety when using needles:

- Know the location of your needles on the surgical field at all times.
- Attach or remove the needle from a syringe using a clamp or other instrument, NOT your hands.
- Never recap a needle using your hands; use the "scoop method" or a recapping device.
- Pass the syringe and needle using a "neutral zone;" avoid hand-to-hand passing.
- Discard a dirty needle by placing it needle-side down into a sharps holder (AccuCount or similar box). At the end of the case, discard the sharps holder into a puncture-proof sharps disposal bucket.
- If the needle is equipped with a safety shield, trigger the safety shield over the needle at the end of the case before disposing of it. *Remember:* On some needles, if you trigger the safety shield, it cannot be retracted; therefore, the needle cannot be used again. That is why I recommend waiting until the end of the case to trigger the device.

## OTHER SUPPLIES

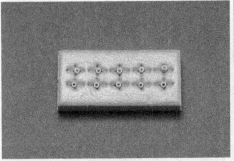
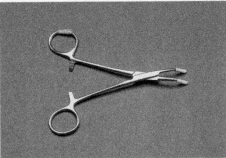

**Name:** suture boots

**Alias:** shods

**Use:** protect sutures from damage by serrated instrument jaws—facilitates grasping and tagging

**Features:** soft plastic; fit onto the tips of mosquitos (Halstead) or Crile clamps

**Additional Information:** come in packages of 10; may be included as part of the count

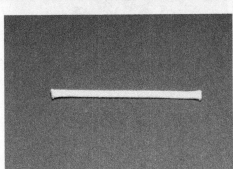
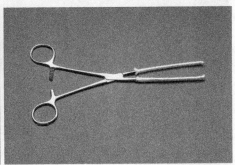

**Name:** clamp cover

**Alias:** none

**Use:** covers the blades of clamps to protect delicate tissue

**Features:** available in wide or narrow; may be made of cotton or rubber

**Additional Information:** dipping into saline before applying to the clamp blade makes the cover easier to put on and makes it wet and ready to use; may be included as part of the count

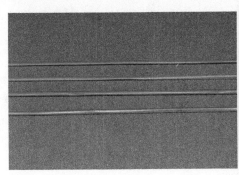
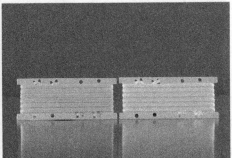

**Name:** vessel loops

**Alias:** none

**Use:** retract vessels during surgery

**Features:** available in red (arteries), blue (veins), white (nerves), and yellow (tendons)

**Additional Information:** available in narrow or wide; may be included as part of the count

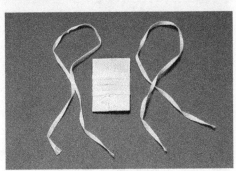

**Name:** umbilical tape

**Alias:** cotton tape

**Use:** ties off umbilical cord; retracts or ties vessels

**Features:** soft; nontraumatic to vessels or tissue

**Additional Information:** may be included as part of the count; should be moistened with saline before use

**Name:** Raney clips

**Alias:** scalp clips

**Use:** retracts scalp tissue out of the way during cranial surgery; aids in hemostasis of the scalp

**Features:** plastic; single-patient use

**Additional Information:** need to be loaded onto a manual applier for use, also available in disposable multiload clip appliers

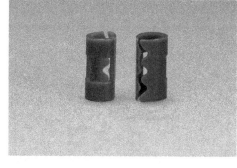 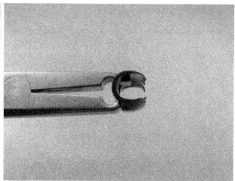

**Name:** medication labels

**Alias:** none

**Use:** labels medication and solution containers on the field

**Features:** may be blank or preprinted

**Additional Information:** self-stick backing allows for application directly to the containers

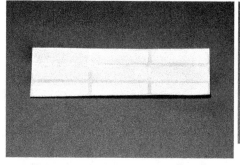 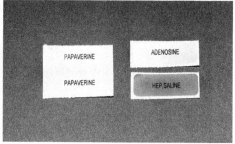

**Name:** umbilical cord clamp

**Alias:** cord clamp

**Use:** clamps off the umbilical cord after birth

**Features:** clamp tip facilitates closure and secure hold

**Additional Information:** single-patient use; have open on Mayo stand before delivery during a C-section

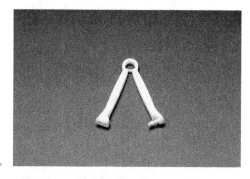

**Name:** ruler

**Alias:** none

**Use:** measures wounds, grafts, implants, and so on

**Features:** markings in inches and centimeters

**Additional Information:** available in paper (single-patient use) or metal (resterilizable)

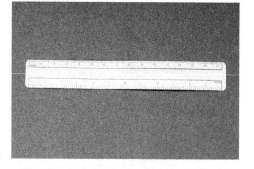

**Name:** surgical markers

**Alias:** marking pen

**Use:** marks the skin

**Features:** available with a medium or fine point; some have rulers marked on the side

**Additional Information:** single-patient use

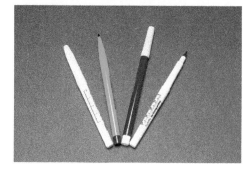

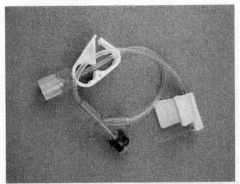

**Name:** winged infusion set
**Alias:** port access needle, Huber needle
**Use:** accesses implanted ports for infusion of fluids or medication
**Features:** noncoring so that it will not damage the port
**Additional Information:** available in a variety of gauge sizes; single-patient use

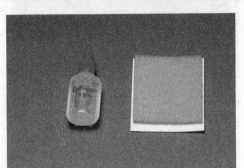

**Name:** defogger kit
**Alias:** none
**Use:** defogs camera and scope lenses
**Features:** comes with liquid and sponge applicator
**Additional Information:** single-patient use

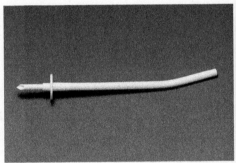
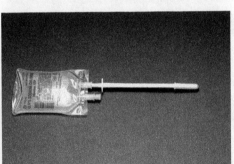

**Name:** decanting cannula
**Alias:** none
**Use:** pours fluid from a sterile IV bag to a container on the sterile field
**Features:** has a spiked end to insert into the port on the bottom of the bag
**Additional Information:** care must be taken not to contaminate the tip while pouring

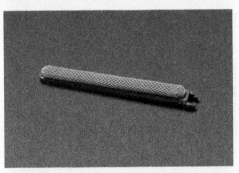

**Name:** Hydrajaw insert
**Alias:** Fogarty insert
**Use:** pads the jaws of Fogarty clamps to minimize tissue damage
**Features:** has clips on the inner side to attach to the clamp jaws; outer side padded; some are made of rubber filled with silicone
**Additional Information:** none

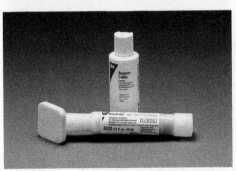

**Name:** remover lotion
**Alias:** DuraPrep Remover
**Use:** removes excess DuraPrep solution from the skin after surgery
**Features:** easy to apply
**Additional Information:** rub onto skin and remove with a dry, clean towel or sponge

**Name:** water-soluble jelly

**Alias:** K-Y Jelly, Surgilube

**Use:** lubricates tubes and catheters before insertion into body orifices

**Features:** water soluble; easy to clean off excess

**Additional Information:** comes sterile in a variety of containers (from small packets to large tubes); spike on cap is used to puncture tube seal

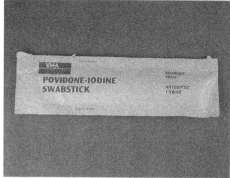

**Name:** povidone-iodine swab

**Alias:** Betadine swab, prep swab

**Use:** cleansing small areas of skin

**Features:** swab impregnated with povidone-iodine, thus eliminating the need for a separate container of solution

**Additional Information:** available in packages of one to three swabs; cannot be used on a patient who has an iodine allergy

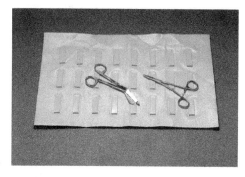
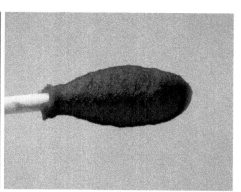

**Name:** magnetic drape

**Alias:** magnetic instrument mat

**Use:** keeps metal instruments from slipping off the draped patient and onto the floor

**Features:** rows of magnets that hold the metal instruments

**Additional Information:** available in a variety of styles and sizes

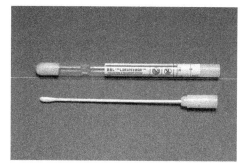

**Name:** culture tube

**Alias:** culturette

**Use:** obtains and contains fluid sample to send for culture

**Features:** sterile swab is used to obtain culture, which is placed in the tube containing culture media

**Additional Information:** swab and inside of media tube are sterile; care must be taken not to contaminate either when placing the swab back into the tube

**Name:** Whitacre spinal needle

**Alias:** none

**Use:** creates a pathway for the introduction of regional anesthetics into the spinal canal; can be used to inject medication into deep or hard-to-reach areas (e.g., the cervix)

**Features:** pencil-point tip; 3.5 to 5.5 inches long

**Additional Information:** available in 18 to 27 gauge; available in regular or high-flow style

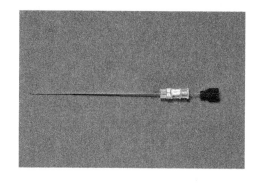

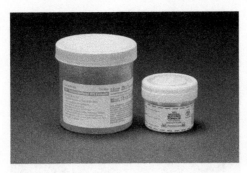

**Name:** specimen containers

**Alias:** none

**Use:** contain and preserve tissue specimens sent to the laboratory

**Features:** some containers are prefilled with preservative; some containers do not contain any preservative and can be used for frozen section specimens as well. If you are sending a specimen that requires a preservative in a dry container, preservative must be added and the container properly labeled

**Additional Information:** both styles come in a variety of sizes to accommodate most specimens

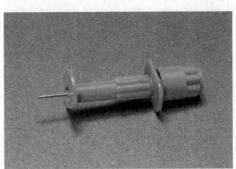

**Name:** Jamshidi needle

**Alias:** bone marrow needle

**Use:** injects fluid or medication into the bone marrow (intraosseous infusion); aspirates bone marrow for biopsy; harvests bone graft from the iliac crest

**Features:** top cap twists off to expose a Luer-lock connection

**Additional Information:** available in several gauges (8 to 17) and lengths

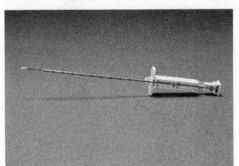

**Name:** Tru-cut biopsy needle

**Alias:** none

**Use:** obtains tissue samples from organs for examination

**Features:** centimeter markings to aid in depth measurement

**Additional Information:** available in several gauges (14 to 27); available in 3-, 4.5-, and 6-inch lengths

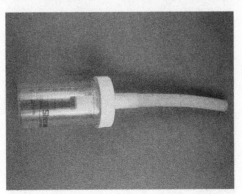

**Name:** sputum trap

**Alias:** Luki trap

**Use:** collects sputum specimen

**Features:** attaches to suction to collect the specimen directly into the container

**Additional Information:** marked in cubic centimeters to allow for estimating specimen volume

**Name:** urine strainer

**Alias:** none

**Use:** strains urine specimen to check for the presence of stones, gravel, or tissue

**Features:** Micro-Mesh captures any stones or sediment

**Additional Information:** many styles and types available

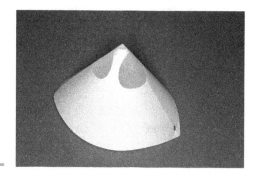

**Name:** biohazard bag

**Alias:** specimen bag

**Use:** contains specimen container sent to the laboratory; protects personnel if leakage occurs

**Features:** resealable; leak-proof if sealed properly; marked with biohazard symbol

**Additional Information:** available in a variety of sizes

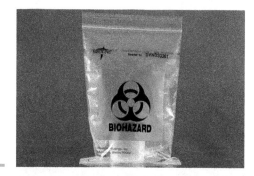

**Name:** tongue blade

**Alias:** tongue depressor

**Use:** holds tongue, allowing visualization of mouth and pharynx; stirs medication mixtures

**Features:** comes packaged as sterile or unsterile

**Additional Information:** none

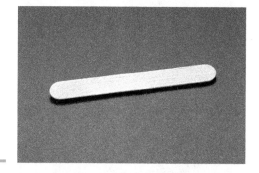

**Name:** cotton-tip applicator

**Alias:** cotton swab

**Use:** applies medication to small areas; dabs blood or fluid from small areas

**Features:** comes packaged as sterile or unsterile

**Additional Information:** available in several lengths and sizes

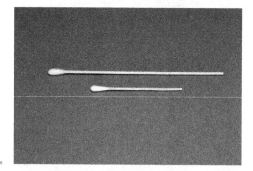

**Name:** isolation bag

**Alias:** none

**Use:** isolates a body part (e.g., foot or bowel) away from the operative area

**Features:** sterile bag with a drawstring closure

**Additional Information:** if using the bag to isolate an organ such as the bowel, add sterile saline to keep the organ moist while it is outside the body

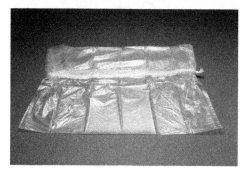

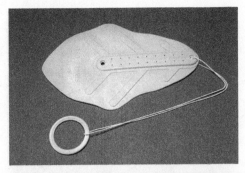

**Name:** Glassman viscera retainer

**Alias:** fish

**Use:** protects the viscera while suturing

**Features:** the body portion is inserted between the viscera and the peritoneum; when the wound is almost closed, the retainer is removed by pulling on the tail portion

**Additional Information:** single use

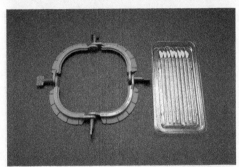

**Name:** Lone Star retractor system

**Alias:** none

**Use:** retracts soft tissue; used in vaginal and rectal surgery

**Features:** hooks are placed on the soft tissue then attached to the retractor frame

**Additional Information:** available in several sizes and styles; hooks and frame come separately so you need to make sure you have both packages; single-patient use

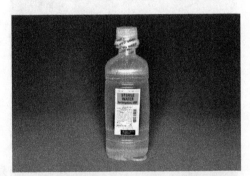

**Name:** sterile water

**Alias:** none

**Use:** fills Pleur-evacs, Blanketrols, or other medical equipment requiring water; soaks surgical instruments

**Features:** noncorrosive

**Additional Information:** available in several sizes; 500 cc and 1,000 cc are the most common

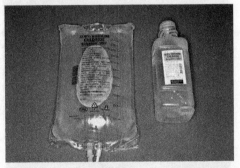

**Name:** normal saline

**Alias:** none

**Use:** irrigates wounds or body cavities

**Features:** isotonic solution

**Additional Information:** corrosive to stainless steel; do not use for soaking instruments; available in several sizes; 500 cc and 1,000 cc are the most common

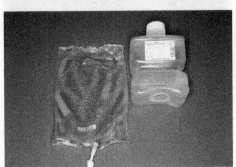

**Name:** glycine 1.5%

**Alias:** none

**Use:** irrigate body cavities during procedures requiring use of resectoscope/cautery

**Features:** nonconducting

**Additional Information:** comes in 3,000-cc bag

**Name:** surgical nerve locator
**Alias:** nerve stimulator
**Use:** locates and stimulates nerves intraoperatively
**Features:** direct current stimulator; adjustable 0.5 mA to 2.0 mA
**Additional Information:** single-patient use; handheld; battery powered

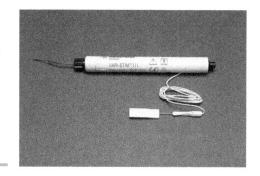

**Name:** suture bag
**Alias:** garbage bag
**Use:** disposal of suture wrappers, cut-off pieces of suture and other waste items intraoperatively
**Features:** self-sticking tabs make it easier to hang on the back table
**Additional Information:** none

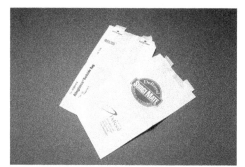

**Name:** handheld cautery
**Alias:** none
**Use:** cauterization of fine vessels or tissue (e.g., in hand surgery)
**Features:** battery powered; tip heats up
**Additional Information:** single-patient use

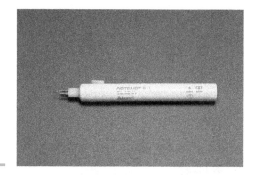

**Name:** blade knife handle
**Alias:** Beaver Blade handle
**Use:** holds knife blades
**Features:** available in long or short handle lengths
**Additional Information:** for use with series 50, 60, 70 blades

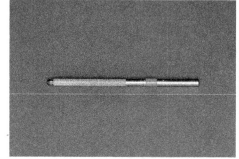
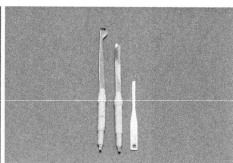

**#10 Blade:** generally used for skin incisions
**#11 Blade:** for small "puncture" incisions (e.g., in a hook phlebectomy, arthroscopic, or endoscopic procedures)
**#12 Blade:** curved with a cutting surface on the inside; used in oropharyngeal surgery (e.g., tonsils, uvulopalatopharyngoplasty)
**#15 Blade:** used for cutting small vessels and tissue, plastic surgery skin incisions, and hand procedures

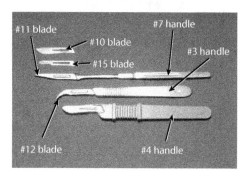

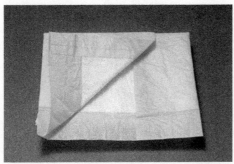

**Name:** incontinence pad

**Alias:** Chux, prep pad, bed protector pad

**Use:** absorbs fluids; used to protect the bed linen from prep solutions or body fluids

**Features:** absorbent top backed by a fluid-proof backing

**Additional Information:** available in many sizes and styles

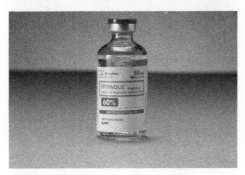

**Name:** Hypaque

**Alias:** diatrizoate

**Use:** contrast media used for intraoperative radiography

**Features:** clear; available in several strengths; 60% is the most commonly used

**Additional Information:** make sure ALL bubbles are out of the syringe before handing it to the surgeon; bubbles can resemble a stone on the x-ray image; make sure fluid is properly labeled with name and strength; use only with extreme caution in iodine-sensitive patient

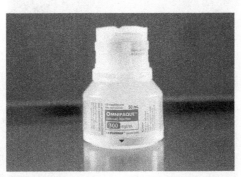

**Name:** Omnipaque

**Alias:** Iohexol

**Use:** contrast media for intraoperative angiography (also used for myelography and arthrography)

**Features:** clear; available in several strengths (180, 240, 300, and 350); 350 is the most commonly used for intraoperative angiography

**Additional Information:** make sure ALL bubbles are out of the syringe before handing it to the surgeon; bubbles can resemble a stone on the x-ray image; make sure fluid is properly labeled with name and strength; use only with extreme caution in iodine-sensitive patient

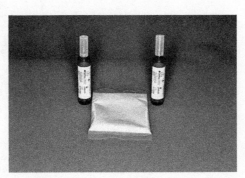

**Name:** polymethyl methacrylate

**Alias:** bone cement

**Use:** cements prostheses in place during total joint arthroplasty

**Features:** comes as a powder with one to two vials of liquid; mix only with the liquid polymer that comes with it

**Additional Information:** has strong vapors; excessive exposure can be potentially hazardous for staff; mix using a closed cement mixing system to decrease fumes; pregnant women should not be in the OR during the mixing of bone cement

**Name:** polymethyl methacrylate with gentamycin

**Alias:** antibiotic bone cement

**Use:** cementing prostheses in place during total joint arthroplasty; used for patients at higher risk for infection (e.g., diabetic patients or those with a history of infection)

**Features:** comes as a powder with one to two vials of liquid; mix only with the liquid polymer that comes with it

**Additional Information:** has strong vapors; excessive exposure can be potentially hazardous for staff; mix using a closed cement mixing system to decrease fumes; pregnant women should not be in the OR during the mixing of bone cement; not for use in patients with a sensitivity to gentamycin

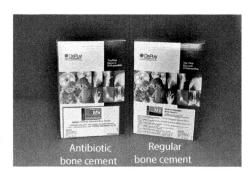

**Name:** Esmarch

**Alias:** none

**Use:** exsanguinates the extremity before surgery

**Features:** latex free; comes in a roll for easy application

**Additional Information:** extremity is always wrapped starting at the distal point and moving toward the proximal end; available in 3-, 4-, or 6-inch width; available sterile or nonsterile

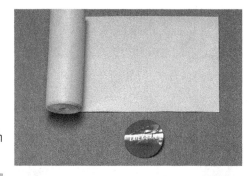

**Name:** TUR system with flow pouch

**Alias:** none

**Use:** provides constant, high-pressure irrigation during transurethral resection procedures

**Features:** 2,000-cc reservoir pouch; dual spikes allow two bags of irrigation fluid to be hung simultaneously

**Additional Information:** none

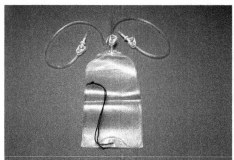

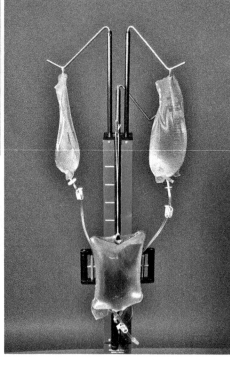

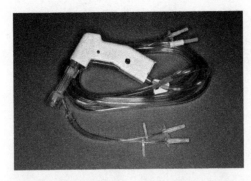

**Name:** Simpulse SOLO irrigator

**Alias:** pulsed lavage irrigator

**Use:** irrigating surgical sites during orthopedic procedures

**Features:** battery operated; no external power source needed; variable power control at located at the trigger; pistol grip

**Additional Information:** is a dual irrigation/ suction system

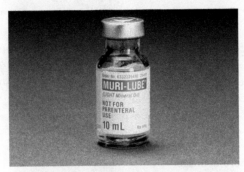

**Name:** sterile mineral oil

**Alias:** none

**Use:** lubricates skin before using a dermatome for skin grafting

**Features:** sterile

**Additional Information:** single-patient use

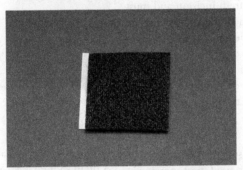

**Name:** scratch pad

**Alias:** tip cleaner

**Use:** removes char and tissue from electrocautery tip

**Features:** adhesive backing allows it to stick to drape or cautery holster

**Additional Information:** may be included as part of the count (refer to institutional policy)

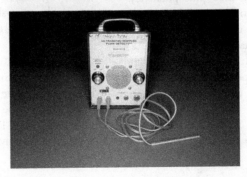

**Name:** Doppler

**Alias:** none

**Use:** assesses blood flow in arteries

**Features:** detachable cord so that cord can be sterile and box left unsterile; adjustable volume

**Additional Information:** a nonsterile probe can be used preoperatively and postoperatively; have a sterile one available intraoperatively; there are many models available

**Name:** ultrasonic gel

**Alias:** none

**Use:** provides an acoustically correct medium for the transmission of ultrasonic waves; provides lubrication for the probe to glide over the skin

**Features:** hypoallergenic; nonirritating to skin; nonstaining

**Additional Information:** available in sterile packets or unsterile bottles (depending on your intended use)

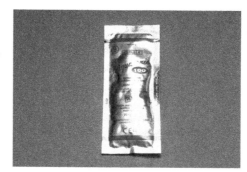

## SURGICAL WOUND DRESSINGS

A surgical dressing is placed over the surgical wound site immediately after the incision is closed. The main purpose of the dressing is to protect the surgical incision from contaminants in the environment, but dressings also can give the wound extra support, protect it from trauma, provide skin closure, apply pressure, debride it, or absorb drainage.

Surgical dressings are placed over a fresh incision and must be sterile to protect the wound from microbial contamination. When applying the dressing, it should be handled by the edges to avoid contaminating the part placed over the wound. If the person applying the dressing has been wearing two pairs of sterile gloves during the procedure, the outer gloves should be removed and the dressing applied with the clean inner gloves.

### Gauze Sponges

As the name implies, gauze sponges are squares of sterile gauze. They are the most common dressing used postoperatively. Gauze sponges are used mainly for protection of the wound and absorption of body fluids. These dressings are made to be low lint to prevent lint from contaminating the wound. They are absorbent and wick blood and fluids into their layers to keep the wound dry. Gauze sponges come in a variety of sizes. The most common sizes are 4 × 4 inches and 2 × 2 inches (Fig. 3–27).

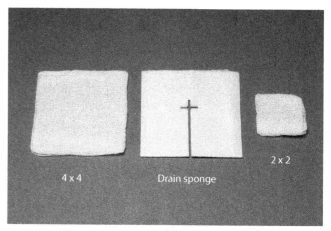

FIGURE 3-27 2 × 2, 4 × 4, and drain sponges.

Another type of gauze sponge is referred to as a *drain sponge*. A drain sponge is a 4 × 4-inch gauze sponge with a cross shape cut into it. The cross-shaped cutout is placed around the drain, allowing the dressing to fit snuggly and the drain to protrude.

### Abdominal Dressing

The abdominal dressing (also known as the *ABD pad*) is a thick, absorbent gauze used to cover large wounds (Fig. 3–28). The ABD pad can be used as a stand-alone dressing or as an outer dressing when large amounts of drainage are expected. These dressings are available in 5 × 9-inch and 8 × 10-inch sizes.

### Eye Pad and Eye Shield

The eye pad is an oval gauze dressing that is applied over the patient's closed eyelid after ophthalmic surgery (Fig. 3–29). The purpose of this dressing is threefold: to keep the eyelid closed to allow the eye to rest, to absorb any drainage from the eye, and to keeping medications from seeping out of the eye.

The eye shield is a rigid, raised oval shield that is placed over the eye or eye dressing. The shield protects the eye from trauma or pressure postoperatively. Shields can be made of rigid plastic or metal. The edge of the oval that rests on the patient's face is covered with a soft material to prevent skin damage.

> ### WATCH OUT! Dressings Versus Surgical Sponges
>
> Dressing materials do NOT have a radiopaque strip because they are not intended for use inside the body (see Fig. 3–27). Many dressing materials look similar to Ray-Tec sponges, and they easily could be confused. Dressing material should be kept in a separate area on the back table or not opened until the final surgical sponge count has been completed. Institution policy varies; check your institution's policies and procedures.
>
> Ray-Tec sponges should not be used as dressings. On a postoperative radiograph, the radiopaque strip would be visible and could look like a Ray-Tec sponge was left inside the patient.

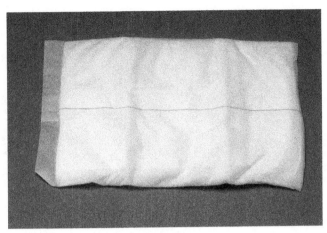

FIGURE 3-28 Abdominal dressing.

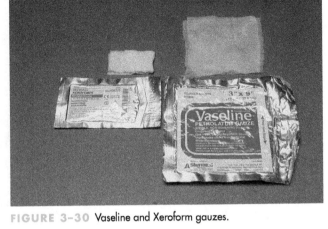

FIGURE 3-30 Vaseline and Xeroform gauzes.

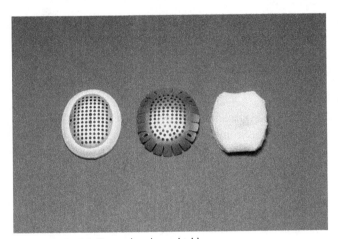

FIGURE 3-29 Eye pad and eye shield.

## Nonadhering Dressings

Occlusive dressings are made of a fine mesh material that has been impregnated with a petroleum-based substance (e.g., Vaseline) to provide an airtight and watertight seal. The two most common types of occlusive dressing are Vaseline gauze and Xeroform gauze (Fig. 3–30).

The petroleum-based substance on the dressing prevents it from sticking to the wound whereas the mesh allows drainage. This type of dressing is often used over a suture line to protect it and to maintain a moist environment to help healing. It also can be used around a chest tube insertion site to prevent outside air from entering the chest through the stab-wound site.

Vaseline dressings are available in sheets or rolls. Sizes range from 1 × 8 inches to 6 × 36 inches. The most common sizes of Xeroform dressings are 1 × 8 inches and 5 × 9 inches.

### Adaptic

Adaptic is one brand of nonocclusive gauze that has been impregnated with a petroleum-based substance. It does *not* provide a watertight or airtight seal. Adaptic does, however, provide a nonadhering layer that wicks drainage away from

the wound and allows the dressing to be removed without sticking (Fig. 3–31). Adaptic is available in three sizes: 3 × 3 inches, 3 × 8 inches, and 3 × 16 inches.

### Telfa

Telfa is a brand of absorbent gauze that is bonded on both sides with a nonadherent material to prevent it from sticking to the wound. It allows air to reach the wound and wicks the drainage away from the wound (Fig. 3–32). Telfa is available in three sizes: 2 × 3 inches, 3 × 4 inches, and 6 × 10 inches.

Telfa also can be used as a mat for tissue specimens. The nonadherent covering keeps the specimen from sticking, thus preserving the tissue integrity. Scrubbed personnel often place small tissue specimens on a piece of Telfa to keep them from becoming lost.

### Film Dressing

Film dressing is a thin, transparent, waterproof dressing (e.g., Tegaderm). It is used as an outer dressing for wounds from which large amounts of drainage are not expected or as a stand-alone dressing over intravenous (IV) sites. The clear film

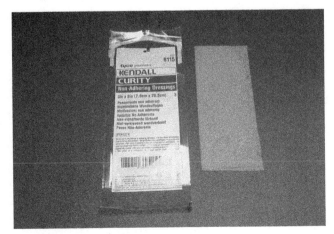

FIGURE 3-31 Adaptic.

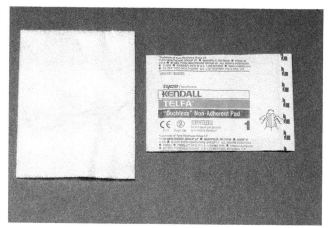

FIGURE 3-32 Telfa.

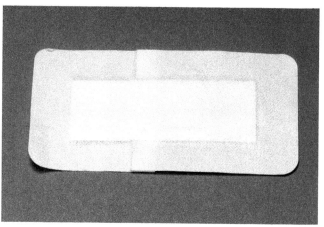

FIGURE 3-34 Island dressings.

allows visualization of the dressing or IV site underneath it (Fig. 3–33). Tegaderm is available in sizes ranging from 2¾ × 2¾ inches to 8 × 12 inches.

## Island Dressings

Island dressings combine a nonadherent gauze dressing with a nonirritating adhesive border. The built-in adhesive border allows these dressings to adhere directly to the skin, negating the need to use tape or a wrap to secure them (Fig. 3–34). These dressings are used on wounds from which large amounts of drainage are not expected. Two of the most common brand names are Covaderm and Primapore. These dressings come in a variety of shapes (e.g., square, round, and rectangular) and sizes.

## Dressing Wraps

Dressing wraps come in either loosely woven gauze, nonwoven gauze, or elastic material. Generally used to secure a dressing or splint in place, the wraps conform to the contours of the patient's body, allowing freedom of movement. They also can be used to help apply pressure to a wound or to pack a large wound.

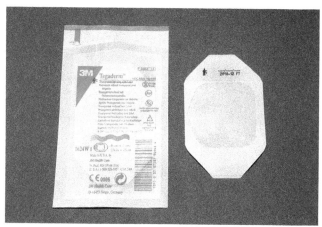

FIGURE 3-33 Film dressing.

Kerlix (six-ply loosely woven gauze) is available as a 4½-inch × 4-yard or 2¼-inch × 3-yard roll (Fig. 3–35). Kerlix is also available as a dressing sponge impregnated with an antimicrobial substance.

Kling (nonwoven gauze) is available in 1-, 2-, 3-, 4-, or 6-inch widths.

An Ace bandage (also known as an *Ace wrap*) is a roll of elastic bandage commonly used to provide support to a sprain or strain of a joint (Fig. 3–36). It also can be used to secure a dressing or to hold a splint in place.

The elastic in the bandage allows it to stretch to conform to the area and provide limited freedom of movement. Ace bandages can be secured with tape, although most come with metal fasteners or Velcro closures. Available sizes are 2-, 3-, 4-, and 6-inch widths.

## Self-Adherent Wraps

Self-adherent wraps are made of a blend of nonwoven fibers and elastic to allow for stretch. They contain a cohesive material so that the bandage can stick to itself but not to skin or other materials (Fig. 3–37). These bandages are used to secure dressings or splints in place. The two most common brand names for this type of dressing are Coban and Flex-wrap. Self-adherent wraps are available in widths ranging from 1 to 6 inches.

**WATCH OUT!** **Wrapping Bandages**

Use caution when wrapping any bandage (regardless of material) in a circular fashion that encompasses the entire diameter of an extremity or other body part. The bandage should fit snuggly so that it does not slide off, but it should NOT be wrapped so tight that it causes circulatory problems.

After wrapping the bandage, check the areas distal to the bandage for signs of impaired circulation: cyanosis, skin coolness, skin mottling, or patient complaints of numbness or tingling.

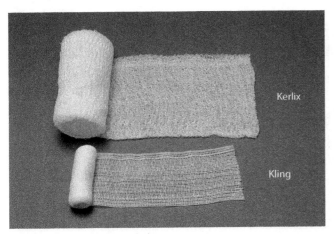

FIGURE 3-35 Kerlix and Kling.

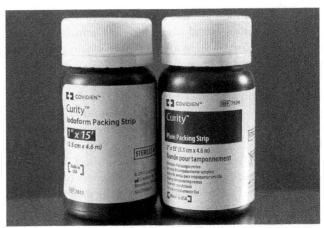

FIGURE 3-38 Plain and iodoform packing strip.

The packing is usually made of a long strip of gauze material that is plain or impregnated with antimicrobial substances such as iodoform or silver. Creams (e.g., estrogen cream or hemorrhoid cream) may be used to coat plain packing for use after specific types of surgery. Packing material is available in widths ranging from ¼ inch to 4 inches.

## Liquid Chemical Dressings

### Collodion

Collodion is a thick, yellow liquid consisting of pyroxylin mixed with alcohol and ether (Fig. 3–39). As the solvent evaporates, collodion dries to form a waterproof film over the wound. This type of dressing is used on small wounds from which drainage is not expected. It is highly flammable and has a strong odor.

Collodion is applied over the dry suture or staple line using a cotton-tipped applicator. A thin layer is applied and left open to the air to dry. Once dry, the film provides protection from environmental contaminants and water.

### Liquid Skin Adhesives

Topically applied liquid adhesives are designed to close small, superficial lacerations and surgical incisions. In addition

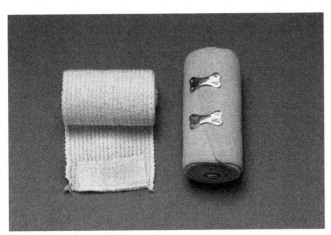

FIGURE 3-36 Ace wrap.

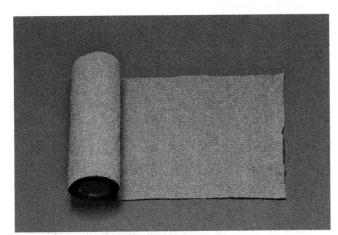

FIGURE 3-37 Self-adherent wraps.

## Packing

Packing material is packed inside the wound to provide support, to provide hemostasis, or to allow wound drainage and healing (Fig. 3–38). The packing is used for boils, abscesses, fistulas, and other draining or tunneling wounds as well as packing nasal passages, the rectum, and the vagina.

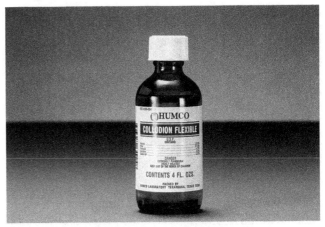

FIGURE 3-39 Collodion.

to wound closure, they also provide a chemical film barrier for protection. Brand names include Dermabond, Marathon, New-Skin, and LiquiBand. These adhesives come in small ampoules with an applicator (Fig. 3–40). The ampoule is squeezed to saturate the applicator with adhesive. A thin layer of adhesive is applied to the wound and allowed to dry, and then another layer is applied (application techniques may vary with brand; always follow the manufacturer's instructions).

Before use, it is important to check patient allergies to make sure it is appropriate to use these adhesives (e.g., Dermabond contains formaldehyde and cannot be used on patients with formaldehyde allergies).

## Adhesive Tapes

Medical adhesive tape (also known as *surgical tape*) is the most common method of securing dressings. Available in many types and widths, it is an easy and inexpensive way to keep dressings in place. Listed are the most common types of adhesive tape (Figures 3–41 and 3–42):

- *Paper tape:* Hypoallergenic. Leaves very little adhesive residue when removed and is gentle on the skin. Used

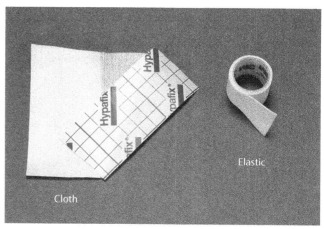

FIGURE 3–42  Elastic and cloth tapes.

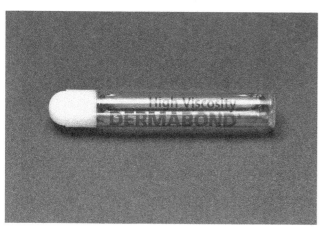

FIGURE 3–40  Dermabond.

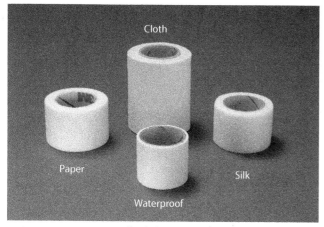

FIGURE 3–41  Paper, silk, cloth, and waterproof tapes.

on patients with adhesive sensitivities or patients who have friable (fragile) skin. Good for use when repeated dressing changes are anticipated on sensitive skin. Used by some anesthesia personnel to tape eyelids shut during general anesthesia. Tends not to stick well when wet. Available in ½-, 1-, 2-, and 3-inch widths.

- *Silk tape:* "Silk-like tape." Most commonly used, general-purpose adhesive tape. Hypoallergenic adhesive leaves tape residue after removal. Available in ½-, 1-, 2-, and 3-inch widths.

- *Elastic tape:* Cotton elastic tape designed for use for pressure dressings or support strapping of orthopedic injuries. Conforms to knees, shoulders, and elbows. Allows for wicking of moisture away from the skin. Has a rubber-based adhesive. Available in 1-, 2-, 3-, and 4-inch widths.

- *Plastic tape:* Flexible, contouring, clear plastic tape that allows viewing of the wound site. Used for securing dressings, IV catheters, or tubes. Available in 1-, 2-, or 3-inch widths.

- *Fabric tape:* Porous and nonabsorbing fabric used to secure dressings, tubes, and cannulas. Nonirritating adhesive allows skin underneath it to breathe. Available in 1-, 2-, 4-, 6-, and 8-inch widths.

- *Foam elastic tape:* Elastic foam material used for compression dressing or dressing in hard-to-secure areas. Stretches in all directions. Waterproof and hypoallergenic. Available in 1-, 2-, 3-, and 4-inch widths.

- *Cloth tape:* Nonwoven polyester tape. Easy-to-tear, hypoallergenic, general-purpose tape. Has moderate stretch to allow for movement and swelling. Available in 1-, 2-, 3-, 4-, 6-, and 8-inch widths.

- *Waterproof tape:* Zinc oxide–based tape. Waterproof, oil resistant, and gentle to all skin types, it will remain intact for long periods of time, even when wet. Conforms easily to body contours. Used to secure dressings or tubes. Used by some anesthesia personnel to secure endotracheal tubes. Available in ½-, 1-, and 2-inch widths.

## Casting Material (Rigid Dressings)

### Plaster

Plaster bandages are made from cotton material that is impregnated with plaster of Paris. To apply, you dip the material in water and wrap it in place. The plaster hardens as it dries, creating a hard shell that provides support and protection to the surgical or fracture site. Plaster-casting material is both strong and easy to manipulate, making it a popular choice for creating casts. The disadvantage to plaster is that it becomes mushy and loses its shape and supporting ability when it becomes wet. It is also heavier than fiberglass, making it uncomfortable for some patients. Plaster-casting material is available in rolls (for applying casts) or strips (for making splints) ranging from 2 to 6 inches wide (Fig. 3–43).

### Fiberglass

Fiberglass casting material has become popular because it is lightweight and holds its shape better than plaster when it is exposed to moisture. These bandages consist of a knitted fiberglass bandage impregnated with polyurethane. To apply, you dip the fiberglass material in water and wrap it into place. As it dries, it forms a protective and supportive shell around the surgical or fracture site. Fiberglass dries more quickly than plaster and, as it hardens, the chemical reaction causes the casting material to become warm. It is a good idea to tell the patient that as the cast dries, it will feel warm. Fiberglass casting material is available in rolls (for applying casts) or precut (for making splints) of various sizes and widths (Fig. 3–43).

## Undercast Padding

Undercast padding, such as Webril or stockinette, is soft-cotton padding applied to the skin before a cast or pneumatic tourniquet is fitted to provide protection (Fig. 3–44). It contours to the body and stays in place without shifting or sagging. The padding is not waterproof; therefore, if the patient gets the cast wet, the padding could absorb some of the water and hold it next to the skin, causing skin irritation or breakdown.

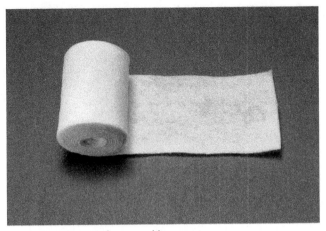

FIGURE 3-44 Undercast padding.

Webril is available in rolls ranging from 2- to 6-inch widths.

Stockinette is available in several styles that can be used to pad under casting material (to prevent chafing), to drape an extremity for surgery, or to hold a dressing in place. It also can be placed over a device such as a cervical collar to help keep it clean. When the stockinette becomes soiled, slip it off and either wash it or apply a new one.

As the name implies, stockinette is a round tube of soft-cotton material that is applied by slipping it onto the extremity or torso like you would put on a stocking (Fig. 3–45). It is stretchy, lightweight, and breathable. Stockinette comes in a tubular roll and is available in widths ranging from 1 to 12 inches.

## Miscellaneous

### Skin Closure Tapes

Commonly referred to by the brand name *Steri-Strips* (3M company), skin closure tapes are polyester-reinforced strips of material with a hypoallergenic adhesive backing (Fig. 3–46). They can be used to close a wound or incision or to reinforce a sutured incision line. The most commonly used sizes are ¼- and ½-inch wide.

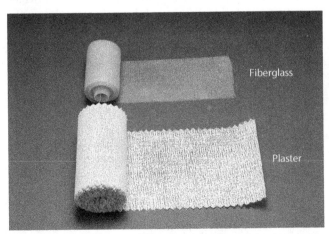

FIGURE 3-43 Plaster and fiberglass casting materials.

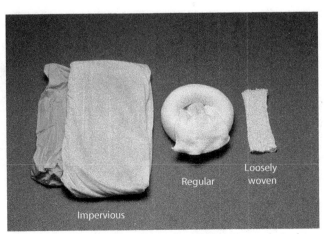

FIGURE 3-45 Regular, impervious, and loosely woven stockinettes.

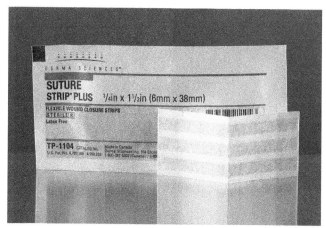

FIGURE 3-46  Skin closure tapes.

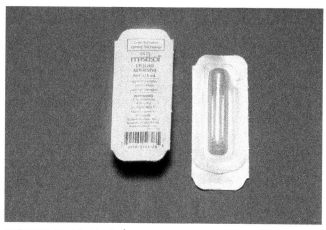

FIGURE 3-48  Mastisol.

## Tincture of Benzoin

Benzoin is an alcohol compound that can be used to help increase the adhesion of Steri-Strips or dressings. Once it is dry, it forms a protective film on the skin. Available in swabs or ⅔-mL ampoules (Fig. 3–47).

## Mastisol

Mastisol is a clear, nonirritating, non-water-soluble adhesive that helps secure dressings for a prolonged period of time. Often, it is used in conjunction with Tegaderm dressings. Mastisol is 7 to 10 times stickier than benzoin. Available in ⅔-mL ampoules and 15-mL and 60-mL bottles (Fig. 3–48).

## Montgomery Straps

Montgomery straps are large adhesive strips that are placed opposite each other. The straps have holes along the inner edge that can be threaded with gauze or twill tape to secure the dressing (Fig. 3–49).

The advantage to Montgomery straps is that the dressing can be accessed and changed without having to change the adhesive. Generally, these are used for large wounds for which frequent dressing changes are expected. Available in 7¼ × 11⅛-inch sizes, they can be cut to the desired length.

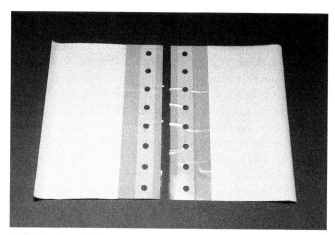

FIGURE 3-49  Montgomery straps.

## Ostomy Appliances

Ostomy appliances (also known as *stoma bags* or *ostomy bags*) are available in many sizes and styles depending on the desired use and patient preference. These appliances have an opening near the top where the ostomy effluent drains into the bag, and many have a reclosable opening at the bottom of the bag to allow for emptying. The bags may be one piece, in which the adhesive seal that goes around the stoma is built into the bag, or two pieces, in which the adhesive seal is separate and the bag attaches to it (Fig. 3–50). The adhesive seal is circular; on some styles, it can be cut to fit the stoma, and some models it is a fixed size. The most common ostomy appliances are used for patients with urostomies, ileostomies, and colostomies.

Many institutions employ an ostomy nurse who is responsible for helping patients preoperatively and postoperatively with fitting the appliance, caring for the stoma, and learning to live and cope with an ostomy. These nurses are a valuable resource for the perioperative team.

## Vacuum-Assisted Closure Dressings

Vacuum-assisted closure (VAC) dressings, also called negative pressure wound therapy, are designed to apply

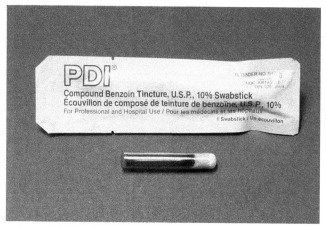

FIGURE 3-47  Benzoin.

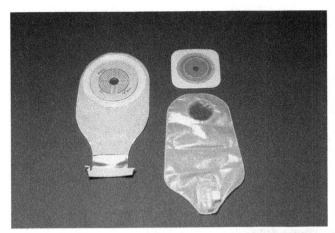

FIGURE 3–50 One-piece (left) and two-piece (right) ostomy bags.

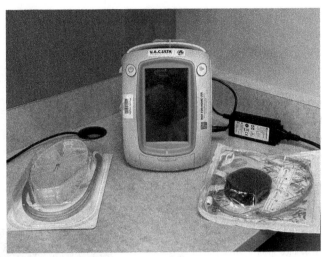

FIGURE 3–51 Machine canister (left), vacuum machine (middle) and foam dressing (right).

negative pressure to chronic wounds to help accelerate the healing process. For example, VAC dressings are used for chronic ulcers, skin grafts, flaps, traumatic wounds, and partial-thickness burns.

There are two parts to the VAC dressing: the vacuum machine and the foam sponge dressing. The foam sponge is placed into the open wound, the wound is sealed with an adhesive drape, and the sponge's hose is attached to the vacuum machine's hose (Fig. 3–51). Negative pressure is then applied to the wound using the machine.

VAC dressing sponges are available in two different foam materials. GranuFoam is designed to remove exudate and assist in wound granulation. Vers-Foam is a nonadherent material that helps promote graft survival, helps protect underlying structures, and can be used in wounds with tunnels or undermining.

VAC foam sponges are available in various sizes to fit hands, heels, and abdomen, although they can also be used for wounds in other parts of the body. The vacuum machine is available in a floor model (larger size) or a small, portable model that comes with a case and carrying strap. For more information, see www.KCI1.com.

## SPLINTS

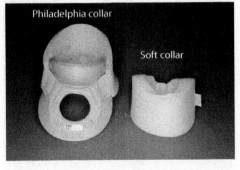

Philadelphia collar

Soft collar

**Name:** Philadelphia collar

**Alias:** rigid cervical brace

**Use:** supports neck post–cervical injury or surgery

**Features:** rigid foam construction; two pieces: front and back

**Additional Information:** available with hole in the front for tracheostomies or with solid front; available in extra-small through large sizes; collar height varies from 2.25 inches (extra-small) through 5.25 inches (large)

**Name:** soft cervical collar

**Alias:** none

**Use:** supports minor cervical injuries or acts as a transition collar between a more rigid collar and no collar

**Features:** soft, 1-inch-thick foam; easily contours to neck

**Additional Information:** available in small, medium, large, and extra-large sizes; collar height varies from 3 inches (small) to 4.25 inches (extra-large)

**Name:** knee immobilizer

**Alias:** knee splint

**Use:** immobilizes knee in a straight position post injury or surgery

**Features:** Velcro straps for easy adjustment; padded inside; cutout area fits over knee

**Additional Information:** available in 12 through 26-inch lengths; available in sizes extra-small through universal

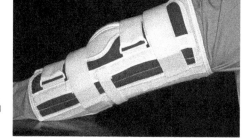

**Name:** hip abduction pillow

**Alias:** none

**Use:** provides hip abduction following hip surgery

**Features:** foam pillow; foam straps help to keep it positioned correctly

**Additional Information:** available in small (12.5-inch base × 18-inch length) or large (17-inch base × 24-inch length)

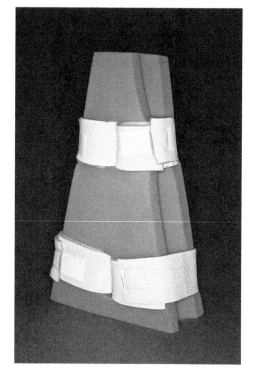

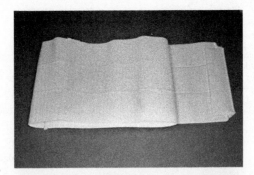

**Name:** abdominal binder

**Alias:** none

**Use:** provides postoperative abdominal support

**Features:** stretchable to accommodate a variety of abdominal girths; Velcro closure

**Additional Information:** available in small, medium, large, and universal sizes

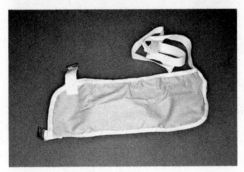

**Name:** sling

**Alias:** none

**Use:** provides support to arm and limits mobility post trauma or surgery

**Features:** adjustable shoulder strap; padded arm rest to support arm

**Additional Information:** many styles of sling are available; many slings have a swathe without the waist strap; most types are available in adult and pediatric sizes

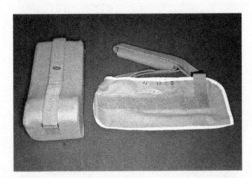

**Name:** sling and swathe

**Alias:** shoulder immobilizer

**Use:** immobilizes shoulder post trauma or surgery

**Features:** arm is placed in sling, and strap goes around waist to hold the arm close to the body; adjustable waist and shoulder straps

**Additional Information:** many styles of sling and swathe are available; most are available in sizes small through extra-large; some have padded waist and shoulder straps

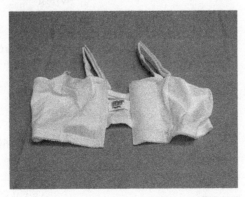

**Name:** postsurgical bra

**Alias:** breast support

**Use:** holds dressings in place; provides compression and support after breast surgery

**Features:** front closure; expandable fabric to allow for swelling

**Additional Information:** available in sizes extra-small to XX-large

**Surgical Session Review**

1) Which type of sponge should *never* be used as a dressing?
   a. Ray-Tec
   b. Topper
   c. Drain sponge
   d. ABD pad

2) All of the following statements are true about sponges *except*
   a. Used sponges should be discarded off the field into a proper receptacle
   b. Once initial count is done, it is OK to remove sponges from the room
   c. When setting up your back table, similar sponges should be kept together
   d. Never handle soiled sponges with your bare hands

3) Ray-Tec sponges come in a package containing _____ sponges.
   a. 5
   b. 8
   c. 10
   d. 12

4) Peanut sponges may also be known as
   a. Kittners
   b. Dissectors
   c. Cherries
   d. Tonsil sponges

5) Cottonoids would most likely be used during which type of surgery?
   a. Gynecological
   b. Neurosurgical
   c. Bowel
   d. Obstetrical

6) Which of the following is a hemostatic?
   a. Saline
   b. Collodion
   c. Bone wax
   d. Chlorhexidine

7) An insulin syringe is marked in _____.
   a. cc (cubic centimeters)
   b. μg (micrograms)
   c. mg (milligrams)
   d. Units

8) During which of these surgical procedures would you expect to have a blue bulb syringe on your sterile field?
   a. Bowel resection
   b. Cesarean section
   c. Hysterectomy
   d. Total hip replacement

9) Which of these needles would have the largest diameter?
   a. 16
   b. 18
   c. 25
   d. 27

10) A needle cannot be placed on the tip of a _____ syringe.
   a. Luer-lock
   b. Toomey
   c. Catheter tip
   d. Glass

11) _____ is a type of liquid dressing.
   a. Coban
   b. Adaptic
   c. Collodion
   d. Tegaderm

12) Ioban *cannot* be used on a patient with a(n) _____ allergy.
   a. Iodine
   b. Latex
   c. Wheat
   d. Sulfa

13) DuraPrep contains both iodophor (Betadine) and
   a. Chlorhexidine
   b. Detergent
   c. Alcohol
   d. Soap

14) Specimens of a frozen section should be sent to the laboratory in
   a. A suction trap
   b. A specimen container with formalin
   c. A dry specimen container
   d. A culture tube

15) Another name for a Glassman viscera retainer is a(n):
    a. Isolation bag
    b. Fish
    c. Swab
    d. Blade

16) Raney clips are used to hold _____ tissue.
    a. Bowel
    b. Bone
    c. Scalp
    d. Spine

17) The surgeon is performing a transurethral resection of the prostate using a resectoscope. Which of the following solutions will most likely be used for intraoperative irrigation?
    a. Glycine
    b. Sterile water
    c. Sterile saline
    d. Iodophor

18) You are scrubbed on a vascular procedure, and intraoperative angiography is anticipated. Which of the following will you most likely have on your sterile field?
    a. Indigo carmen
    b. Methylene blue
    c. Omnipaque
    d. Gentian violet

19) Polymethyl methacrylate is also known as
    a. Bone wax
    b. Heparin
    c. Thrombin
    d. Bone cement

20) Sterile mineral oil would most likely be used during which type of procedure?
    a. Open reduction internal fixation of an ankle
    b. Skin graft
    c. Appendectomy
    d. Cholecystectomy

# 4 Tubes, Drains, and Catheters

## DRAINS

Drains are placed in the surgical wound to remove blood, fluid, air, or, in some cases, pus. This allows the wound to heal without formation of fluid pockets, air pockets, or hematomas.

Drains can be *passive,* meaning that they use gravity to drain the wound, either into an attached container or into the dressing. Passive drains are simple and generally are used in situations when minimal drainage is expected. Drains also can be *active,* meaning that they drain the wound using negative pressure (suction). Active (or suction) drains are used for moderate or large amounts of drainage. They always require the use of a collection device to create the negative pressure. All drains are disposable, single-patient-use items.

### Passive Drains

#### Penrose

The Penrose drain is a soft tube of rubber or silicone placed into a wound to create a conduit for drainage to reach the body surface (Fig. 4–1). It is not connected to a collection device; instead, it drains the fluid directly into the dressing.

Penrose drains can be moistened with saline and used to retract delicate structures (e.g., the esophagus or spermatic cord) during surgery. They are available in 12-, 18-, and 36-inch lengths but can easily be cut to the desired length. Available widths are ¼, ⅜, ½, ⅝, ¾, ⅞, and 1 inch.

The *cigarette drain* is similar to the Penrose drain, but it is used less often. Unlike a Penrose drain, this drain has a gauze strip in the center of the tube.

### Biliary T-Tube

As the name implies, the T-tube is a latex tube shaped like the letter T. It is placed in the biliary tract after surgery to facilitate drainage of bile from the common bile duct. This type of drain is often used during open gallbladder or common bile duct surgeries. The T-tube is attached to a *bile bag* (Fig. 4–2), which collects the bile for visualization and measurement. T-tubes come in sizes ranging from 5 Fr to 24 Fr. They usually have an 11- to 12-inch stem with a 5- or 12-inch crossbar but can be cut to the desired size.

### Tympanostomy Tube

A tympanostomy tube (also known as a *pressure equalization* or *PE tube*) is used to treat recurrent ear infections by ventilating and equalizing pressure in the middle ear and by allowing drainage to escape. It is inserted through a small incision in the tympanic membrane (ear drum) called a *myringotomy.* There are several styles of tubes; the most popular being the *grommet.* The *button* and *bobbin* are other types of tympanostomy tubes (Fig. 4–3). These drains are extremely small (only millimeters) and are made of plastics such as Teflon or silicone. The tubes must be handled carefully with micro alligator forceps.

### Active Drains

#### Jackson-Pratt Drain

A Jackson-Pratt (JP) drain is a thin radiopaque tube with multiple drainage holes that is connected to clear plastic tubing (Fig. 4–4). The drain part is placed inside the wound, and the plastic tubing is on the outside of the body. The tubing is

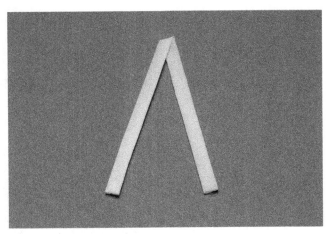

FIGURE 4–1 Penrose drain.

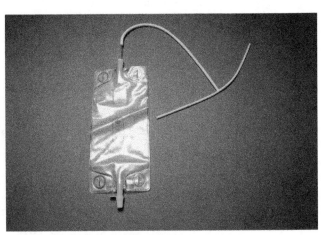

FIGURE 4–2 T-tube and bile bag.

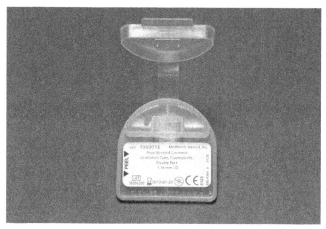

FIGURE 4-3 Tympanostomy tube.

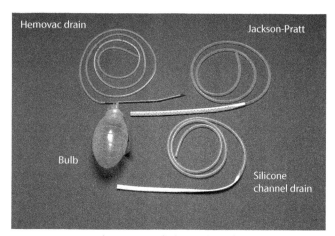

FIGURE 4-4 Jackson-Pratt and silicone channel drains and bulb reservoir.

connected to a separate collection device known as a *bulb reservoir*. The drain is connected, the empty bulb is squeezed to get the air out, and the reservoir cap is closed. This creates gentle suction that pulls fluid and blood out of the wound.

A JP drain can be left in the wound for as little as 24 hours or up to several weeks. It is removed once the wound drainage subsides. The cap on the reservoir can be opened to allow for emptying the drainage.

JP drains can be used after many types of surgery, including general, orthopedic, plastic, neurological, gynecological, cardiovascular, and head and neck procedures. They are available in 7-mm, 10-mm, and 15-mm diameters.

The most common size reservoir is 100 cc, but the 400-cc size is available for incisions when a great deal of drainage is expected. The 400-cc size has dual inlet ports to allow for hooking up two drains.

## Silicone Channel Drains

A silicone channel drain is a radiopaque drain that consists of four channels along the sides and a solid core center (see Fig. 4-4). The drain comes attached to silicone tubing. This drain works similar to a JP drain in that the drain is placed in

the wound, and the tubing is outside the body. The drain is attached to a *bulb reservoir* (see Fig. 4-4) in the same fashion as the JP drain.

Silicone channel drains can be used after a variety of surgeries, including orthopedic, cardiovascular, plastic, neurological, gynecological, head and neck, and general procedures. This type of drain is available in a flat or round shape. The flat drain is available in 7 mm or 10 mm. The round style is available in 10 mm, 15 mm, 19 mm, or 24 mm.

## Spring Action Drain

The spring action drain (commonly referred to by the brand name Hemovac) consists of a round collection reservoir with three springs inside it that attaches to a multiholed silicone drain (Fig. 4-5). The drain is attached to the collection reservoir, both sides of the reservoir are squeezed down nearly flat, and the reservoir cap is closed to create the vacuum (negative pressure). Spring action collection devices have an antireflux valve to prevent backflow of fluid into the patient. The collection reservoir has a capacity of 400 cc.

## TLS Evacuated Tube Drain

The TLS evacuated tube drain consists of a silicone drain that is attached to clear glass vacuum test tubes (Fig. 4-6). The drain

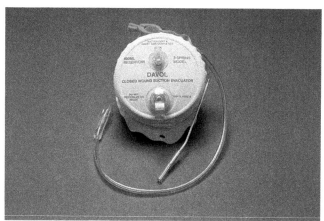

FIGURE 4-5 Spring action drain.

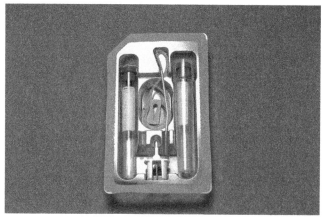

FIGURE 4-6 TLS evacuated tube drain.

kit comes with the drain and two 15-mL tubes. Extra tubes are available separately. These drains are designed for use after surgery of the neck, craniofacial surgery, or surgery of the extremities, in which small amounts of drainage are expected.

Drains are available in 7 mm or 10 mm with holes down the center or on the sides.

## Chest Drain

Chest tube drainage systems are used for treatment of pneumothorax (spontaneous or traumatic) or for reexpansion of the lung(s) and reestablishment of proper pleural cavity pressures after cardiothoracic surgery. Chest tubes are inserted into the chest cavity and attached to a water seal collection device, such as a Pleur-evac.

### Chest Tubes

Chest tubes are flexible, clear plastic drains that are inserted at the end of surgery to drain air, fluid, blood, or pus into the collection device. Depending on the circumstances, more than one chest tube may be required on the same side, or they may be required bilaterally. Chest tubes have holes (known as *eyes*) in the end that is inserted into the chest. These holes allow for flow of drainage into the tube. The other end of the tube is attached to the collection device hose adapter (Fig. 4–7). Chest tubes come with a sharp metal trocar that can be used to insert the chest tube. Whether or not the trocar is used depends on the circumstances and surgeon preference.

Chest tubes are generally secured in place with a purse-string suture to enable easier wound closure upon removal of the tube.

*Caution:* Chest tubes should NOT be "stripped" to maintain patency. Stripping of chest tubes can cause pressures of −400 cm or higher!

Chest tubes are available in a variety of diameters. The size used depends on patient size and circumstances. Generally, a smaller tube (18 to 22 Fr) is used to treat an adult with a pneumothorax, whereas a larger tube (26 to 32 Fr) is used in the presence of a hemothorax (blood) or empyema (pus).

### Pleur-evac

The Pleur-evac is a widely used chest drainage system (Fig. 4–8). This device consists of a three-chambered collection unit (originally modeled after the old three glass bottle system) that has two hoses: one attaches to the patient's chest tube and the other attaches to suction.

If the device is facing you, the chamber on the right is the chest drainage collection unit. The hose on the top of this chamber attaches to the patient's chest tube to allow blood and/or fluid to drain directly into the chamber. This chamber is marked in milliliters (mL) to allow for measurement of drainage. The outside surface of this chamber can be written on to record the date and time when the drainage is checked to track the patient's total drainage output.

The middle chamber is the water seal chamber. This chamber allows air to exit the pleural space with exhalation and prevents air from entering the pleural space with inhalation. This chamber must be filled with sterile fluid up to the 2-cm water level marking. To maintain this water seal, the Pleur-evac needs to be kept in an upright position and the water level monitored (fluid can evaporate and may need to be refilled). If there is no air leak, the water level in this chamber should rise with inspiration and fall with expiration, reflecting normal pressure changes in the pleural cavity. Exceptionally high negative pressure readings can be caused by respiratory distress, crying, decreased or disconnected

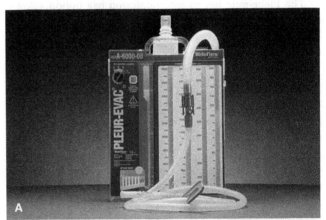

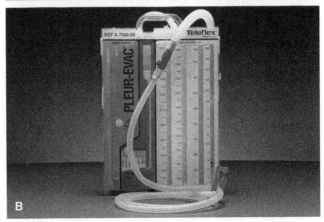

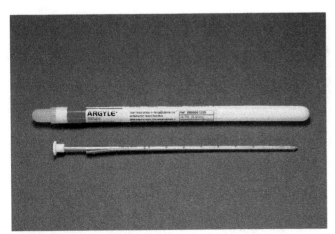

FIGURE 4-7  **Chest tube with trocar.**

FIGURE 4-8  (A) Dry Pleur-evac. (B) Wet Pleur-evac.

suction, or stripping the chest tube. High pressures are indicated by a rising water level in the small arm of the chamber.

The left-hand chamber is the suction-control chamber. In some models, the chamber is "wet," requiring it to be filled to a specified line with sterile fluid. In other models, the suction-control chamber does not require fluid and thus is "dry." The dry models have several advantages over the older "wet" models:

1. There is no fluid bubbling; therefore, they are much quieter (a plus for patient and roommate for whom the continuous bubbling could be irritating).
2. There is no fluid that can evaporate, causing decreased suction levels.
3. Higher suction levels can be achieved.
4. They are easier to set up.

There is a small, or "mini," version of the dry unit available when minimal drainage is expected. The small version allows for greater ease of mobility and ambulation.

The hose on the top of the suction-control chamber is connected to the suction. Pleur-evacs come with a preset level of −20 cm of water for suction but can be set to −10 cm, −15 cm, −30 cm, and −40 cm (refer to manufacturer's instructions). Conditions in which the suction may need to be adjusted higher (−30 cm or −40 cm) include empyema, a large air leak from the lung surface, or anticipated problems with lung reexpansion.

The Pleur-evac has an autotransfusion bag option, allowing for blood to be collected and reinfused back to the patient. The autotransfusion bags contain a 200-micron filter that filters out impurities in the blood.

## Flutter Valve Chest Drain

The flutter valve chest drain (Fig. 4–9) is a mobile device that may be used in place of a traditional water seal drainage system such as the Pleur-evac in certain circumstances. The system consists of rubber flutter leaflets encased in a plastic chamber with adapters on both ends. The proximal adapter is attached to the patient's chest tube while the distal one is attached to

tubing leading to a plastic drainage bag or regulated suction, if desired. The device is easily portable and can function in any position.

The uses of the device include treatment of spontaneous pneumothorax, recurrent pleural effusion, open thoracotomy, and traumatic hemopneumothorax.

## Ventricular (Cerebrospinal Fluid) Drains

### External Ventricular Drain

An external ventricular drain (EVD) is used to drain cerebrospinal fluid (CSF) from the brain ventricles resulting from certain brain injuries or tumors. The CSF is drained into a clear bag that is calibrated in milliliters, allowing for fluid visualization and measurement (Fig. 4–10).

The external drains can also be used to take pressure measurements using a special transducer. The transducer is set up externally to the body and placed at the level of the ventricles using a laser level to assure accuracy.

Pressure measurements are used to monitor intracranial pressure (ICP). An increase in ICP can be an indication of a potentially life-threatening condition, such as an obstructive tumor, serious head injury, or intracranial bleeding.

### Ventricular Shunt

A ventricular shunt (see Fig. 4–10) is an internal drain that shunts the excess CSF from the ventricles to either the peritoneum (ventriculoperitoneal shunt) or the heart atrium (ventriculoatrial shunt). These devices are used to treat hydrocephalus.

Hydrocephalus is an accumulation of an excessive amount of CSF in the ventricles. This condition can be congenital (present at birth) or acquired. Congenital hydrocephalus can be caused by infection (e.g., rubella), congenital malformations, or hemorrhaging in the brain. Acquired hydrocephalus can happen at any age and may be caused by hemorrhage, trauma, tumor, cysts, or infection (e.g., bacterial meningitis or abscess formation).

There are many types of shunts; you need to be familiar with the types that your institution uses. As with any implant, these

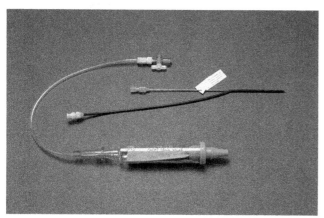

FIGURE 4–9 Flutter valve chest drain.

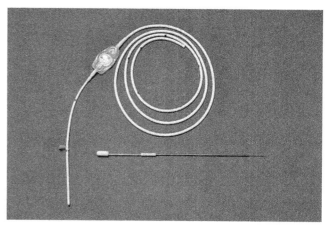

FIGURE 4–10 Ventricular drain and shunt.

shunts should be handled as little as possible and kept away from lint and dust. Absolute adherence to aseptic technique is essential. One of the major complications of this type of shunt is infection, which can lead to patient death.

## Postoperative Autotransfusion Drains

Autotransfusion is the reinfusion of the patient's own blood or blood products. The patient may donate blood or blood products before having surgery, or blood may be collected intraoperatively or postoperatively and then reinfused. The postoperative blood collection and reinfusion devices are covered in this section.

The postoperative collection drains are the simplest autotransfusion devices. These devices are closed collection systems that use a three-spring evacuator (similar to a Hemovac drain) or controlled wall suction to suction blood from the surgical wound postoperatively and collect it for possible reinfusion back to the patient. These devices contain filters within the collection chamber to filter out clots and debris. They have access ports to allow for the addition of anticoagulant medication.

The advantages to these drains are that they are easy to set up and use; they are closed systems, thus decreasing the chance of staff exposure to blood; and they are relatively inexpensive compared with other reinfusion technology. The transfer of the fluid into the reinfusion bag is easily accomplished with the push of a button or lever, and you only need one device per patient. (They can be used to collect and reinfuse fluid multiple times.) The disadvantages are that they can be used postoperatively only (not intraoperatively), and they have a smaller collection capacity than some other devices.

As with any medical device, you must make sure you are familiar with the autotransfusion device and how to use it *before* using it on your patient. If you are unfamiliar with the device, check your institution's procedure for its use and the manufacturer's instructions. Although there are many manufacturers of these devices, the following are two examples of commonly used autotransfusion drains. Both systems collect blood and reinfuse it back to the patient after orthopedic surgery.

### SureTrans

Manufactured by Davol, the SureTrans system (Fig. 4–11) creates suction with a spring action evacuator (similar to a Hemovac) that is attached to the collection reservoir. The 800 mL collection reservoir is clear to allow for visualization and measuring of blood and contains a filter and blood transfer button. The button allows the blood to go from the reservoir to the 1,000-mL blood bag. The blood is reinfused—according to institutional policy—from the blood bag, allowing the evacuator to continue to collect drainage at the same time.

### ConstaVac CBCII System

Manufactured by Stryker, the ConstaVac CBCII system consists of a clear 800-mL reservoir that contains a filter for

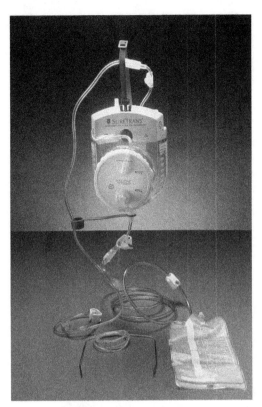

**FIGURE 4–11** SureTrans system.

blood collection and a reinfusion bag (Fig. 4–12). The drain is attached to the reservoir, which has a variable vacuum setting. Depressing the lever transfers the blood from the reservoir to the blood bag. The blood is reinfused—according to institutional policy—from the blood bag, allowing the evacuator to continue to collect drainage at the same time.

## GASTROINTESTINAL TUBES

### Nasogastric Tubes

Nasogastric tubes are inserted through the nose into the back of the throat, down the esophagus, and into the stomach. These tubes are used most commonly to decompress the stomach but can be used for gastric lavage (in drug overdoses), for enteral feedings, or to obtain specimens for analysis. Nasogastric tubes are for short-term use (usually less than 6 weeks). Prolonged usage could lead to necrosis of the nasal septum.

The Salem sump tube is the most widely used nasogastric tube. It is made of polyvinyl chloride (PVC) plastic. This tube is double-lumened to allow for suction drainage and air ventilation. The drainage lumen is usually connected to continuous low suction. The ventilation lumen helps to keep the tube away from the stomach wall and to decrease the chance of damage to the mucosa. The ventilation port can be used if irrigation is necessary. A radiopaque line runs the length of the tube to allow for radiographic conformation of placement. Salem sump tubes are available in 24-inch length (for pediatric patients) and 36- and 48-inch lengths (Fig. 4–13). The available diameters range from 6 Fr to 18 Fr.

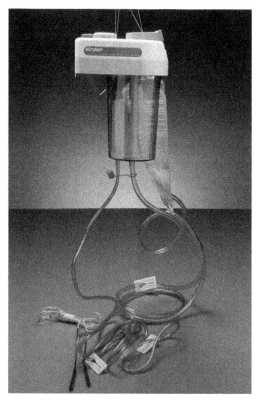

FIGURE 4–12 ConstaVac CBC system.

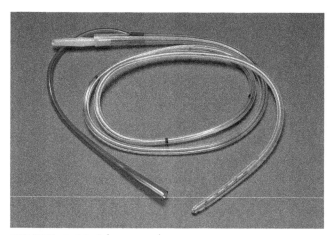

FIGURE 4–13 Salem sump tubes.

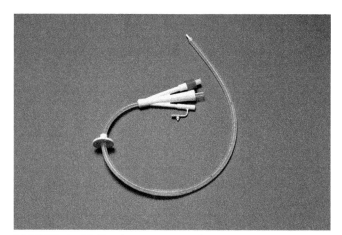

FIGURE 4–14 Regular gastrostomy tube.

## Gastrostomy Tubes

A gastrostomy tube is placed, endoscopically or surgically, directly into the patient's stomach. These tubes can be temporary or permanent. They are used for patients who cannot swallow correctly or continually aspirate food, for people who cannot take in enough food by mouth to keep well nourished, and for infants with birth defects of the mouth or esophagus. The tubes can be used to instill tube feedings and medication or to aspirate air and stomach contents.

Gastrostomy tubes come in a variety of styles but have some common features (Fig. 4–14). All of them have a balloon at the distal tip that is inflated to keep them in place. They all

have at least one port to allow instillation of enteral feedings, fluids, or medications. Some tubes have two or more ports so that feedings do not have to be interrupted to give medications or to allow for gastric decompression. Gastrostomy tubes are made of silicone and have a radiopaque strip to allow for radiographic confirmation of placement. The feeding port is flexible to accommodate a variety of catheter-tip syringes. The most common sizes of these tubes are 12-Fr (pediatric) through 24-Fr diameters.

One common style of gastrostomy tube is known as a *feeding peg* or *button*. This tube fits closely to the skin surface, making it less noticeable under clothing. It is generally used if long-term or permanent use is anticipated. Feeding pegs are available in 14-Fr through 24-Fr diameters and a variety of stoma lengths (1.5 to 4.0 cm) to accommodate most patients.

## URETHRAL CATHETERS

Urethral catheters come in two major categories: indwelling *(retention)* and straight *(nonretention)*. Generally, urethral catheters are used to drain urine from the bladder, but indwelling catheters can be placed in a cavity as a drain, and nonretaining catheters can be used as irrigation devices in ducts or body cavities.

The 8-Fr catheter is a very narrow catheter generally used for small children; 32-Fr is a large-diameter catheter. The most common adult sizes of catheters are 14 Fr, 16 Fr, and 18 Fr.

In the past, all urethral catheters were made of rubber. Because of the growing concern over latex exposure and the increasing number of people who are latex allergic, most styles of catheters are now made with nonlatex material (usually silicone).

This section covers the types and uses of the most common indwelling and straight urethral catheters.

### Indwelling (Retention) Catheters
#### Foley Catheters

When we think of an indwelling urethral catheter, the Foley catheter is the one that comes to mind. It is the most

## General Catheterization Guidelines

There are several important things to remember before inserting any urethral catheter:
- Before opening the catheter or catheter kit, check the patient's allergies. If the patient has a latex sensitivity or allergy, make sure you have a nonlatex catheter.
- Urethral catheterization is a STERILE procedure. Be sure to maintain strict aseptic technique when handling and inserting a catheter. Failure to maintain asepsis could result in a urinary tract infection for the patient and possibly increased hospital stay or other complications.
- Catheters are for one-time use. If you contaminate the catheter while trying to insert it or if the catheter selected is the wrong size, get a new one.

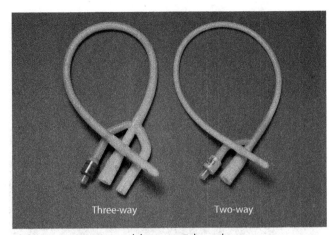

FIGURE 4-16 Two-and three-way Foley catheters.

common one in use. A Foley catheter has a balloon at one end that can be inflated to hold the catheter in place. The balloon has either a 5-cc or a 30-cc capacity (Fig. 4–15). The 5-cc balloon is used simply to hold the catheter in place. A Foley with a 30-cc balloon is used to maintain hemostasis (e.g., after transurethral resection of the prostate [TURP]).

Foley catheters can have a two-way or a three-way system (Fig. 4–16). The two-way system has one port to inflate the balloon and one to hook up a drainage bag. The three-way catheter has two drainage hookups—one for instilling irrigation fluids and one for a drainage bag—as well as a port to allow for balloon inflation. The three-way Foley is used when continuous or intermittent bladder irrigation is desired.

Foley catheters have several uses:

- Long-term drainage of the bladder
- Decompression of the bladder during surgery to decrease the chance of bladder injury
- Continuous bladder irrigation
- Blood clot evacuation
- Measurement and tracking of urinary output
- Possible drainage of a body cavity (e.g., can be used as a chest tube)

### Malecot Catheters
The Malecot catheter is another type of self-retaining urethral catheter. Instead of using a balloon, the tip of the Malecot has either two or four wings that expand out to hold it in place (Fig. 4–17). The most common Malecot catheter sizes are 12 Fr through 18 Fr. Other uses for Malecot catheters include being inserted into the stomach to be used as a feeding tube, into a wound or body cavity to be used as a drain, or inserted percutaneously into the kidney for drainage.

### Pezzer Catheter
The Pezzer catheter, also known as a *mushroom catheter*, has a tip that resembles a mushroom cap that holds the catheter in place (Fig. 4–18). The tip has two holes to allow for drainage. Pezzer catheters are available in sizes 14 Fr through 32 Fr. Similar to other self-retaining catheters, the Pezzer can be used for bladder drainage, as a feeding tube, or as a wound drain.

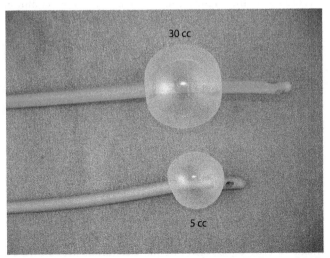

FIGURE 4-15 Foley catheters with 5-cc and 30-cc balloons inflated.

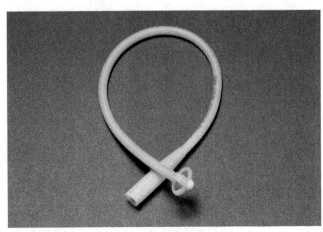

FIGURE 4-17 Four-wing Malecot self-retaining catheter.

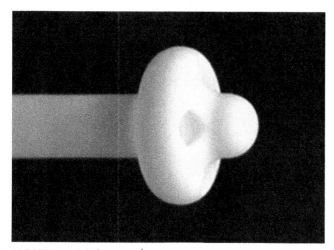

FIGURE 4-18 *Pezzer catheter.*

## Urinary Drainage Bags

All self-retaining catheters need to be attached to a drainage bag. There are two types of bags: a small leg bag that is often used during the day when the person is up and about and a larger bag that is used when the patient is in the hospital or in bed at night (sometimes referred to as a *nighttime bag*).

The leg bag attaches around the upper leg with two straps—one at the top of the bag and one at the bottom (Fig. 4–19A).

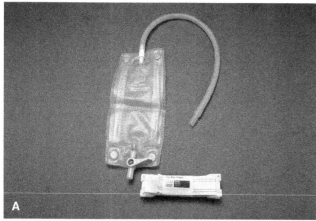

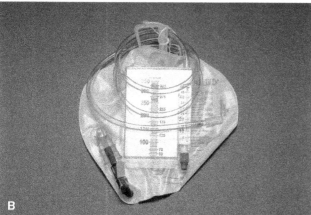

FIGURE 4-19 (A) Urinary leg bag. (B) Urinary drainage bag with a urometer attached.

It allows the person greater freedom because the bag is worn under clothing to conceal it from view when the person is out in public or participating in activities. Leg bags have a capacity of anywhere from 450 cc to 1,300 cc; the most common sizes are 600 cc to 800 cc, which need to be emptied more frequently than the larger nighttime bags. Most leg bags have a hard plastic valve at the bottom for ease of emptying.

The larger bag (or nighttime bag) is the bag most frequently used in the operating room (OR). The self-retaining catheter is attached to the bag to allow the bladder to continuously drain. Urinary output and color can be monitored during the procedure and postoperatively. This type of bag is less convenient if the patient is going to be going home with an indwelling catheter because it cannot be concealed under clothing and must be carried around by hand. Patients who go home with an indwelling catheter and leg bag will also have this larger drainage bag to use at night so that they do not have to wake up to empty it.

The larger bags are available in 2,000-cc to 4,000-cc capacity, with or without a urometer attached (Fig. 4–19B). A urometer is a 350-cc to 500-cc device that allows for more careful monitoring of urinary output over shorter time intervals. For example, the anesthesia provider may need to monitor the hourly urine outputs of a patient undergoing major surgery. The urine first flows into the urometer, and the volume is recorded before the urine is emptied into the larger bag.

## Nonretaining (Straight) Catheters

Nonretaining catheters, also known as *straight catheters,* are used temporarily to drain the bladder or to irrigate a duct. These catheters do not have balloons or wings to hold them in place. Drainage bags are unnecessary because the catheter does not stay in. The straight catheter is inserted, the bladder is drained, and the catheter is immediately removed. They may be inserted at the beginning of the surgical procedure to drain the bladder when an empty bladder is desirable but ongoing bladder decompression is unnecessary.

Similar to indwelling catheters, straight catheters are sized according to the French gauge system. The most common sizes are 14 Fr and 16 Fr for adults, 10 Fr for children, and 8 Fr for toddlers and some infants.

### Coudé Catheter

A Coudé catheter is available in both self-retaining and nonretaining styles. This type of catheter has a curved, stiff tip that makes it easier to insert if the patient has an enlarged prostate or urethral stricture (Fig. 4–20). This type of catheter is often used when attempts to insert a regular catheter are unsuccessful.

### Robinson Catheter

The Robinson catheter *(straight catheter)* is the most common nonretaining catheter. The tip is soft and rounded, with two opposing eyes for drainage (Fig. 4–21). Robinson catheters are made of latex or silicone. The most common sizes are 12 Fr through 18 Fr.

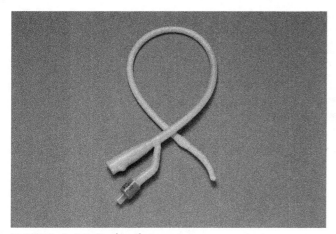

FIGURE 4-20 Coudé catheter.

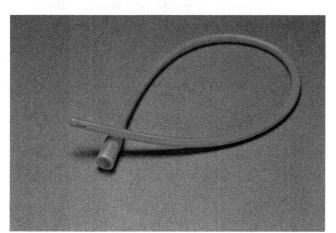

FIGURE 4-21 Robinson catheter.

## Ureteral Catheters

Ureteral catheters are narrow tubes inserted into the ureters with the use of a cystoscope. These catheters can be used to bypass a tumor or kidney stone, provide drainage of the ureter, keep the ureter open, instill contrast media, allow stones to pass, block the ureters during radiological procedures, or obtain specimens. Ureteral catheters may be inserted before open abdominal surgery to identify the ureter, thus decreasing the chance of injury to it.

Ureteral catheters are very narrow, generally ranging from 3-Fr to 6-Fr diameter (Fig. 4–22). They are marked in centimeters to allow the surgeon to gauge how far they have been inserted. These catheters come in a variety of tip shapes: whistle, cone, open end, spiral, round, angled, and wedge (similar to a Pezzer tip). The type of catheter the surgeon selects depends on the purpose for which it is being used. For example, a wedge tip may be used during a retrograde pyelogram, whereas an open-end tip is used for drainage or navigating a tortuous ureter.

## Ureteral Stents

Some patients have the ureteral catheter left in place postoperatively to allow for healing. This is known as a *stent*, and it can

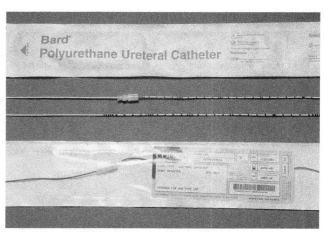

FIGURE 4-22 Different types of ureteral catheters.

be attached to a urinary drainage bag. Two of the most common types are the J stent and the pigtail (Figs. 4–23 and 4–24). The ends of both catheters have a spiral shape, which helps to hold them in place in the ureter. The length of time a stent is left in place depends on how long the healing process takes; it can be anywhere from days to months (or even years). If the stent is to be left in for the long term, the patient may need to come back into surgery periodically to have it changed.

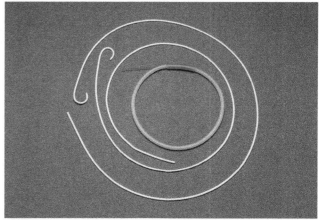

FIGURE 4-23 J stent.

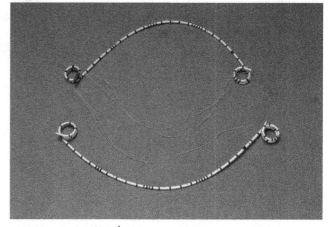

FIGURE 4-24 Pigtail stent.

Many stents come with a tether attached. A tether is a long strand of material attached to the stent that aids in the manipulation or removal of the stent. The surgeon may choose to leave the tether attached (in which case it is often secured to the inside of the upper thigh) or cut it off.

## Cystostomy Tube

The cystostomy tube is used when less-invasive methods of urine drainage such as transurethral catheterization are not possible. The surgeon inserts the tube through the patient's abdominal wall and into the urinary bladder. The tubes come in sizes 8 Fr to 14 Fr.

## Nephrostomy Tube

A nephrostomy tube is a narrow plastic tube usually less than 5 mm in diameter. The tube is placed percutaneously into the kidney to allow for temporary drainage of urine. This procedure is done with the use of fluoroscopy in the OR interventional radiology suite.

## Surgical Session Review

1) The _____ drain does not have an attached fluid collection device.
   a. Pleur-evac
   b. Hemovac
   c. Penrose
   d. TLS

2) The flutter valve device is used to drain air from the
   a. Abdomen
   b. Chest
   c. Knee joint
   d. Pelvic cavity

3) The nephrostomy tube is placed
   a. Percutaneously
   b. Transurethrally
   c. Transcytopic
   d. Intra-abdominally

4) The Malecot is a type of
   a. Nasogastric tube
   b. Knee drain
   c. Ventricular drain
   d. Urinary catheter

5) The urologist is having trouble catheterizing an elderly male patient because of an enlarged prostate. Which type of catheter is the doctor most likely to ask you to have available?
   a. Robinson
   b. Three-way Foley
   c. Coudé
   d. Salem

6) A cystostomy tube is placed into which of the following structures?
   a. Kidney
   b. Ureter
   c. Bladder
   d. Urethra

7) The SureTrans drain is most likely to be used after what type of surgery?
   a. Craniotomy
   b. Total knee
   c. Radical neck
   d. Total abdominal hysterectomy

8) A TLS drain could be used after surgery on all of these areas *except* the
   a. Foot
   b. Face
   c. Breast
   d. Knee

9) A JP drain is another name for a
   a. Jackman-Pratt
   b. Jackson-Pratt
   c. Jackson-Prett
   d. Jackman-Prett

10) A Salem sump is a common type of
   a. Urinary catheter
   b. Tracheostomy tube
   c. Nasogastric tube
   d. Endotracheal tube

11) The ventricular shunt is used to drain excess
   a. Blood
   b. CSF
   c. Urine
   d. Gastric juices

12) J and "double pigtail" are types of
   a. Wound drains
   b. Foley catheters
   c. Ureteral stents
   d. Chest tubes

# 5 Sutures and Suture Needles

## SUTURE TERMS

When you are looking at sutures, it is important that you understand the following key terms:

*Absorbable:* This suture is capable of being absorbed by tissue in a given time frame, allowing the tissue time to heal itself. The time frame varies with each type of absorbable suture.

*Nonabsorbable:* This suture resists absorption by tissue. Used when a permanent suture is required or when the suture will be removed later (e.g., on the outside of the body).

*Monofilament:* This suture consists of a single strand. This type of suture does not easily harbor bacteria and glides through tissue smoothly. The drawback to monofilament suture is that it can be harder to handle and does not hold a knot as well as a multifilament suture.

*Multifilament:* This suture consists of more than one strand. The strands are either braided or twisted together. Multifilament suture is easier to handle, holds knots better, and has greater flexibility and tensile strength than monofilament suture. The disadvantage to multifilament is that it can harbor bacteria and therefore should not be used in the presence of infection.

*Braided:* The strands are intertwined.

*Twisted:* The strands are twisted in the same direction.

*Coated:* This suture is coated to ease handling and help reduce tissue drag (friction).

*Natural:* This suture is made from naturally occurring plants or tissue (e.g., cotton suture).

*Synthetic:* This suture is made from manufactured materials (e.g., nylon suture).

*Memory:* This suture has "memory," which means it springs back into curls when removed from the package. The scrub person needs to hold each end and give it one gentle pull outward before handing it to the surgeon.

## SUTURE SIZES

Sutures come in a variety of sizes (known as the *gauge*). Suture gauges range from 5 (heaviest suture) down to 11-0 (thinner than a strand of hair).

5  4  3  2  1  0  2-0  3-0  4-0  5-0  6-0  7-0  8-0  9-0  10-0  11-0

←——————————————————————————————————→

Heavy                                            Very Fine

The gauge of suture that a surgeon chooses depends on the thickness and type of tissue being sutured. The heavier sutures are used to approximate bone or are used to put retention sutures in an abdominal midline incision. Sutures that are 2 to 5 gauge are used for tendon repair or high-tension structures in orthopedic surgeries. Sutures that are 0 or 1 gauge are generally used on thick tissue (e.g., on abdominal muscle or fascia, during orthopedic surgery). Sutures in the 4-0 to 7-0 range generally are used in plastic surgeries or in cardiovascular and vascular surgery. Sutures in the 8-0 to 11-0 range generally are used for surgery of the eye or in microsurgery procedures (e.g., microvascular, vasovasostomy) (Fig. 5–1).

## COMPARISON OF SUTURE MATERIALS

Sutures are either absorbable or nonabsorbable. They are composed of various materials, natural and synthetic, which make them suitable for certain procedures or tissues. Tables 5–1, 5–2, and 5–3 allow you to compare suture materials made by various manufacturers. Table 5–2 lists the absorbable sutures' approximate wound support times to allow for further comparisons.

## COMPONENTS OF SUTURE PACKAGING

You can judge some things by their covers. Figures 5–2 through 5–5 show the information found on the outer packaging of the suture material produced by four major suture

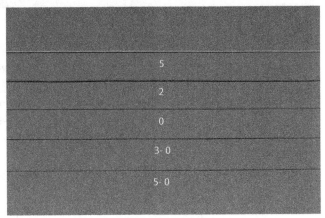

**FIGURE 5-1** Suture thickness comparison.

115

### TABLE 5–1 Nonabsorbable Sutures

| SUTURE MATERIAL | COVIDIEN PRODUCT | ETHICON (A JOHNSON & JOHNSON COMPANY PRODUCT) |
| --- | --- | --- |
| Monofilament nylon | Dermalon; Monosof | Ethilon |
| Braided nylon | Surgilon | Nurolon |
| Braided polyester (uncoated) | Surgidac | Mersilene |
| Braided polyester (coated) | Ti Cron | Ethibond |
| Monofilament polybutester | Novafil | — |
| Monofilament polybutester (coated) | Vascufil | — |
| Monofilament polypropylene | Surgipro; Surgipro II | Prolene |
| Hexafluoropropylene VDF | — | Pronova Poly |
| Monofilament steel | Steel | Surgical Stainless Steel |
| Multistrand steel | Flexon | Surgical Stainless Steel |
| Silk | Sofsilk | Silk; Perma-Hand |

### TABLE 5–2 Other Nonabsorbable Sutures

| SUTURE MATERIAL | SUTURE NAME AND MANUFACTURER |
| --- | --- |
| Monofilament nylon (ophthalmic) | Alcon Nylon suture (made by Alcon) |
| Twisted silk (ophthalmic) | Silk suture (made by Alcon) |
| Monofilament polypropylene (ophthalmic) | Polypropylene suture (made by Alcon) |
| Braided polyester (ophthalmic) | Polyester suture (made by Alcon) |
| Monofilament suture coated with polycaprolate | BioSorb and BioSorb C (made by Alcon); BioSorb C also available as a braided suture |
| Monofilament PTFE (polytetrafluoroethylene) | Gore-Tex (made by Gore Medical) |

### TABLE 5–3 Absorbable Sutures

| SUTURE MATERIAL | COVIDIEN PRODUCT | ETHICON (A JOHNSON & JOHNSON COMPANY PRODUCT) |
| --- | --- | --- |
| Gut fiber | Plain Gut (7–10 day wound support) | Surgical Gut Plain (7–10 day wound support) |
| Gut fiber with chromium salt | Chromic Gut; Mild Chromic Gut (10–14 day wound support) | Surgical Gut Chromic (21–28 day wound support) |
| Synthetic monofilament polyglyconate | Maxon, Maxon Plus (6–week wound support) | — |
| Monofilament synthetic polyester (polyglytone 6211) | Caprosyn (10–day wound support) | — |
| Coated glycolic acid polymer | Dexon II, Dexon S (3–week wound support) | — |

## TABLE 5–3    Absorbable Sutures—cont'd

| SUTURE MATERIAL | COVIDIEN PRODUCT | ETHICON (A JOHNSON & JOHNSON COMPANY PRODUCT) |
| --- | --- | --- |
| Monofilament polyester | Biosyn (3–week wound support) | — |
| Monofilament polydioxanone | — | PDS (up to 6-weeks' wound support) |
| Monofilament poliglecaprone | — | Monocryl (7–14 day wound support) |
| Braided copolymer of lactide and glycolide | Polysorb (3–week wound support) | — |
| Braided polyglactin 910 | — | Vicryl Rapide (7–10 day wound support) |
| | | Vicryl (2–3 week wound support) |

Sources: www.jandjmedicaldevices.com; www.syneture.com; www.Alcon.com.

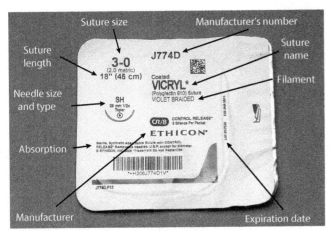

FIGURE 5–2 Ethicon suture package components.

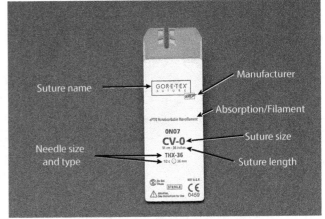

FIGURE 5–4 Gore Medical suture package components.

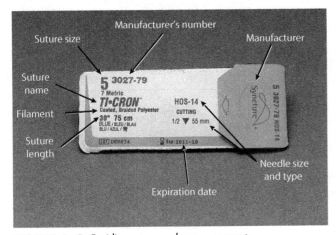

FIGURE 5–3 Covidien suture package components.

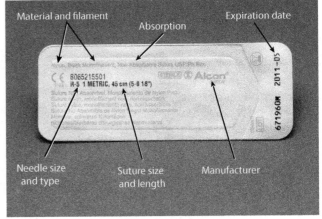

FIGURE 5–5 Alcon suture package components.

manufacturers. The packaging will always list the following components:

- Suture name
- Filament

- Suture size and length
- Needle size and type
- Absorption
- Manufacturer
- Expiration date

## SUTURE SUPPLIES

**Name:** needle counter

**Alias:** foam block needle counter

**Use:** holds used suture needles, knife blades, and other sharps

**Features:** numbered foam insert; sticky surface on opposite side for blades

**Additional Information:** putting only one suture needle in each numbered space enables the count to be accomplished more efficiently; some needle counters have metal magnetic strips instead of foam blocks to hold the sharps

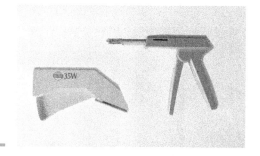

**Name:** skin stapler

**Alias:** none

**Use:** closes skin incisions

**Features:** comes in regular and wide widths

**Additional Information:** available in a variety of styles

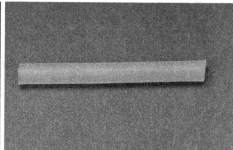

**Name:** retention suture bolster

**Alias:** bolster

**Use:** sheaths the retention suture to avoid cutting the patient's skin

**Features:** may be made of rubber or plastic

**Additional Information:** 6 per package

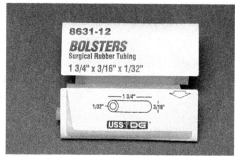
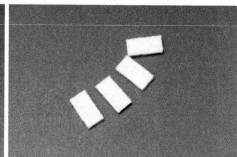

**Name:** pledgets

**Alias:** none

**Use:** exert pressure over small holes to prevent bleeding and promote clotting; prevent suture from tearing the tissue; used in some vascular procedures

**Features:** nonabsorbable

**Additional Information:** available in several sizes (3 × 7 mm pictured); fold the pledget in half and put the suture through the top half of the fold

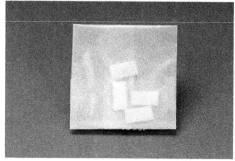

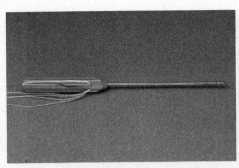
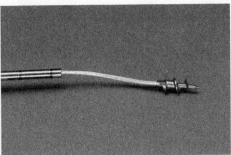

**Name:** corkscrew suture anchor

**Alias:** none

**Use:** repairs of bones and joints

**Features:** corkscrew-shaped anchor, two nonabsorbable polyester sutures (one green and one white)

**Additional Information:** comes as a disposable self-contained unit; comes in several sizes

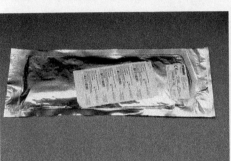
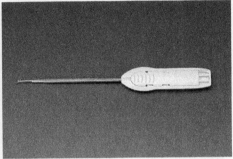

**Name:** Mitek anchor

**Alias:** none

**Use:** repair of anterior cruciate ligament, meniscuses, and rotator cuff

**Features:** absorbable anchor with sutures attached

**Additional Information:** comes as a disposable self-contained unit; comes in a variety of sizes, depending on the intended use

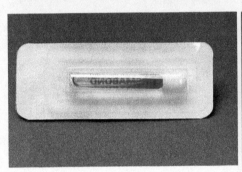
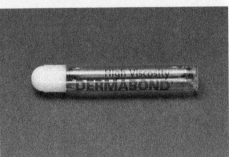

**Name:** surgical skin adhesive

**Alias:** Dermabond, SurgiSeal, Octylseal

**Use:** approximates wound edges

**Features:** provides a flexible, antimicrobial, water-proof barrier

**Additional Information:** should not be used on patients who have formaldehyde sensitivity

**Name:** UltraTape™ and Ultrabraid™

**Alias:** none

**Use:** repairing tendons and ligaments; attaching soft tissue to bone

**Features:** nonabsorbable; polyethylene fiber; available attached to an anchor for shoulder repairs

**Additional Information:** 5 mm wide

(Photo used with permission from Smith + Nephew Inc.)

| Brand | | Type | USP size/Width |
|---|---|---|---|
| ULTRABRAID° | | Round suture | 2-0 |
| LOOPED SUTURE | | Round suture | #2 suture |
| ULTRABRAID | | Round suture | #5 suture |
| MINITAPE° | | Tape | 1.4mm width |
| ULTRATAPE° | | Tape | 2mm width |

**Name:** Endoknot

**Alias:** none

**Use:** endoscopic surgery

**Features:** straight taper needle attached to one end; the other end is attached to a scored plastic tubing that acts as a handle; 42 inches long

**Additional Information:** available in 0 Vicryl, 0 PDS II, 0 Ethibond

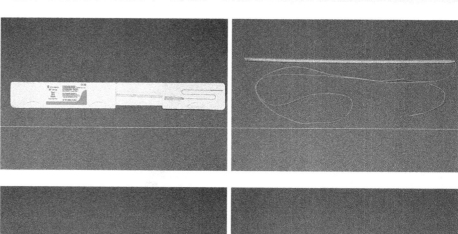

**Name:** Endoloop

**Alias:** looped suture

**Use:** pedicle ligation during endoscopic procedures

**Features:** needleless; comes in a single unit pack; 18 inches long

**Additional Information:** available in 0 Vicryl, 0 PDS II, 0 Ethibond, 0 Monocryl

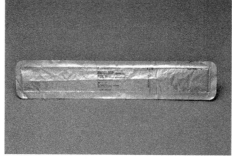
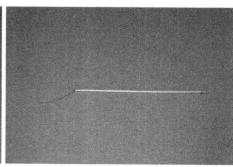

## ABSORBABLE SUTURES

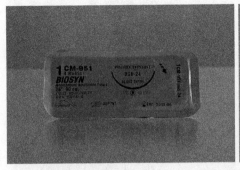
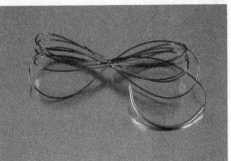

**Name:** Biosyn

**Alias:** none

**Use:** general tissue approximation and ligation; ophthalmic surgery

**Features:** monofilament

**Additional Information:** available in sizes 6-0 to 1

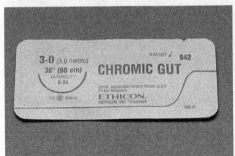
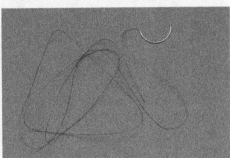

**Name:** chromic gut

**Alias:** surgical gut

**Use:** approximates general tissue; not for use in cardiovascular or neurosurgical procedures

**Features:** made from collagen, which comes from beef or sheep intestines; packaged in alcohol and water to prevent suture from drying out; treated with chromium salts to delay absorption; do not use in patients with chromium allergies

**Additional Information:** available in sizes 7-0 to 3; suture has "memory"

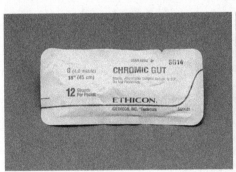
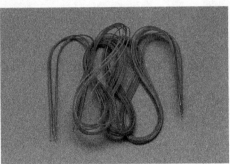

**Name:** chromic gut ties

**Alias:** surgical gut ties

**Use:** allows general tissue ligation; do not use in cardiovascular or neurosurgical procedures

**Features:** made from collagen, which comes from beef or sheep intestines; packaged in alcohol and water to prevent suture from drying out; treated with chromium salts to delay absorption; do not use in patients with chromium allergies

**Additional Information:** available in sizes 3-0 to 0; available in 18- and 54-inch lengths; tie has "memory"

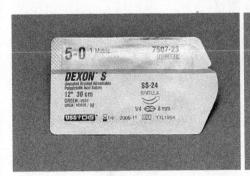
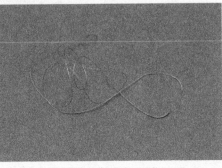

**Name:** Dexon S

**Alias:** none

**Use:** general tissue approximation; not for use in cardiac or neurosurgery

**Features:** Can be braided, twisted, or monofilament

**Additional Information:** available in sizes 8-0 to 2; may be undyed or green color

**Name:** Maxon

**Alias:** none

**Use:** general soft tissue repair

**Features:** monofilament

**Additional Information:** available in a variety of sizes and with a variety of needles; suture has "memory"

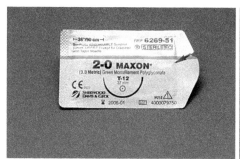
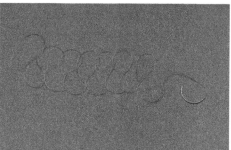

**Name:** Monocryl

**Alias:** none

**Use:** approximation of soft issue; not used for cardiovascular, neurological, or ophthalmic tissue

**Features:** absorbable; monofilament; undyed or violet; tensile strength gone in 28 days

**Additional Information:** available in a variety of sizes (6-0 to 2); available with a variety of needles; suture has "memory"

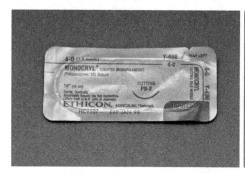
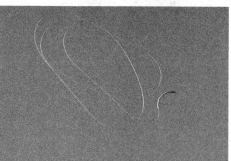

**Name:** PDS II

**Alias:** none

**Use:** allows soft tissue approximation except for adult cardiovascular or neural tissue; not for use in microsurgery

**Features:** monofilament; clear or violet; absorption is complete within 6 months

**Additional Information:** available in sizes 9-0 to 2; suture has "memory"

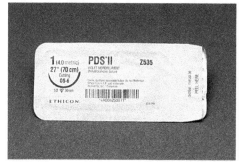
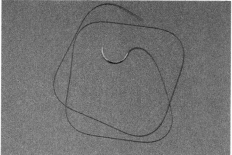

**Name:** plain gut

**Alias:** none

**Use:** general tissue approximation; not for use in cardiovascular or neurosurgical procedures

**Features:** absorbable; made from collagen, which comes from beef or sheep intestines; packaged in alcohol and water to prevent suture from drying out

**Additional Information:** available in sizes 7-0 to 3; suture has "memory;" also available as ties

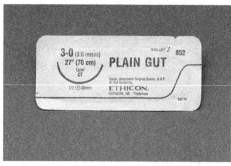
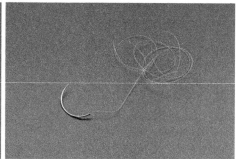

**Name:** Vicryl Rapide

**Alias:** none

**Use:** closure of skin and mucous membranes in cases in which 7 to 10 days of wound support is needed

**Features:** braided; tensile strength completely gone in 10 to 14 days; undyed

**Additional Information:** available in sizes 5-0 to 1

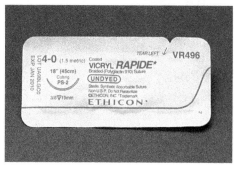
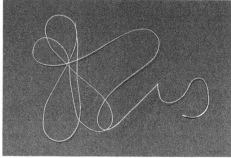

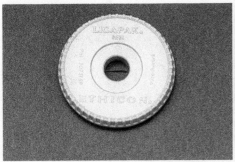
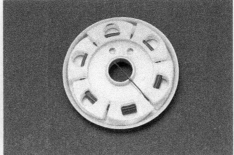

**Name:** Vicryl reel

**Alias:** Ligapak

**Use:** ligates blood vessels or structures

**Features:** braided; number of holes in the bottom of the reel indicates size (2 holes = 2-0, 4 holes = 4-0, and so on)

**Additional Information:** available in 2-0, 3-0, and 4-0 sizes; reel must be accounted for in your surgical count

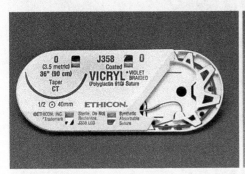
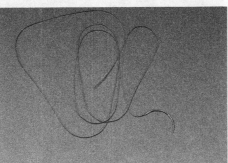

**Name:** Vicryl suture

**Alias:** none

**Use:** general soft tissue approximation

**Features:** braided; tensile strength gone in 5 weeks

**Additional Information:** one of the most commonly used sutures; available in undyed or dyed (violet); sizes range from 8-0 through 2

## NONABSORBABLE SUTURES

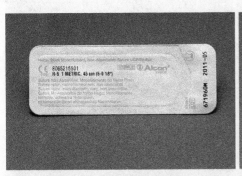
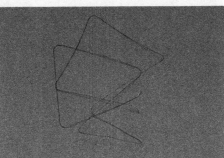

**Name:** Alcon ophthalmic suture

**Alias:** none

**Use:** ophthalmic suturing

**Features:** monofilament; black nylon

**Additional Information:** double armed to allow for suturing in a circle; need to use Castroviejo or other microsurgery needle holder to handle

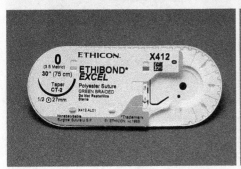
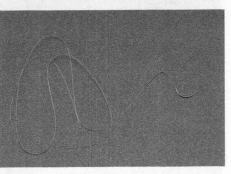

**Name:** Ethibond

**Alias:** none

**Use:** sutures general soft tissue

**Features:** nonabsorbable; braided polyester

**Additional Information:** available in sizes 7-0 through 5; large diameter may be used for retention sutures; also available as ties

**Name:** Ethilon

**Alias:** nylon suture

**Use:** closes skin; eye surgery

**Features:** monofilament; nylon fiber

**Additional Information:** available in black, green, or undyed; available in sizes 11-0 to 2

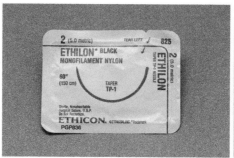 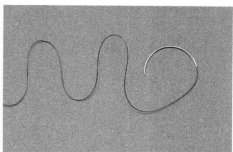

**Name:** Gore-Tex suture

**Alias:** none

**Use:** cardiovascular surgery, suturing in vascular grafts, hernia repair

**Features:** monofilament

**Additional Information:** available in several sizes; often comes double armed to allow for suturing in a circle around blood vessels

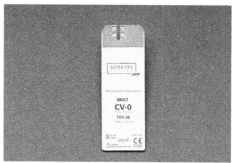 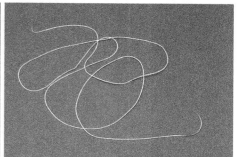

**Name:** Mersilene

**Alias:** none

**Use:** general tissue approximation

**Features:** braided; nonabsorbable; may be undyed or green

**Additional Information:** available in sizes 11-0 and 10-0 (for use in ophthalmic and microsurgery procedures) and 6-0 to 5; also available as ties

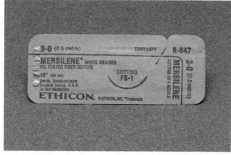 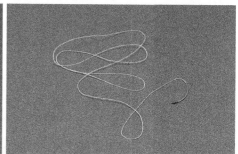

**Name:** Novafil

**Alias:** none

**Use:** general tissue approximation

**Features:** monofilament

**Additional Information:** available in sizes 7-0 to 2, blue in color

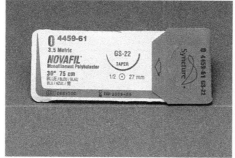 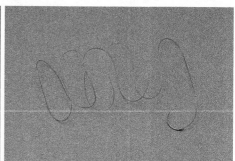

**Name:** Nurolon

**Alias:** none

**Use:** general tissue approximation, including cardiovascular, neurological, and ophthalmological procedures

**Features:** braided; nylon fiber

**Additional Information:** available in sizes 6-0 to 1

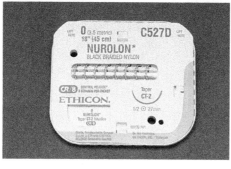 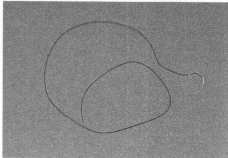

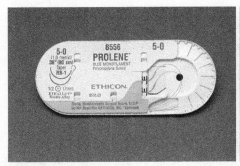

**Name:** Prolene

**Alias:** none

**Use:** general tissue approximation and ligation; often used in vascular surgery

**Features:** monofilament; may be clear or blue

**Additional Information:** available in sizes 10-0 to 2; suture has "memory;" smaller sizes available as double armed to allow for suturing in a circle around blood vessels

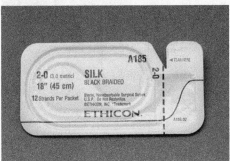
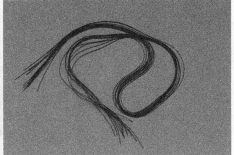

**Name:** silk ties

**Alias:** none

**Use:** ligates blood vessels or structures

**Features:** braided; black

**Additional Information:** available in a variety of sizes (4-0 to 0 are the most common); come in 18-, 30-, and 60-inch lengths or on reels

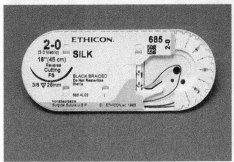
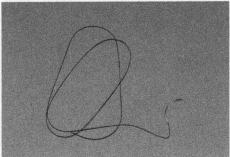

**Name:** silk suture

**Alias:** none

**Use:** general tissue approximation and ligation secures drains

**Features:** braided; black

**Additional Information:** comes in a variety of sizes (9-0 to 5); 2-0 silk is the most commonly used size for securing drains

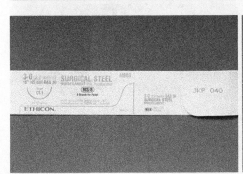
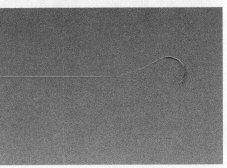

**Name:** stainless steel suture

**Alias:** surgical steel

**Use:** sternal closure, hernia repair, abdominal wound closure, tendon and cartilage repair

**Features:** should not be used in patients with stainless steel, nickel, or chromium allergies

**Additional Information:** available in sizes 10-0 to 7

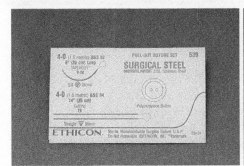
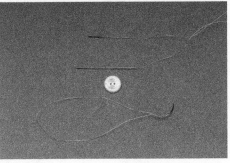

**Name:** stainless steel suture set

**Alias:** surgical steel

**Use:** hernia repairs; orthopedic procedures

**Features:** nonabsorbable, stainless steel suture material

**Additional Information:** comes with two sutures, one on a Keith (straight needle) and one on a tapercut needle; set includes a polypropylene button that can be used as a suture bolster

**Name:** Supramid Extra II

**Alias:** none

**Use:** used in plastic surgery, orthopedics, endodontics

**Features:** nylon fiber (composed of several fine nylon fibers enclosed in an outer smooth nylon shell)

**Additional Information:** comes as a looped cable; available in sizes 4-0 to 8

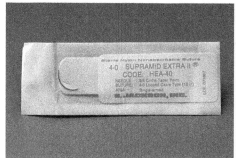
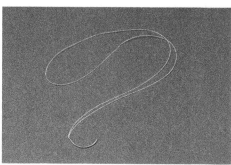

**Name:** Tevdek

**Alias:** none

**Use:** making pursestring sutures in the aorta of adults; orthopedic procedures

**Features:** braided; green

**Additional Information:** available in a variety of sizes

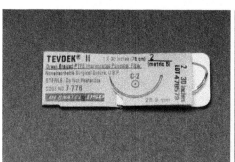
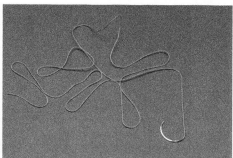

**Name:** Ti Cron

**Alias:** none

**Use:** sutures heavy tissue (mainly in orthopedic surgery)

**Features:** braided; coated polyester; blue

**Additional Information:** available in a variety of sizes (2 and 5 are most popular sizes)

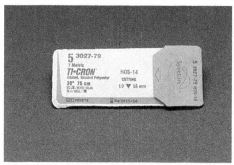
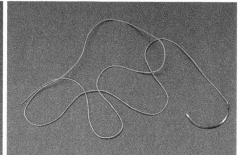

**Name:** Vicryl ties

**Alias:** none

**Use:** ligates blood vessels or tissue

**Features:** braided; violet

**Additional Information:** available in 18-, 27-, and 30-inch lengths; available in a variety of sizes

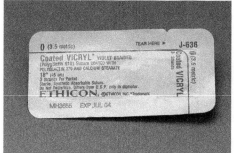
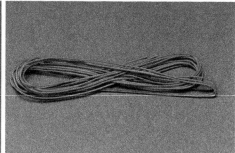

## SUTURE NEEDLE

A needle is required to pass the suture material through tissue. Needle selection is based on the type of tissue being sutured, the type of procedure being performed, and the surgeon's preference. Needles can be straight or curved, with curved being the more common. The body (Fig. 5–6) makes up most of the needle. This is the part that is held in the needle holder. Depending on the surgery, type of tissue, and surgeon preference, the needle holder generally is placed on the distal half to one-third of the body.

The swedged end (see Fig. 5–6) is where the suture is attached (by the manufacturer). Most sutures are made this way. One common type of swedged end is the controlled release or

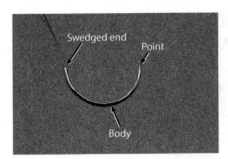

FIGURE 5-6 Parts of a suture needle.

The free needle does not have a suture attached. This needle has an eye, like a sewing needle, through which a suture can be threaded.

There are several different types of suture needle points. Each point was designed with a specific purpose in mind. The point or tip (see Fig. 5–6) is the first part of the needle to enter the tissue. The three most common types of tips are cutting, taper, and blunt. Cutting needles generally are used to close skin or secure drains, taper needles generally are used on tissue inside the body cavity, and blunt needles usually are used to suture organs (e.g., the liver). The following describes the features and general uses for each type of needle point.

"pop off." Once the surgeon has placed the suture, he or she can give the needle a tug and it "pops off," leaving only the needle in the needle holder. The other common type is permanently swedged to the needle, requiring that the needle be cut off the suture.

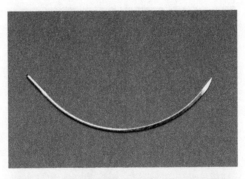

**Name:** conventional cutting needle
**Features:** three cutting edges; the third one is located on the inside concave curvature of the needle
**Use:** closes skin or secures drains

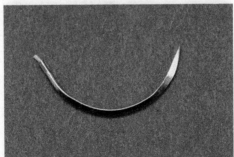

**Name:** reverse cutting needle
**Features:** three cutting edges; the third one is located on the outer convex curvature of the needle
**Use:** designed for use on tough tissue (muscle, skin, or fascia)

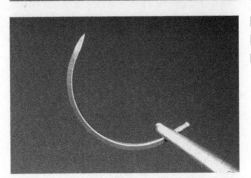

**Name:** heavy body reverse cutting needle
**Features:** heavy needle body; ½- circle curvature
**Use:** closes muscle, fascia, bone, skin, and cartilage

**Name:** premium X-cutting needle
**Features:** four-sided plastic surgery cutting edge
**Use:** closes cuticle and subcuticle

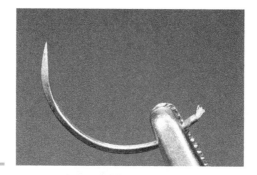

**Name:** spatula (side-cutting) needle
**Features:** flat on top and bottom; eliminates the tissue cutout of a cutting point
**Use:** designed for use in ophthalmic procedures

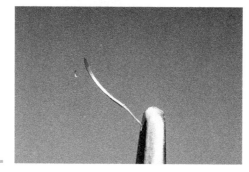

**Name:** taper needle
**Features:** pierces and spreads tissue without cutting it; used in easily penetrated tissue; very common needle point
**Use:** can be used on most tissues inside the body cavity

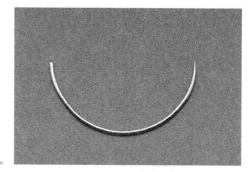

**Name:** taper cut (trocar point) needle
**Features:** combines the features of a reverse cutting point and taper point
**Use:** sutures dense, fibrous tissue

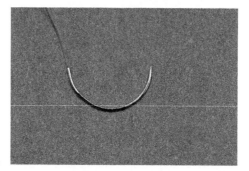

**Name:** blunt needle
**Features:** dissects the tissue rather than cutting it
**Use:** sutures friable tissue such as liver and kidney

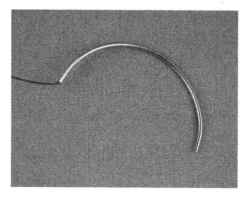

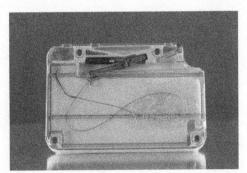

**Name:** endoscopic needle

**Features:** taper point

**Use:** used in laparoscopic procedures

(Sources of information: www.jandjmedicaldevices.com; www.Alcon.com.)

## WATCH OUT! Suture Needle Safety Tips

**When handling suture needles, several safety precautions must be taken to minimize the risk of needlestick injury to oneself or others.**

- Load the suture needle directly onto the needle holder; do not pick it up with your fingers to load it.
- When possible, load needles just before use to avoid open needles on the back table or Mayo stand.
- Put your needles and needle holders in the same place on your back table or Mayo stand each time you set up and during surgery. By putting them in the same place every time, you know where they are and are less apt to accidently get stuck when you reach for other instruments.
- Know where your needles are at all times. Know the location of needles on the surgical field, your Mayo stand, and back table. If the surgeon says, "needle back" or "needle down," look to see where he or she placed it (especially if your institution does not use a neutral zone).
- Use a neutral zone for passing and receiving suture needles. A neutral zone is a designated area when the scrubbed person places the loaded needle holder. The surgeon (or assistant) picks up the loaded needle holder from the designated area. When the surgeon or assistant is done with the suture, he or she places the used needle and needle holder back in the neutral zone. The scrubbed person takes the used needle and holder back from the neutral zone; there is no hand-to-hand passing. This helps avoid the chance of being stuck during hand-to-hand passing. Note: Check your institution's policies and procedures.
- Place all used needles in a puncture-proof foam or magnetic needle counter. Placing each used needle in a counter keeps them in one place, makes it easier to count needles, and lessens the likelihood of being stuck by a stray needle.
- At the end of the case, dispose of all needles and the needle counter in a puncture-proof biohazard waste box.

## INDIVIDUAL SUTURE NEEDLES

The two major manufacturers of suture material are Ethicon (a Johnson & Johnson company) and Covidien. The suture needles described in this section contain the name the manufacturer gave the needle as well as comparable needles (where applicable) made by the other manufacturer.

**Name:** BB needle
**Alias:** blue baby needle
**Comparable needle:** CV, CVF (Covidien)
**Use:** used in cardiovascular surgery
**Features:** taper point
**Additional Information:** ⅜ circle shape

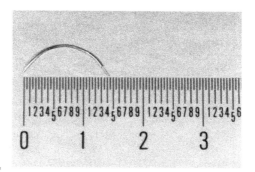

**Name:** BP needle
**Alias:** blunt point needle
**Comparable needle:** BGS-28 (Covidien)
**Use:** used to perform blunt dissection of friable tissue (e.g., liver, kidney, cervix, intestine, spleen)
**Features:** blunt taper point
**Additional Information:** ½-circle shape; available in a variety of sizes

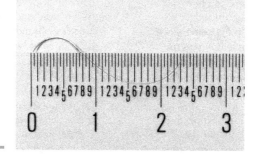

**Name:** BV needle
**Alias:** blood vessel needle (Covidien)
**Use:** sutures fine blood vessels
**Features:** taper point
**Additional Information:** ⅜-circle shape; usually comes as a double-armed suture (two needles: one on each end of the suture)

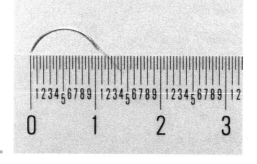

**Name:** C needle
**Alias:** cardiovascular needle
**Comparable needle:** CV, CVF (Covidien)
**Use:** used in cardiovascular surgery
**Features:** taper point
**Additional Information:** ½- circle shape

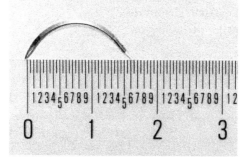

**Name:** CE needle
**Alias:** cutting edge needle
**Use:** approximates skin; sutures dense, thick tissue
**Features:** cutting point
**Additional Information:** ½-circle shape; available in a variety of sizes

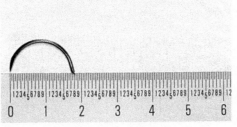

**Name:** CP needle
**Alias:** cutting point needle
**Comparable needle:** GS-10, GS-11, GS-12 (Covidien)
**Use:** approximates skin
**Features:** cutting point
**Additional Information:** ⅜ -circle shape; available in a variety of sizes

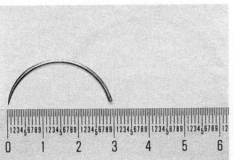

**Name:** CT needle
**Alias:** circle taper needle
**Comparable needle:** GS-24 (Covidien)
**Use:** sutures easily penetrated tissue (e.g., abdominal viscera and peritoneum)
**Features:** taper point; available on some sutures as a controlled-release ("pop off") needle
**Additional Information:** ½-circle shape; available in a variety of sizes

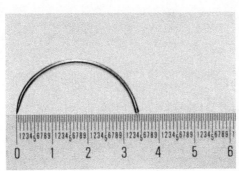

**Name:** CTX needle
**Alias:** circle taper extra-large needle
**Comparable needle:** GS-25 (Covidien)
**Use:** installs sutures in easily penetrated tissue
**Features:** pierces and spreads tissue without cutting
**Additional Information:** ½-circle shape; used in large areas or on large viscera

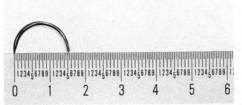

**Name:** Davis Tonsil needle
**Alias:** none
**Use:** installs sutures in the throat and mouth
**Features:** taper point; closed eye; free needle (does not come with suture attached)
**Additional Information:** ½-circle shape

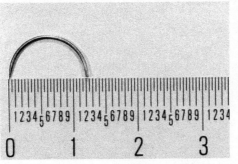

**Name:** Ferguson needle
**Alias:** none
**Use:** taper point (round body)
**Features:** delicate tissue approximation; free needle (does not come with suture attached)
**Additional Information:** ½-circle shape

**Name:** FS needle
**Alias:** for-skin needle
**Comparable needle:** C (Covidien)
**Use:** closes skin; sutures drains in place
**Features:** reverse cutting point
**Additional Information:** ⅜-circle shape; available in a variety of sizes

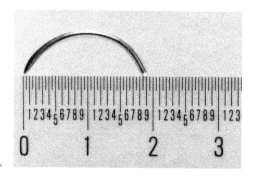

**Name:** FSL needle
**Alias:** for-skin large needle
**Comparable needle:** C-17 (Covidien)
**Use:** closes skin in large wounds
**Features:** reverse cutting point
**Additional Information:** ⅜-circle shape; available in a variety of sizes

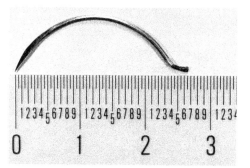

**Name:** G needle
**Alias:** Grieshaber ⅜ (circle) needle
**Comparable needle:** HE (Covidien)
**Use:** closes skin
**Features:** micropoint cutting point
**Additional Information:** ⅜ circle shape

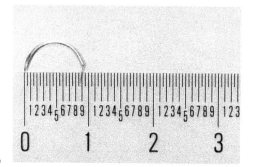

**Name:** GS needle
**Alias:** Grieshaber spatula
**Use:** sutures easily penetrated tissue (e.g., abdominal viscera and peritoneum)
**Features:** spatula point; pierces and spreads tissue without cutting
**Additional Information:** ½-circle shape

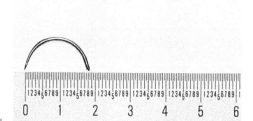

**Name:** HE needle (Covidien)
**Alias:** none
**Comparable needle:** G
**Use:** used for general tissue approximation
**Features:** reverse cutting point
**Additional Information:** ⅜-circle shape

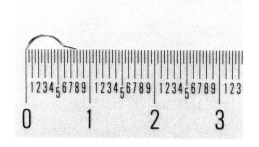

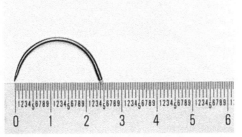

**Name:** HGS needle (Covidien)
**Alias:** heavy Grieshaber
**Comparable needle:** MO
**Use:** sutures heavy tissue
**Features:** taper point
**Additional Information:** ½-circle shape; available in a variety of sizes

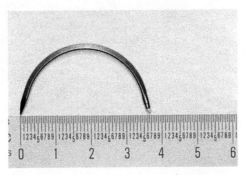

**Name:** HOS needle (Covidien)
**Alias:** heavy orthopedic surgery needle
**Comparable needle:** OS
**Use:** approximates heavy soft tissue (e.g., meniscal repair)
**Features:** reverse cutting point
**Additional Information:** ½-circle shape

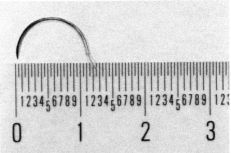

**Name:** J needle
**Alias:** conjunctive needle
**Comparable needle:** C-22, C-26 (Covidien)
**Use:** used in ophthalmic procedures; sutures delicate tissue
**Features:** reverse cutting tip
**Additional Information:** ½-circle shape; available in a variety of sizes

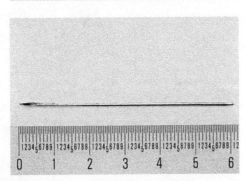

**Name:** Keith needle
**Alias:** straight needle; KS needle
**Comparable needle:** SC-2 (Covidien)
**Use:** closes skin of abdominal wounds
**Features:** cutting point
**Additional Information:** available in varying lengths and sizes

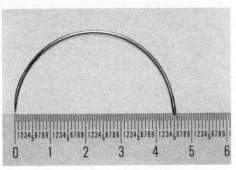

**Name:** LH needle
**Alias:** large half (circle) needle
**Use:** passes through dense or thick dermal tissue
**Features:** cutting point
**Additional Information:** ½-circle shape

**Name:** LR needle

**Alias:** larger retention needle

**Comparable needle:** GS-18 (Covidien)

**Use:** inserts retention sutures

**Features:** large, heavy needle for penetrating multiple layers of tissue; cutting point

**Additional Information:** bolsters may be used if the surgeon is placing retention sutures

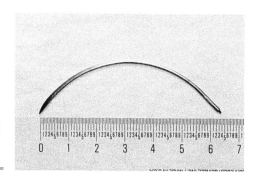

**Name:** Martin uterine needle

**Alias:** none

**Use:** installs sutures through uterine or other heavier tissue

**Features:** cutting edge; closed eye; free needle (does not come with suture attached)

**Additional Information:** ½-circle shape

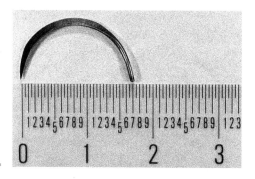

**Name:** Mayo Catgut needle

**Alias:** none

**Use:** works for general tissue approximation (not for use on heavy tissue)

**Features:** taper point; closed eye; free needle (does not come with suture attached)

**Additional Information:** ½-circle shape

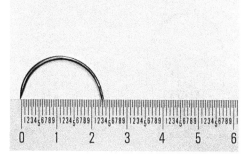

**Name:** Mayo Intestinal Needle

**Alias:** none

**Use:** sutures bowel; used in general tissue approximation

**Features:** taper point; closed eye

**Additional Information:** free needle (does not come with suture attached)

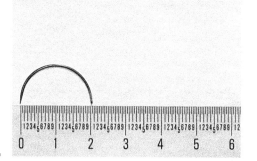

**Name:** MH needle

**Alias:** medium half (circle) needle

**Comparable needle:** CV-300, V-26 (Covidien)

**Use:** used for general tissue approximation

**Features:** taper point

**Additional Information:** ½-circle shape

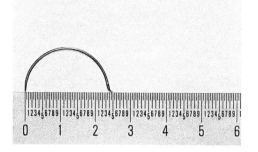

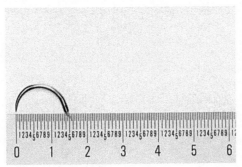

**Name:** MO needle
**Alias:** Mayo needle
**Comparable needle:** HGS (Covidien)
**Use:** sutures dense tissue in gynecological surgery, hernia repair, and general tissue closure
**Features:** taper point with a heavier, flatter body
**Additional Information:** ½-circle shape; available in a variety of sizes

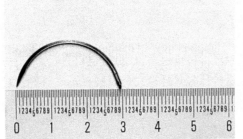

**Name:** OS needle
**Alias:** orthopedic surgery needle
**Comparable needle:** HOS (Covidien)
**Use:** sutures heavy tissue (ligaments, tendons)
**Features:** reverse cutting tip
**Additional Information:** ½-circle shape; available in a variety of sizes

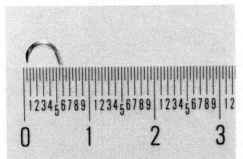

**Name:** P needle (Covidien)
**Alias:** plastic needle
**Comparable needle:** P
**Use:** used in cosmetic surgery
**Features:** reverse cutting point
**Additional Information:** ⅜-circle shape; available in a variety of sizes

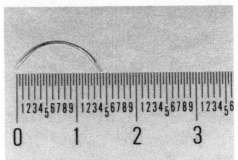

**Name:** PC needle
**Alias:** precision cosmetic needle
**Comparable needle:** PC-10 (Covidien)
**Use:** closes skin in cosmetic surgery
**Features:** fine point; precision reverse cutting needle
**Additional Information:** narrow needle body taper

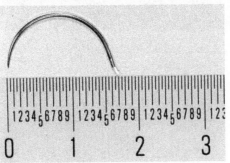

**Name:** PH needle (Gore Medical)
**Alias:** none
**Use:** used in cardiac or vascular surgery
**Features:** piercing point
**Additional Information:** ½-circle shape; available in a variety of sizes; usually comes on a double-armed, Gore-Tex suture (two needles: one on each end of the suture)

**Name:** PS needle
**Alias:** plastic surgery needle
**Comparable needle:** P (Covidien)
**Use:** approximates tissue in plastic surgery
**Features:** fine point; reverse cutting point
**Additional Information:** ⅜ -circle shape; available in a variety of sizes

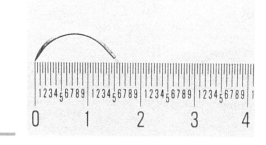

**Name:** RB needle
**Alias:** renal (artery) bypass needle
**Comparable needle:** CV, CVF (Covidien)
**Use:** sutures tissue in urological procedures
**Features:** taper tip
**Additional Information:** ⅝ -circle shape

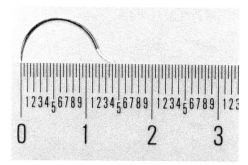

**Name:** S needle
**Alias:** spatula needle
**Comparable needle:** SS (Covidien)
**Use:** sutures delicate tissue; ophthalmic surgery
**Features:** flat on top and bottom with side-cutting edges to separate or split through thin layers of tissue (spatula point)
**Additional Information:** available in a variety of sizes

**Name:** SBE needle
**Alias:** slim blade needle
**Use:** sutures delicate structures
**Features:** taper point needle
**Additional Information:** ½-circle shape; taper point pierces and spreads tissue without cutting it

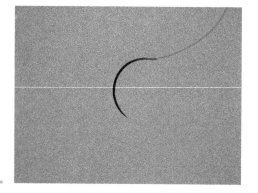

**Name:** SH needle
**Alias:** small half (circle) needle
**Comparable needle:** CV-24, CV-25 (Covidien)
**Use:** sutures easily penetrated tissue
**Features:** taper point
**Additional Information:** ½-circle shape; available in a variety of sizes

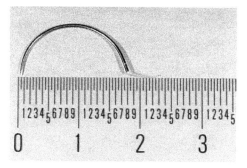

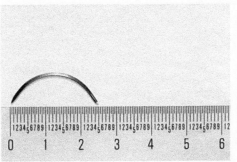

**Name:** T needle
**Alias:** taper needle
**Use:** passes sutures through large areas or wounds
**Features:** taper point
**Additional Information:** ½-circle shape; available in a variety of sizes

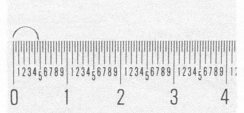

**Name:** TG needle
**Alias:** transverse ground needle
**Comparable needle:** SE (Covidien)
**Use:** used in ophthalmic procedures
**Features:** flat on top and bottom with side-cutting edges to separate or split through thin layers of tissue (spatula point)
**Additional Information:** ⅜-circle shape

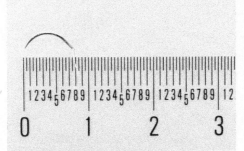

**Name:** TT needle (Gore Medical)
**Alias:** none
**Use:** used in cardiac or vascular surgery
**Features:** taper point
**Additional Information:** ⅜-circle shape; available in a variety of sizes; usually comes on a double-armed, Gore-Tex suture (two needles: one on each end of the suture)

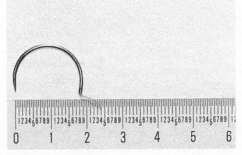

**Name:** UR needle
**Alias:** urology needle
**Comparable needle:** GU (Covidien)
**Use:** sutures around or under structures during urology procedures
**Features:** taper point
**Additional Information:** ⅝-circle shape; available in a variety of sizes

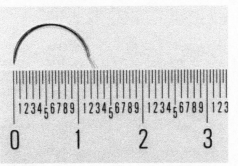

**Name:** V tapercut needle
**Alias:** tapercut surgical needle
**Comparable needle:** KV (Covidien)
**Use:** puts sutures in dense, thick tissue
**Features:** three cutting edges extend from the point (known as a trocar point); more uniform cutting
**Additional Information:** comes in a variety of circle types (½ circle, ⅜ circle, etc.) and sizes

**Name:** X needle
**Alias:** exodontal needle
**Comparable needle:** C-23 (Covidien)
**Use:** used for dental surgery
**Features:** reverse cutting point
**Additional Information:** ½-circle shape

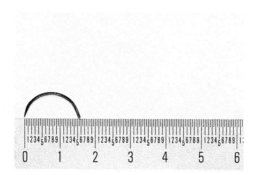

 **Surgical Session Review**

1) The surgeon is finishing cardiac bypass surgery and is ready to close the sternum. Which suture is he or she most likely to use?
   a. Nylon
   b. Prolene
   c. Stainless steel
   d. Monocryl

2) The surgeon wishes to put retention sutures into a large midline abdominal wound. Which suture would be the most appropriate to have ready?
   a. 4-0 nylon
   b. 5 Ethibond
   c. 5-0 Prolene
   d. 5-0 Vicryl

3) Used needles and sharps should be placed in a _____.
   a. Sterile towel
   b. Needle counter
   c. Paper trash bag
   d. Kidney basin

4) _____ is a liquid, topical skin adhesive.
   a. Dermabond
   b. DuraPrep
   c. Duralon
   d. Dermabrade

5) Which of the following is made of nylon fiber?
   a. Monocryl
   b. Prolene
   c. Vicryl
   d. Ethilon

6) Which suture does NOT have memory?
   a. Maxon
   b. Prolene
   c. Chromic
   d. Vicryl

7) During eye surgery, which of the following sutures would most likely be used?
   a. 4 Ethilon
   b. 2 Ethilon
   c. 2-0 Ethilon
   d. 9-0 Ethilon

8) Which suture is absorbable?
   a. Stainless steel
   b. Ethilon
   c. Vicryl
   d. Prolene

9) Another name for a straight needle is a _____ needle.
   a. Kevin
   b. Keith
   c. LH
   d. CT

10) The "PS" in PS needle stands for
   a. Pointed straight
   b. Plain suture
   c. Plastic surgery
   d. Pointed suture

11) The surgeon requests a taper-point needle. Which of
the following would be appropriate to hand him?
a. CP needle
b. CT needle
c. CE needle
d. OS needle

12) An RB needle is usually used during what type of
procedures?
a. Cardiovascular
b. Gynecological
c. Urological
d. Obstetrical

13) An MH needle has a _____ circle shape.
a. ¼
b. ⅜
c. ½
d. ⅝

14) The needle designed specifically for suturing in the
throat (tonsils) is a
a. Davis
b. Ferguson
c. Martin
d. Mayo Catgut

15) The S needle has a _____ point.
a. Cutting
b. Taper
c. Reverse Cutting
d. Spatula

16) What type of needle would most likely be used to place
retention sutures into a large abdominal wound?
a. PC
b. LR
c. Martin
d. PS

17) Which of these suture sizes is the heaviest (thickest)?
a. 3
b. 0
c. 2-0
d. 3-0

18) Gore-Tex suture is
a. Monofilament
b. Multifilament
c. Braided
d. Polyfilament

19) All of the following statements about sharps safety are
true *except*
a. Use a neutral zone when passing sharps
b. Know where your needles and sharps are located at
all times
c. Load needles as far in advance of use as possible
d. At the end of the case, dispose of all needles in a
puncture-proof container

20) A needle without a suture attached is called a(n)
_____ needle.
a. Swedged
b. Free
c. Orphaned
d. Solo

# 6 Microscopes

The need to magnify things to allow for better visualization started with the invention of the magnifying glass around 1262. The first microscopes were invented in the late 16th century and were used mostly in private research. The first documented use of a monocular microscope in the operating room was in 1921 by ear, nose, and throat (ENT) surgeon Dr. Carl Nylen. Dr. Gunnar Holmgren introduced the binocular microscope in 1922, allowing for the ability to see better with improved depth of field. Microscopes did not really gain a lot of momentum in the operating room until the 1950s, when improvements in design and optics allowed their use in a variety of specialties. Today's modern microscopes allow surgeons to perform many and varied procedures on microscopic structures.

## COMPOUND (OPERATING) MICROSCOPE

This type of microscope is commonly used in the operating room (OR) for a variety of microsurgical procedures (Fig. 6–1). Many procedures require that the surgeon be able to reattach or reanastomose tiny structures that would be hard to see with the naked eye. The microscope makes this job easier by magnifying the surgical field. A structure as fine as a hair can look like a piece of rope when magnified under a microscope.

Some examples of procedures using a microscope include the following:

- *Urology:* Vasovasotomy (reanastomosis of the vas deferens)
- *Neurosurgery:* Removal of small tumors or vascular anomalies; microscopic disc (back) surgery
- *Reimplantation and plastic surgery procedures:* Suturing of tiny nerves and blood vessels
- *Gynecological surgery:* Tubal reanastomosis
- *Ear, nose, and throat* (ENT): Middle ear surgery
- *Eye surgery:* Vitrectomy, corneal transplant, cataract
- *Vascular:* Reanastomosis or repair of tiny blood vessels
- *Dental:* Restorative surgery, endodontics (e.g., root canal)

Microscopes may be mounted in one of four ways—on casters, mounted on a wall, mounted on a ceiling, or set on a tabletop. The most popular models are mounted on casters so they can be moved around and positioned as needed.

Regardless of the mounting system, microscopes all have the same components. The lens system (Fig. 6–2) consists

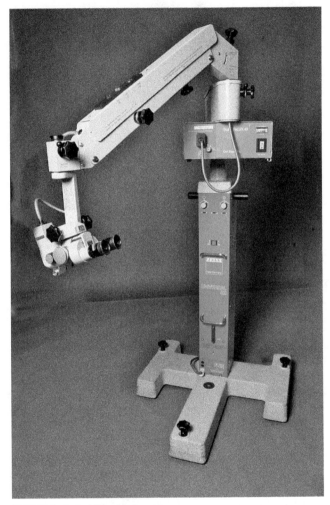

**FIGURE 6–1** Microscope.

of two types of lenses: *objective* and *ocular*. *Ocular lenses* are proximal lenses or eyepieces that the surgeon looks through. The ocular lens magnifies the field of view. *Objective lenses* are the distal lenses. Objective lenses provide magnification and establish the working distance from the surgical field. In order to figure out how much magnification is being used, multiply the magnification of the objective lenses by the magnification of the ocular lenses. For example:

300 (magnification of objective lens) × 10 (magnification of ocular lens) = 3000 (total magnification)

The lens system has a focus control to allow the surgeon to sharpen the view of the surgical field. The focus control may

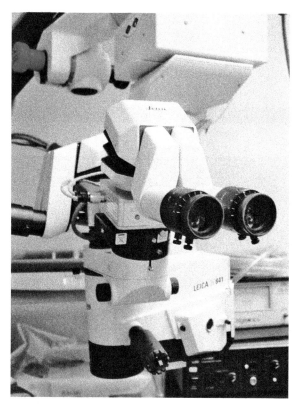

FIGURE 6-2 Lens system.

be hand operated with knobs or controlled by a foot pedal, depending on the microscope model.

Every microscope has an illumination (lighting) system that allows for visualization of the field. This lighting system is usually fiberoptic, incandescent or halogen light. It is referred to as the *coaxial illuminator*. A *paraxial illuminator* is made up of light tubes that contain bulbs and focusing lenses. This system allows light to focus as the working distance of the scope is changed.

Microscopes come equipped with a zoom lens to allow for changes in magnification of the field. If these systems are operated by foot pedals, it is important to make sure that the foot pedal is within easy reach of the surgeon's foot.

One important accessory is the *beam splitter*. The beam splitter transmits the image seen by the primary ocular to the secondary (or assistant's) ocular and produces an identical image so that the assistant can see exactly what the surgeon is seeing. The beam splitter also can be used with a camera to allow the picture to be projected onto a monitor for viewing by the entire team.

## Microscope Care and Handling

Microscopes are very delicate pieces of machinery. The lenses can be easily scratched or damaged, fiberoptics can be broken, or the internal components could be jarred loose or broken. You can follow the tips listed in the box for proper handling and moving of microscopes.

---

**TIPS** | **Microscope Care and Handling**

- Never place your fingers on the lenses.
- Clean the lenses with a cleaner recommended by the manufacturer or with lens paper.
- Wipe down the microscope casing before and after the procedure, following your institution's procedures for equipment decontamination.
- Cover the microscope while it is being stored. This will help to protect the lenses from scratches as well as keep dust from collecting on the casing. Store in a clean, dry area to avoid fungus growth on the optics. Store the microscope with the lens caps in place.
- If the surgeon is going to be using a foot pedal, cover it with a clear, plastic bag–type drape so surgical fluids do not get into it and cause the electronics to malfunction.
- Check all cords and plugs for fraying. If a cord or plug is damaged, do not use the microscope. Get a replacement microscope and have biomedical engineering check the damaged one.
- When moving the microscope, secure the arm so that it cannot swing outward and hit a doorway or wall.
- Never move the microscope by holding onto the head. Always move it by holding onto the center of the vertical column with two hands.
- Make sure the brakes work before moving the microscope up to the surgical field.
- Check the focus knobs and zoom control before the case to make sure they are working properly.
- Balance the microscope before use. The manufacturer's instructions should be followed for this procedure.
- Be familiar with the operation and troubleshooting of the microscope before the case.
- Make sure the head control knob is secure before surgery.
- If the microscope has an X-Y carrier, make sure it is centered before positioning the microscope at the surgical field.

Refer to the manufacturer's instructions if you have questions.

## IMPROVEMENTS OVER THE YEARS

Operating microscopes have seen a great many improvements since they first entered the operating room:

- Good magnification without significant anomalies.
- Adequate illumination without excessive heat (LED illumination).
- Good stability without sacrificing flexibility.
- Modern cameras attached to them allow surgical procedures to be recorded in high-definition quality.
- With attachments, it is possible for one or two assistants to visualize the same surgical field as the surgeon.

- Controls for releasing the brakes and adjusting magnification can be placed on handles or on a pedal.
- 3D 4K imaging.
- The ability to augment images with digital imagery.

These improvements, and improvements in technology, will make microscopes an indispensable piece of equipment for many years to come.

 **Surgical Session Review**

1) The first documented use of the microscope in the operating room occurred in what year?
   a. 1920
   b. 1921
   c. 1922
   d. 1923

2) Who used the first binocular microscope in the operating room?
   a. Nylen
   b. Pasteur
   c. Holmgren
   d. Lister

3) The proximal lenses that the surgeon looks through are called the _____ lenses.
   a. Monocular
   b. Objective
   c. Ocularmotor
   d. Ocular

4) The distal lenses are known as the _____ lenses.
   a. Binocular
   b. Monocular
   c. Objective
   d. Ocular

5) Which of the following surgeries would you most likely NOT find the surgeon using a microscope for?
   a. Root canal
   b. Total knee replacement
   c. Vasovasotomy
   d. Finger reimplantation (reattachment)

6) Which accessory makes it possible for the assistant to see the same image through his/her lenses as the surgeon is seeing?
   a. Beam splitter
   b. Coaxial illuminator
   c. Paraxial illuminator
   d. LED illuminator

7) When moving a microscope, where should you hold onto it to minimize the possibility of damage?
   a. The head
   b. The ocular lenses
   c. The center of the vertical column
   d. The X-Y carrier

8) The most popular mounting system for operating microscopes is:
   a. Casters
   b. Wall
   c. Ceiling
   d. Tabletop

9) If the magnification of the objective lens is 400 and the magnification of the ocular lens is 10, what is the total magnification?
   a. 400
   b. 4,000
   c. 410
   d. 4,500

# 7 Lasers

Lasers were first used for surgery in the 1960s. Similar to all technology, lasers have vastly improved since their inception, allowing them to play a major role in many surgical specialties.

The acronym *LASER* stands for Light Amplification by the Stimulated Emission of Radiation. Lasers work with light waves. Waves of light stimulate atoms to produce more waves of light until millions of waves of light produce an intense beam. This intense beam is used to vaporize or cut tissue or to control bleeding.

There are several factors that determine how deeply the beam penetrates into the tissue. These factors are power, color, wavelength, duration of tissue exposure, and tissue consistency.

When laser light hits a surface (e.g., tissue), any of the following things can occur:

- *Reflection:* The direction of the beam is changed after it contacts a surface; the beam can be intentionally reflected to treat hard-to-reach areas or reflection can inadvertently happen and pose a safety hazard.
- *Scattering:* The beam can disperse in all directions, causing a decrease in intensity; the beam spreads over a large area.
- *Absorption:* The beam alters or disrupts the tissue in some way.
- *Transmission:* The beam is transmitted through tissue without thermally affecting it.

In order to produce these light waves, the laser needs an energy source or medium. It is this medium that gives each type of laser beam its distinct properties. Media can include gas, solid, liquid, or semiconductor. The two media most commonly found in surgery are gas (i.e., argon, carbon dioxide, and krypton) and solid (i.e., holmium, neodymium: yttrium-aluminum-garnet [Nd:YAG], potassium-titanyl-phosphate [KTP], and ruby). The laser is named after the medium that it contains.

## PARTS OF A LASER

There are five main components to a laser system:

- Excitation source (also known as the energy pump): Supplies the energy to the laser head, producing the laser light. Gas lasers use electricity as the source whereas solid medium lasers use flash lamps.
- Delivery system: The instrument or attachment (such as the laser fiber) that transmits laser energy to the tissue.
- Laser head (also known as the optical resonator): This part contains the active laser medium and the mirrors.
- Control panel: Contains the touch-screen controls for operating the laser.
- The ancillary or accessory equipment: Includes the vacuum pump, cooling system and outer cover, or console. These vary according to the laser type.

## TYPES OF LASERS

The laser the surgeon chooses depends on the tissue on which it is to be used and the desired effect on that tissue. The next several paragraphs cover the most common types of lasers used in surgery, their effect on tissues, and some of the types of surgery for which each is used.

### Carbon Dioxide Laser

The *carbon dioxide* laser is the medical laser most commonly used in surgery (Fig. 7–1). The beam from this laser is strongly absorbed by water, which constitutes a large portion of soft tissue, making the carbon dioxide laser suitable for a wide variety of surgeries. The absorption does not depend on tissue pigment; therefore, it can be used on light or dark tissue. The beam can be focused into a thin beam to cut tissue, similar to a conventional scalpel, or defocused to vaporize, ablate, or shave tissue. This type of laser also can be used to coagulate bleeding vessels.

Unlike other lasers, the *action* on the tissue is directly visible as the laser is being used. The beam itself, however, is invisible and requires a helium-neon beam (which is red) to make it visible for aiming purposes. The carbon dioxide laser has a wide variety of uses in many surgical specialties, including laparoscopic gynecological surgeries, wart ablation, laryngectomy,

---

## Characteristics of LASER Beams

Even though they are produced by different media (e.g., gas, solid, dye excimer), all laser beams have certain common characteristics:
- Coherent: The peaks and troughs of the light wave are all exactly the same; the waves all travel in the same direction.
- Monochromatic: The light waves have all the same wavelength or color.
- Parallel (collimated): The light waves all move in narrow columns and do not spread out as they travel.

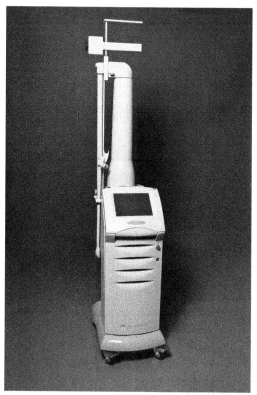

FIGURE 7-1 Carbon dioxide laser.

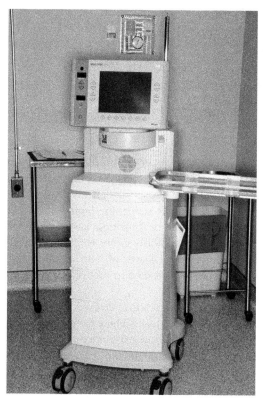

FIGURE 7-2 Argon laser.

benign laryngeal lesions, middle ear procedures, skin lesion removal, breast biopsy, breast reduction, tumor removal from the brain and spinal cord, skin resurfacing (for irregularities or wrinkles), vascular surgeries, and some podiatry surgeries.

## Argon Laser

The *argon* laser produces a visible blue-green beam that is absorbed by red-brown pigmented tissues (e.g., hemoglobin and melanin) (Fig. 7–2). This type of beam is not absorbed by clear tissue, making it useful for retinal surgery because it passes through the cornea, vitreous, and lens of the eye without affecting them.

Argon lasers are used for sealing and coagulation. Other uses for argon lasers include treatment of port wine stains, dark moles or lesions, spider veins on the face, retinopathy, glaucoma, and inner ear surgery.

## Holmium:YAG Laser

A third type of laser used in surgery is the *holmium: YAG* (also referred to as a *holmium* laser) (Fig. 7–3). The acronym YAG stands for *yttrium-aluminum-garnet,* which is used in combination with other mediums in laser therapy.

The holmium laser has a beam outside of the visible range; therefore, an aiming beam is necessary to see where the laser will contact the tissue. The aiming beam may be red or green.

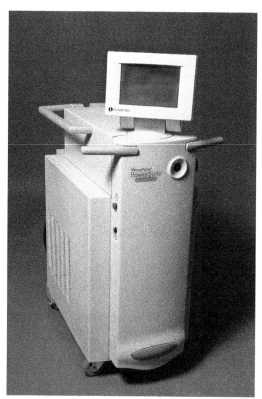

FIGURE 7-3 Holmium laser.

The holmium laser is versatile as it can cut, ablate, coagulate, and contour tissues of all types. It can be used in urology to perform laser lithotripsy on renal stones or to resect prostate tissue; in orthopedics to ablate bone or cartilage; in ear, nose, and throat (ENT) surgery to assist with endoscopic sinus procedures; or in endoscopic spinal surgery to remove a disc. In addition to these applications, it can be used in minimally invasive surgery, gynecological surgery, general surgery, and ophthalmology (to perform laser thermal keratoplasty to treat farsightedness).

## Neodymium:YAG Laser

Neodymium is another medium that is used in conjunction with yttrium-aluminum-garnet to produce a laser beam. Similar to the holmium:YAG laser, the Nd:YAG laser has a beam that is outside the visible range and needs an aiming beam (usually a red helium-neon beam).

This type of laser is absorbed by pigmented tissues and has the greatest ability of any laser to coagulate blood vessels. The Nd:YAG laser can be used in ophthalmology to perform iridotomy or to treat diabetic retinopathy, in cosmetic surgery to remove hair or to treat spider veins, and in dental surgery to perform certain procedures on the soft tissues (e.g., gingivectomy). There are some dual-wavelength Nd:YAG lasers available that can be used for general, orthopedic, ENT, thoracic, and podiatry procedures.

## OTHER TYPES OF LASERS

This section describes lasers that are less common to surgical procedures.

The *excimer* laser uses a combination of an inert gas (e.g., krypton, xenon, or argon) and a reactive gas (e.g., chlorine or fluorine). It emits short bursts of laser light through fiberoptic cables that cause tissue to disintegrate (ablation). This type of laser creates less heat than others, thus making it less damaging to nearby tissues. It is extremely precise, able to remove 0.25 μm of tissue with a single pulse. The main uses for this laser are LASIK (laser-assisted in situ keratomileusis) eye surgery, photorefractive keratotomy, and some dermatology procedures.

The *ruby* laser has been replaced by the *Alexandrite* laser. Alexandrite has proven to be a more efficient medium. This type of laser is used to remove tattoos, liver spots, freckles, and port wine stains.

The *KTP* (potassium-titanyl-phosphate) laser produces a green light that is used to cut tissue, treat vascular lesions (leg veins), and remove red and orange tattoo pigment. This type of laser is capable of producing a very tiny beam, making it suitable for use in microscopic surgery. It is used to treat rosacea and port wine stains and in ENT, general, urology, and gynecological surgeries.

*Tunable dye* lasers emit a pulsed laser beam by exposing certain dyes or vapors to argon laser light. The dye absorbs the light and produces a broad-spectrum light that is tuned to select a beam of a particular color (wavelength). Tunable lasers are used to destroy vascular (e.g., port wine stains, rosacea, cherry angiomas) and pigmented (e.g., café-au-lait spots, nevi) lesions. Another use of tunable dye lasers is photosensitive drug therapy (PDT). In PDT, a photosensitive dye is injected about 48 hours before surgery, the dye is metabolized out of normal tissue but remains in malignant tissue, and the laser is used to destroy the malignant tissue.

As laser technology improves, the medical and surgical applications for it broaden. Some of the advantages to laser procedures include shorter hospital stays, less painful recoveries, and less blood in the surgical field (meaning better visualization).

Although they do have advantages, medical lasers are powerful machines capable of doing great harm to patients and personnel if used improperly. The next section covers the general important safety rules to follow when using lasers.

## LASER SAFETY

Because of the intense nature of laser beams, if they are not used properly, they have the potential to cause great harm: fire, electrical shock, and damage to unintended tissues (or persons!).

Three agencies develop and oversee regulations for lasers used in medicine: the Occupational Safety and Health Administration (OSHA), the American National Standards Institute (ANSI), and the Center for Devices and Radiological Health (CDRH). The job of these agencies is to put into place regulations to ensure the safety of patients and staff while lasers are in use.

In addition to these agencies, each institution has policies and procedures to deal with the safe use of lasers within their own facility, including designating a laser safety officer in the operating room (OR) and credentialing those permitted to operate using lasers. The Association of periOperative Registered Nurses (AORN) has published guidelines for laser safety, which many institutions use as a basis for their own laser procedures in the OR. Make sure you know your own institution's policies and procedures.

Although each institution has its own set of policies dealing with laser safety, there are some basic rules that should be followed to ensure safe use of lasers:

- All doorways leading into the room where a laser is in use must be marked with a warning sign stating that a laser is in use (Fig. 7–4).
- Eye tissue is the most vulnerable of all tissues to inadvertent exposure. All personnel who enter the room must wear proper protective eyewear. Each type of laser requires eyewear that protects against that specific type of laser beam. Make sure that the eyewear in the room is specific to the type of laser being used (e.g., eyewear designed for use with a carbon dioxide laser will NOT protect your eyes against inadvertent exposure to a holmium laser beam).

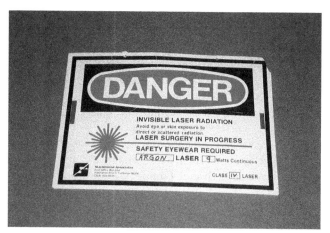

FIGURE 7-4 Laser safety door sign.

- Proper eyewear needs to be hanging on the outer door or just outside the room for use by those who enter the room for any reason.
- The patient's eyes need to be protected against inadvertent exposure. Patients should be fitted with the same eyewear that the staff is wearing (some institutions have protective eye cups for this purpose).
- Regular eyeglasses or goggles are NOT protective eyewear. The eyewear must be specifically designed for the laser in use and cover the tops, bottoms, and sides of the eye to offer complete protection (Fig. 7–5).
- Only personnel knowledgeable in the use and operation of lasers and in laser safety protocols should be allowed to operate the laser. Ongoing education should be in place for staff regarding the safe use of lasers.
- Laser surgery should be performed only by those surgeons credentialed or approved by the institution to do so.
- The foot pedal for turning the laser beam on and off should ONLY be operated by the surgeon holding the handpiece. The pedal should NOT be operated by an assistant, scrub, or nurse.
- All electrical cords should be inspected before surgery. If a cord is found to be frayed or otherwise compromised,

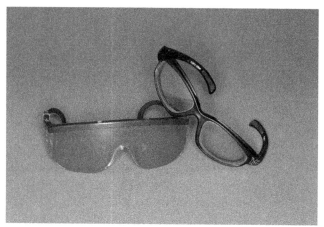

FIGURE 7-5 Laser eyewear.

the laser should NOT be used until it is inspected and repaired by the biomedical engineering department.
- When not in use during surgery, the laser should be placed in "standby" mode.
- There should be a designated laser nurse to operate the machine during the procedure. He or she should stand next to the machine to place it in "standby" mode when not in use and "ready" mode when the surgeon is ready to use it.
- Fire safety precautions must be followed. These include:
  - Allow all prep solutions to dry completely before using the laser.
  - Surround the surgical site with wet towels.
  - Use special laser endotracheal tubes if the laser will be used anywhere near the airway.
  - Use flame-retardant drapes.
  - When not in use, the tip of the laser should be placed on a moist towel, not a dry drape.
  - Oxygen should be delivered at the lowest possible concentration.
  - Water or saline must be available on the surgical field (usually on the back table).
  - Portable fire extinguishers must be readily available (halon extinguishers are recommended).
  - Nonexplosive anesthetics must be used.
  - During anorectal procedures, the rectum must be packed with a sterile water-soaked sponge to prevent a methane gas fire.
  - Liquids should NOT be placed on top of the laser machine (they could spill and cause a fire or electrical short).
- All surfaces in the room must be nonreflective, all tables should be covered or removed from the room, all instruments should be nonreflective (matte finish or ebony), and metal jewelry should not be worn by personnel in the room or entering the room.
- A laser safety officer should be designated to update and enforce laser safety policies.
- To protect against plume exposure, staff should wear specially designated laser masks (these masks are designed to filter smaller particles of matter).
- Smoke evacuators (not just regular suction) should be used to suction and filter the plume that is produced. The filters in these units need to be checked and changed according to manufacturer's instructions.
- When storing the laser, the key should NOT be left in the machine.
- Shades should be pulled to cover room windows (or cover windows with nonreflective material) to prevent beam reflection or, in some cases, beam penetration through the glass to outside the room.

The use of lasers in surgery has become commonplace. It is up to *every* staff member to know their institution's safety protocols and policies and to see that they are followed. The safety of your patients, your coworkers, and yourself depends on it.

## Troubleshooting the Laser

As with any device, troubleshooting starts with the seemingly obvious and simple (see Figs. 7–6 and 7–7):

| PROBLEM | WHAT TO LOOK AT |
|---|---|
| No beam comes out of the fiber. | ■ Is the machine plugged in?<br>■ Is the machine turned on?<br>■ Is the fiber plugged into the machine?<br>■ Is the connection between the fiber and machine tight?<br>■ Is the machine on "ready" (not "standby")?<br>■ Is the foot pedal connected to the machine?<br>■ Does the fiber need to be replaced? |
| The beam is misaligned. | ■ The beam should be checked for misalignment before use according to institution policy. If the beam is misaligned, the machine should be checked by qualified service personnel; the mirrors may have been damaged or moved when the machine was transferred from another location. |
| The beam is not "crisp" (it has a star or scattered look to it). | ■ If using a reusable fiber, the fiber may need to be recut and stripped; see the manufacturer's instructions on how to do this. |
| The laser has low power. | ■ Check all beam delivery optics. Make sure they are free of dust, dirt, and smoke. |
| The power does not come on. | ■ Is the machine plugged in? You may need to try a different wall plug.<br>■ Is the power switch in the "on" position?<br>■ Is the key in the ignition and the ignition turned to "on"?<br>■ Is the "dummy switch" located in the back of the laser missing? |

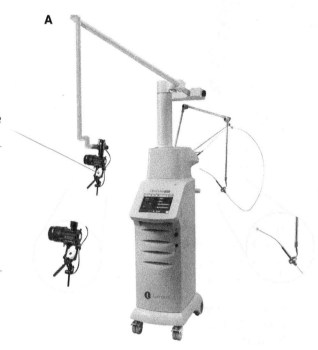
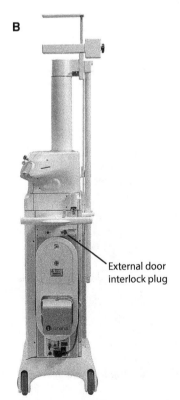

External door interlock plug

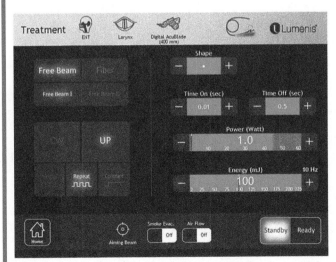

FIGURE 7–6 Laser control panel. Photo courtesy of Boston Scientific Corporation.

FIGURE 7–7 (A) UltraPulse™ DUO CO$_2$ Laser System; (B) External Door Interlock Plug. Photos courtesy of Boston Scientific Corporation.

**Surgical Session Review**

1) All of the following are characteristics of laser light *except*
   a. Monochromatic
   b. Coherent
   c. Polychromatic
   d. Collimated

2) Which factor(s) affect(s) how deep the laser beam penetrates?
   a. Duration of tissue exposure
   b. Power
   c. Wavelength
   d. All of the above

3) Scattering of a laser beam as it hits a surface (e.g., tissue) can cause
   a. An increase in intensity
   b. A narrowing of the beam
   c. A decrease in intensity
   d. The beam to spread over a smaller area

4) The changing of the direction of the laser as it contacts a surface is known as
   a. Scattering
   b. Reflection
   c. Absorption
   d. Transmission

5) The energy source for the laser is known as a *medium*. All of the following can be forms of media *except*
   a. Gas
   b. Solid
   c. Semiconductor
   d. Steam

6) An example of a solid laser medium is
   a. Argon
   b. Holmium
   c. Carbon dioxide
   d. Krypton

7) The most commonly used medical laser is
   a. Carbon dioxide
   b. Argon
   c. Ruby
   d. Holmium

8) Which of the following lasers *do not* require an aiming beam?
   a. Carbon dioxide
   b. Holmium
   c. Argon
   d. Nd:YAG

9) Which of the following is/are potential hazards of laser use?
   a. Fire
   b. Electrical shock
   c. Damage to unintended tissue
   d. All of the above

10) Which agency *regulates* the use of medical lasers in the workplace?
   a. AST
   b. AORN
   c. ANSI
   d. AMA

11) All of the following statements are true about laser protective eyewear *except*
   a. Laser eyewear should be hanging on the outside of the door of the room in case someone needs to enter the room
   b. Each eyewear is specific for a certain type of beam; therefore, you must check to make sure you have the eyewear specific to the laser you are using
   c. Patients do not need to have their eyes protected because they are behind the drape
   d. Regular eyeglasses or goggles are not considered protective eyewear

12) The laser foot pedal should *only* be operated by the
   a. Assistant
   b. Scrub
   c. Circulator
   d. Surgeon holding the handpiece

13) During the procedure, when the laser in not in use, it should be placed in the _____ mode.
   a. Standby
   b. Ready
   c. Coagulating
   d. Cutting

14) Fire safety precautions for laser use include
   a. Using flame-retardant drapes
   b. Using nonreflective instruments
   c. Surrounding the surgical site with wet towels
   d. All of the above

15) All surfaces in the room must be
   a. Reflective
   b. Nonreflective
   c. Sterile
   d. Nonsterile

16) Who is responsible for updating and enforcing laser safety policies?
   a. The surgeon
   b. The physician assistant
   c. The laser safety officer
   d. The hospital CEO

17) The medium and mirrors of the laser are contained in which component?
   a. Cooling system
   b. Delivery system
   c. Laser head
   d. Excitation source

18) The laser machine does not come on. You have checked that the machine is plugged in, the power switch is in the "on" position, the key is in the ignition, and the ignition is in the "on" position. What could be the likely problem?
   a. A hospital-wide power outage
   b. The dummy switch in the back is missing
   c. The fiber is faulty
   d. The fiber needs to be recut

19) One of the main uses for an excimer laser is
   a. Gynecological surgery
   b. Orthopedic surgery
   c. LASIK surgery
   d. Neurosurgery

20) Which type of laser has a beam that is not absorbed by clear tissue, making it useful for retinal surgery?
   a. Carbon dioxide
   b. Argon
   c. Holmium
   d. Ruby

# 8

# Endoscopic Equipment

## ENDOSCOPIC SURGERY

The root word *endo* means "within." The suffix *scopy* means "to view with an instrument." The term *endoscopy* means "using an instrument to view within (a body cavity)." Endoscopy is a general term referring to any procedure that uses an endoscope to view inside a body cavity, but there are several terms that are used to be more specific about which area is being viewed:

- *Anoscopy:* Viewing inside the anus
- *Arthroscopy:* Viewing inside a joint
- *Bronchoscopy:* Viewing inside the lungs (bronchus)
- *Colonoscopy:* Viewing inside the colon
- *Colposcopy:* Viewing inside the vagina and cervix
- *Cystoscopy:* Viewing inside the bladder
- *Duodenoscopy:* Viewing inside the duodenum
- *Enteroscopy:* Viewing the small intestine
- *Esophagoscopy:* Viewing inside the esophagus
- *Esophagogastroduodenoscopy (EGD):* Viewing inside the esophagus, stomach, and duodenum
- *Fluoroscopy:* Viewing inside organs or tissues using x-ray
- *Gastroscopy:* Viewing inside the stomach
- *Hepatoscopy:* Viewing the liver
- *Hysteroscopy:* Viewing inside the uterus
- *Laparoscopy:* Viewing inside the abdominal and pelvic cavities
- *Laryngoscopy:* Viewing inside the larynx
- *Meatoscopy:* Viewing inside the urinary meatus
- *Mediastinoscopy:* Viewing inside the mediastinum (mediastinal space)
- *Pelvioscopy (pelvoscopy):* Viewing inside the pelvis
- *Pharyngoscopy:* Viewing inside the throat
- *Rhinoscopy:* Viewing inside the nose
- *Sigmoidoscopy:* Viewing inside the sigmoid colon
- *Thoracoscopy (pleuroscopy):* Viewing inside the chest (thorax)
- *Tracheoscopy:* Viewing inside the trachea
- *Ureteroscopy:* Viewing inside the ureter
- *Urethroscopy:* Viewing inside the urethra

When a surgical procedure is performed using a scope and very small incisions (known as *stab wound* incisions), it is referred to as *minimally invasive surgery*. Minimally invasive surgery came onto the surgical scene in the 1980s and revolutionized the way surgery is performed. Today, surgeons use minimally invasive techniques to perform a wide range of procedures.

## ADVANTAGES AND DISAVANTAGES OF MINIMALLY INVASIVE SURGERY

There are several advantages to minimally invasive surgery, including smaller incisions (less scarring and less pain), less blood loss, reduced chance of infection, reduced length of hospital stay, reduced time recovering at home, and less time out of work. These advantages can lead to an increase in patient satisfaction. The reduction of time in the hospital and in recovery can lead to an overall cost reduction for the procedure.

It must be stated that not every procedure can or should be performed endoscopically. Some procedures still must be performed as open procedures (e.g., in the presence of a large, infected gallbladder). Often, it is not known until the surgery has begun and the surgeon has had a chance to look inside whether or not the surgery can be safely performed endoscopically. For this reason, every endoscopic case should be set up with the ability to convert to an open case quickly and easily. Most of the time, this means setting up two sets of instruments on the back table: endoscopic instruments and a traditional stringer of instruments to be used for an open case. Other disadvantages or limitations of minimally invasive procedures can include the expense of ongoing staff training, equipment purchase and maintenance, and reduced instrument maneuverability because of working in a small space. In addition, the operative picture on the screen is two dimensional instead of three.

Every minimally invasive procedure requires certain basic equipment: a video viewing system (TV system), a recording system (still pictures or DVD), and a light source for the camera. Procedures involving the abdomen and pelvis require a gas (carbon dioxide) insufflating system. Procedures involving the joints or urinary system require a constant fluid irrigation system. This is usually normal saline, but for some urinary procedures, glycine is used.

The following sections of this chapter cover video towers (including basic troubleshooting); cameras; scopes and equipment (including care and cleaning); and some specifics for arthroscopic, flexible, and rigid scopes.

## VIDEO TOWERS

Minimally invasive procedures require the surgeon to be able to view inside the body cavity where he or she is working. Visualization is done using a camera with the image projected up onto a video system (usually a TV system of some sort).

Although the types of video systems vary from institution to institution, the requirement is the same; scrubbed personnel must be able to view clearly and easily what is going on inside the operative field. The simplest way to accomplish this is to have two TV towers, one on each side of the patient, toward the head of the bed so that personnel on both sides of the operative field can look directly at a monitor (Fig. 8–1).

This setup may vary depending on the procedure and the surgeon. Some procedures may require the use of only one tower at the foot of the bed or, in the case of cystoscopy, there may be one monitor mounted on a movable arm directly over the patient. In any case, the setup needs to meet the requirement of clear and easy viewing by scrubbed personnel.

In addition to the monitor or TV screen, there needs to be a device for recording pictures. The device can be as simple as a printer for still photographs or as advanced as a DVD recording system. The type of system used depends on the institution and the equipment available.

The third basic component of the system is the light source for the camera (Fig. 8–2). The type of light source used is dependent on the camera system being used. It is the responsibility of the operating room (OR) team assigned to the case to ensure that the camera is compatible with the light source.

The last component is the source of insufflation. For procedures of the abdomen and pelvis, insufflation is accomplished using carbon dioxide gas. The gas pressure and rate of gas flow into the abdominal cavity are regulated through the use of an insufflator (Fig. 8–3). The settings on the insufflator vary according to the surgeon and procedure, but a safe flow of gas

## Guidelines for the Recording of Pictures

- Recording surgery is dictated by institutional policies and procedures. Know your institution's policies surrounding the recording of procedures before starting any case in which pictures or video will be shot.
- Usually, for still pictures that are going to be placed in the medical record, a special release is not required because these pictures are part of the medical record and not likely to be viewed by others.
- For video recording that is going to be used for educational purposes, a special release may need to be signed by the patient before surgery. Be sure to check your institution's policy!

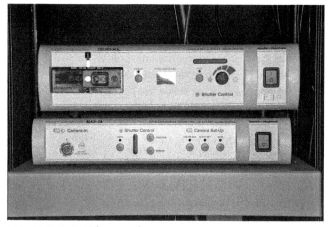

FIGURE 8–2 Light source box.

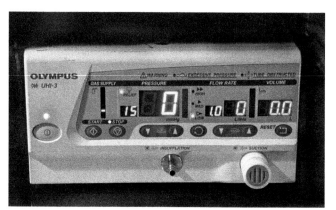

FIGURE 8–3 Insufflator box.

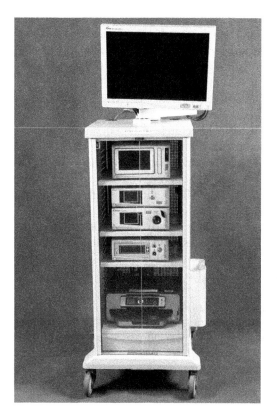

FIGURE 8–1 Video tower.

(start low and then increase as needed) should be used until a pressure of around 15 mm Hg (varies from 12 to 18 mm Hg) is achieved.

*Remember: Always* check the gas level in your carbon dioxide tank before the start of a case. Change the tank if the gas is low or empty. Do not start a procedure with a tank that does not have sufficient gas to complete the case.

When doing endoscopic procedures of the joints or bladder, you will be using fluid rather than gas to expand the cavity for visualization. In most cases, this requires the use of a fluid pump (Fig. 8–4), although some simple urological procedures can be done using a gravity-fed bag. Although different pumps are used for arthroscopic procedures versus urology procedures, the principles are the same: the fluid needs to be pumped into and drained out of the cavity continuously throughout the entire procedure. It is imperative that the circulator (or whoever is in charge of the fluids) makes sure that bags are replaced as soon as they get low; it is not OK for the fluid to run dry. Some pumps have a low fluid warning alarm to alert personnel when the bag is getting low, but do not rely on the alarm. You must be vigilant, watch the fluid level in the bags, and replace them before they run dry.

## Video Tower Setup

As stated earlier, there are a couple of variations of video tower arrangements, depending on the procedure being done and

surgeon preference. The most common setup for general laparoscopic procedures is two video towers, one on each side of the bed, by the patient's shoulders (Fig. 8–5). This allows the operative field to be viewed by scrubbed personnel standing on either side of the patient. The primary monitor is the one attached to the camera box and receives the picture by direct input. The secondary monitor is attached to the primary monitor with a video cable. The towers are not sterile; make sure they are placed at least 12 to 18 inches away from the draped patient.

The second arrangement requires the use of one video tower. This tower may be placed at the foot of the bed or to one side at the head of the bed by the patient's shoulder (Fig. 8–6). The tower is not sterile; make sure it is at least 12

| **WATCH OUT!** | **Potential Fire Hazard** |

- *Caution:* The light source is a source of heat and could be a potential fire hazard!
- When the camera is not in use and is outside the body, place it in *standby* mode.
- A camera with its light source not in standby mode should *never* be placed on the drapes because it could overheat and cause a fire.

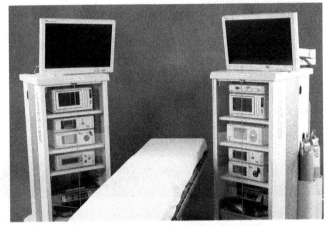

FIGURE 8-5 Two video towers at the head of the bed.

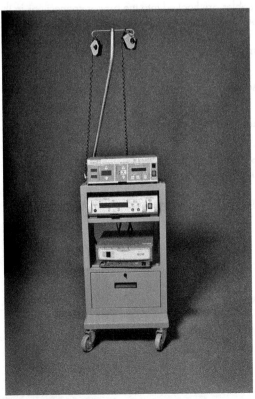

FIGURE 8-4 Fluid pump.

FIGURE 8-6 One video tower at the bottom of the bed.

to 18 inches away from the draped patient. This type of setup is most commonly used for some gynecological and cystoscopic procedures.

All video towers and equipment *must* be checked by the staff assigned to the procedure before bringing the patient into the OR. Equipment must be plugged in, turned on, and checked to make sure it is functioning properly. If it is not functioning properly and cannot be easily fixed, (see Troubleshooting Video Equipment, below), it must be removed from the room and another piece of equipment must be brought in and tested.

At the end of the case, all video towers and equipment should be wiped down with disinfectant, according to your institution's policy, before leaving the room or being used for a subsequent procedure.

Figure 8–7 is one example of how a dedicated endoscopic operating room may be set up.

## ENDOSCOPIC CAMERAS

The invention of cameras that fit onto the eyepiece of rigid endoscopes has revolutionized surgery. The surgeon is no

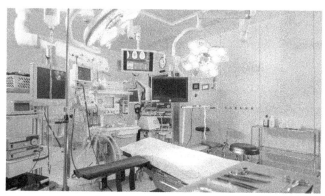

FIGURE 8–7 Endoscopic operating room (gorodenkoff/iStock/ Getty Images Plus).

longer the only one able to visualize the operative field; cameras enable the entire surgical team to watch the procedure and anticipate what might be needed next. In some cases (depending on the institution), a scrub person operates the camera, freeing up both of the surgeon's hands to perform the procedure. Before the invention of endoscopic cameras,

## Troubleshooting Video Equipment

Video equipment and towers are mechanical machines and may, from time to time, not work properly. Here are some simple troubleshooting tips. Always refer to manufacturer's instructions for more in-depth advice.

| PROBLEM | WHAT TO LOOK AT |
|---|---|
| I turn on the video monitor but do not get color bars. (On some monitors, the presence of vertical color bars tells you the monitor is properly hooked up and working.) | ▪ Check to make sure the cables are hooked into the proper connections in the back of the monitor (especially if you have color bars on the primary monitor but not the secondary one).<br>▪ Make sure *all* components of the system are powered on. (Some monitors will not work even if it is the printer that is not turned on.) |
| The picture is blurred or streaked. | ▪ Check the lenses of the scope and camera; they may be dirty or need defogging. |
| The color on the monitor screen is not accurate. | ▪ The camera may need to be rewhite balanced; white balance the camera again. |
| The monitor screen is dark; there is nothing on it. | ▪ Make sure the monitor is plugged in and turned on (check this first).<br>▪ Check cables to make sure they are intact and hooked into the proper connections.<br>▪ Check to make sure the power box is not overloaded with too many devices plugged into it.<br>▪ Check the fuses.<br>▪ Check the connection to the printer to make sure it is properly connected. |
| The still pictures did not print (or are of poor quality). | ▪ Make sure to print the pictures *before* turning off the printer at the end of the case.<br>▪ The printer is out of paper.<br>▪ The paper is in upside down.<br>▪ The cartridge is low or out of ink or toner. |
| The pictures are blurred when printed. | ▪ The camera or scope lens is dirty or fogged up.<br>▪ There was movement by the person operating the camera during picture taking. |

the surgeon would have to use one hand to hold the scope so that he or she could look through the eyepiece.

The camera setup consists of a camera head with a cord and a coupler (Fig. 8–8). In some models, the camera and coupler are one piece. The camera cord attaches to a video box that is attached to the video monitor. Procedures can be documented on video or in still photographs.

The camera head and cord are attached to the endoscope using a coupler. The camera head screws onto the coupler, and the endoscope is attached to the other end using a built-in clamp. The clamp opens to allow you to slip the scope eyepiece into it and then closes around it to hold the eyepiece snugly in place. After attaching the camera and scope to the coupler, check to make sure the connections are tight and neither the camera nor scope is wobbly.

At the end of the case, the camera, cord, and coupler should be cleaned and sterilized according to manufacturer's instructions. *Read the instructions carefully before autoclaving any camera, coupler, or cord.* Not all models can be autoclaved; doing so will result in severe damage (lens breakage, melting of casing, fiberoptic damage).

## Care of Endoscopic Cameras

- Attach the camera and turn it on before surgery to make sure it works. If the light cable is fiberoptic, check

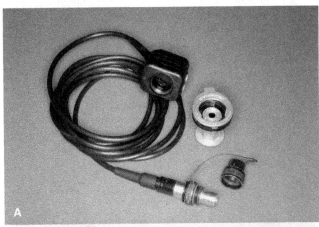

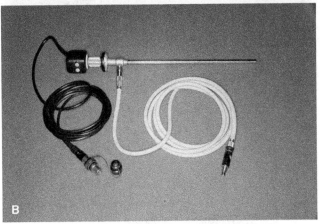

FIGURE 8–8 (A) Camera components. (B) Assembled camera.

it. If the cable contains dark areas where you cannot see light coming through, replace the cable, because these dark areas can indicate broken fibers.

- *Never* place cameras at the bottom of an instrument tray. The weight of the other instruments could damage the camera.
- When you are setting up your table, never place anything else on top of the camera. Cameras are very delicate and another instrument or piece of equipment could easily damage it.
- Coil the camera cord loosely. Coiling the cord too tightly can result in damage and breakage of the fiberoptic fibers.
- Disconnect the cable by grasping the plug, not the cable itself.
- Follow the manufacturer's instructions for cleaning and sterilizing cameras, cords, and couplers. After cleaning, inspect the components for cleanliness and possible damage.
- Never use anything abrasive to clean the camera, lens, or components.

## RIGID SCOPE COMPONENTS

Rigid endoscopes are the oldest type of scope but the most commonly used. Although the scope (sometimes referred to as a *telescope*) is a single instrument, it is composed of several components: the eyepiece (contains the proximal or ocular lens), the light attachment, the shaft, and the distal (or objective) lens.

The proximal end of the scope contains the eyepiece or ocular lens. In most scopes, the proximal end is where the camera attaches to the scope to allow for projection of the image onto the screen.

The light attachment sticks up at a 90-degree angle near the eyepiece at the proximal end of the scope. This is where the light cord (usually a fiberoptic cable) attaches to the scope. The other end of the light cord is passed off to the circulator and attached into the light source box.

The shaft of the scope is the long, thin part of the instrument that is inserted through the trocar into the body cavity. The shaft is very delicate and must be handled with care as it is easily damaged or bent and expensive to repair (see Care of Rigid Endoscopes, on the next page). Shaft diameters vary from 1.9 mm to 10 mm, with 5 mm and 10 mm the most commonly used.

The distal or objective lens is at the end of the shaft. It is used to view and magnify the organs or tissues. Scopes are available with a variety of angles of objective lenses to allow for viewing around structures. The most common objective lenses are the 0-degree (also known as the *forward* or *straight-on*), 12-degree, 30-degree *(forward-oblique)*, 45-degree, and 70-degree.

Objective lenses on the scopes become distorted or fog up due to blood, fluid, or debris. It is important that the scrub personnel have lens defogger available during surgery to clean the objective lens. If the picture becomes unsatisfactory, the scope should be removed from the body cavity, the lens gently wiped clean, the defogger applied, and the scope reinserted through the trocar. If the picture remains unsatisfactory, the camera may need to be removed from the eyepiece and the camera lenses and eyepiece (ocular lens) cleaned.

## Care of Rigid Endoscopes

- Never pick up and hold scopes by the distal end. The weight of the eyepiece could easily bend the shaft.
- Scrubbed personnel must look through the eyepiece before attaching the camera before surgery. If what he or she sees is distorted or cloudy, the eyepiece and objective lens must be cleaned. If cleaning does not clear up the problem, get another scope because one (or both) of the lenses may be damaged and need repair or replacement.
- Before surgery, check the scope shaft for damage, dents, or bends. If the scope is damaged, get another one.
- Attach the camera and turn it on before surgery to make sure it works. If the light cable is fiberoptic, check it. If the cable contains dark areas where you cannot see light coming through, replace the cable because these dark areas can indicate broken fibers.
- *Never* place scopes at the bottom of an instrument tray. The weight of the other instruments could bend or damage the scope. Place the scope in the storage case that it comes in.
- When not in use, set the scope on a flat surface to avoid accidental flexion and damage.
- When you are setting up your table, never place anything else on top of the scope. Scopes are very delicate, and another instrument or piece of equipment could easily damage it.
- When handing the scope to the surgeon or using the scope during a procedure, support the shaft of the scope with one hand to avoid overflexion and possible damage.
- When coiling the light cord, never coil it tighter than 4.72 inches (about the diameter of a 2L soda bottle). Coiling the cord too tightly can result in damage and breakage of the fiberoptic fibers.
- Follow manufacturer's instructions for cleaning and sterilizing scopes. Make sure all lumens and valves are cleaned and rinsed thoroughly before sterilization. After cleaning, inspect the scope for cleanliness and possible damage.

(Some material adapted from Karl Storz Web site.)

## CYSTOSCOPY AND URETEROSCOPY EQUIPMENT

*Cystoscopy* means viewing into the bladder, although this procedure is done typically for more than just "viewing." This procedure can be done for diagnostic purposes (e.g., to find the source of blood in the urine), as part of the treatment of a urological condition (e.g., to remove or resect bladder tumors, remove kidney stones, or resect the prostate), or for ureteral stent insertion.

Cystoscopy can also be done at the end of another procedure to check for inadvertent damage to the bladder.

The cystoscope (also known as a *cystourethroscope*) has several pieces that the scrub person needs to assemble (Fig. 8–9). The *sheath* is the hollow tube that allows for the passage of instruments during the procedure and allows for suction and irrigation. The main (large) channel in the center of the sheath is where the *telescope* is inserted. The side channels allow the insertion of accessory instruments, such as biopsy forceps or graspers. The *obturator* is a rod with a round, blunt tip. The obturator is inserted into the main channel of the sheath and used just during the insertion of the scope. The obturator helps protect urethral tissue from damage. Once the sheath is inserted through the urethra, the obturator is removed and

### Guidelines for the Care of the Cystoscope

- Read the manufacturer's instructions for cleaning and sterilizing the cystoscope. Some cystoscopes and attachments can be autoclaved (steam sterilized) and some cannot. Make sure you know if your scope camera, cords, and so on can be autoclaved before the sterilization process.
- Handle the scope by the *middle* of the shaft. Do not handle it by the ends or it could bend.
- Do not place anything on top of the scope. Do not place it at the bottom of a pan of instruments. For transport, place it in the storage container that it came in.
- Do not coil the cord too tightly; this could damage or break the fiberoptic bundles.
- When setting up your sterile field before the case, check all scopes and accessories for damage (e.g., bending, cracks in the cord casing). Put the scope together and make sure you have all the pieces (e.g., sheath, telescope, obturator, bridge, and instruments). Make sure all instruments are functioning properly.
- When cleaning and sterilizing the cystoscopes after use, make sure all stopcocks are open.

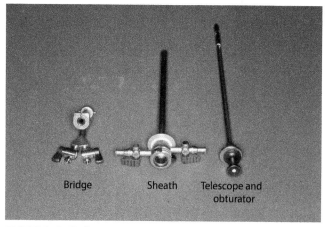

Bridge    Sheath    Telescope and obturator

FIGURE 8–9 Cystoscopy equipment.

the telescope inserted. Similar to all endoscopes, the telescope portion of the cystoscope needs a light cable hooked to it that is attached to a light source. Depending on what procedure is being performed, a *bridge* may need to be attached to the scope to allow for the use of accessory instruments.

Cystoscopes vary in the degree of the angle of the scope's tip. The most common cystoscopes used are 0 degrees, 30 degrees, and 70 degrees. Make sure you have the correct scope for the procedure along with any back-up scopes that may be needed.

Continuous irrigation is necessary for cystoscopic procedures. The solution can be instilled using gravity, although some procedures or institutions may require the use of a pump. Suction with a large volume capacity (e.g., Neptune or large suction carousel) is necessary to handle the continuous outflow of fluid. Normal saline is the irrigation fluid most commonly used for procedures not requiring the use of electrocautery. If the use of electrocautery is anticipated, a *nonelectrolytic* solution, such as 3% sorbitol or glycine, is used. *Nonelectrolytic* means that the fluid is unable to transmit or disperse electricity from the electrode tip. It is the responsibility of the circulator to make sure that the fluid does not run out during the procedure; therefore, he or she must monitor the fluid bags and change them as needed (Fig. 8–10).

Many institutions have a special room dedicated to cystoscopic procedures. This room is equipped with a table that allows for fluoroscopic imaging during the procedure (Fig. 8–11). Lithotomy (legs up in stirrups) is the position of

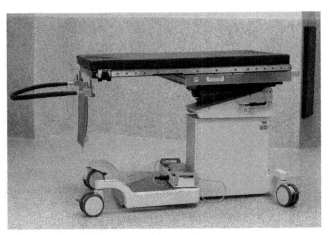

**FIGURE 8-11** Cystoscopy table.

choice for many cystoscopic procedures; therefore, the cystoscopy table must be able to have stirrups attached to it.

Some procedures require the use of laser or fluoroscopy intraoperatively. Turn on the fluoroscopy machine or laser before bringing the patient into the room to make sure the machine is functioning properly. If the use of fluoroscopy is anticipated, make sure there are lead aprons available for all staff to wear (including thyroid shields). If the use of laser is anticipated, make sure that all safety equipment is available and all laser safety precautions are followed (see Chapter 5 for more on laser safety).

## Ureteroscopy

A ureteroscope is a very long, thin scope inserted into the urethra, through the bladder, and into the ureter (Fig. 8–12). Most often this procedure is done for treatment of kidney stones, tissue biopsy, or treatment of urethral stricture, but it can be diagnostic as well. For the treatment of kidney stones, the urologist inserts the ureteroscope up into the ureter until he or she finds the stone(s). Depending on the size and location of the stone(s), the urologist may use a *stone retrieval basket* (Fig. 8–13B) to snare each stone and remove it or may

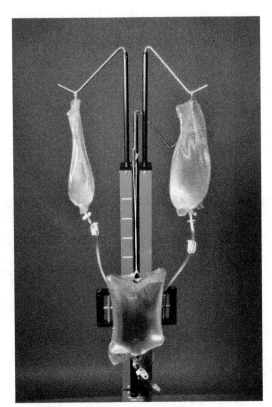

**FIGURE 8-10** Continuous irrigation setup.

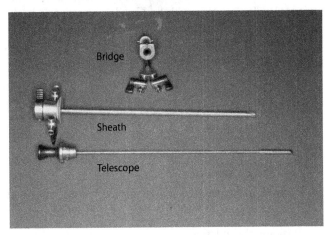

Bridge

Sheath

Telescope

**FIGURE 8-12** Ureteroscope.

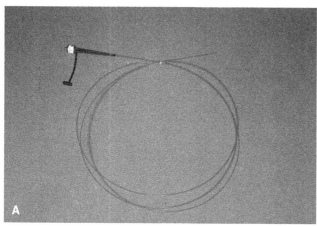

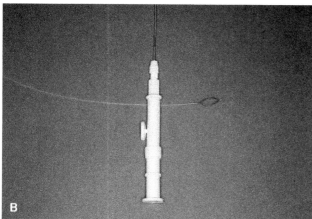

FIGURE 8–13 (A) Laser fiber. (B) Stone retrieval basket.

opt to insert a laser fiber (Fig. 8–13A) and shatter each stone using laser energy.

Ureteroscopes are available in rigid, semirigid, and flexible models. Which type being used depends on surgeon preference and the location of the stone.

As with all scopes, take care when handling the ureteroscope. It is longer than traditional cystoscopes; therefore, you must always be aware of the location of the tip of the scope to avoid inadvertent contamination or damage from the tip hitting against something. Handle the scope with two hands, supporting it in the middle and at the eyepiece end to avoid bending the shaft.

Positioning for ureteroscopy is the same as for cystoscopy; the patient is placed in the lithotomy position on the cystoscopy table.

## RIGID EAR, NOSE, AND THROAT AND THORACIC SCOPES

### Rigid Laryngoscopes for Direct Laryngoscopy

Rigid laryngoscopes are used to see directly within the throat (direct laryngoscopy), usually for one of the following purposes:

- Biopsy throat lesions.
- Diagnose causes of hoarse voice, weak voice, or no voice.
- Identify unknown cause of chronic sore throat.
- Evaluate difficulty swallowing.
- See injuries or obstructions in the throat (e.g., tumors, masses, or strictures).
- Remove foreign bodies from the throat.
- Remove vocal cord polyps.
- Perform laser treatments on throat lesions.

The rigid laryngoscope setup consists of the scope, the light cord or light fibers, and a light source box (Fig. 8–14). Some direct laryngoscopy setups attach to a camera, enabling the entire surgical team to view the throat on a monitor.

The surgeon requires suction and may need flexible biopsy forceps, cup forceps, or graspers, depending on the procedure being performed. If the patient is undergoing a microlaryngoscopy, a suspension device is placed on the patient's chest to hold the rigid laryngoscope, leaving the surgeon's hands free to operate the microscope and instruments. Before the insertion of a rigid laryngoscope, a mouth guard is placed over the patient's upper teeth to protect them from damage.

Patient positioning varies according to institution or surgeon preference, but generally the patient is placed supine with a shoulder roll or doughnut headrest or in a sitting position.

### Rigid Bronchoscopy

Rigid bronchoscopes are long, straight, hollow metal tubes that are inserted into the bronchus (Fig. 8–15), usually for one of the following reasons:

- View airway abnormalities.
- Biopsy tissue or specimens for chronic infections or masses.
- Evaluate abnormal bleeding from the lungs.
- Remove foreign objects lodged in the airway.
- Open the spaces of a blocked airway.
- Treat bronchial stenosis (narrowing) with laser.
- Directly apply medication.

The setup for rigid bronchoscopy is similar to that of rigid laryngoscopy except that the scopes are longer. You need a

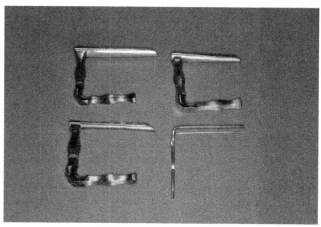

FIGURE 8–14 Rigid laryngoscope.

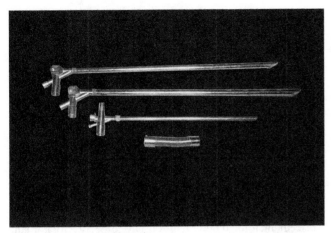

FIGURE 8-15 Rigid bronchoscopes.

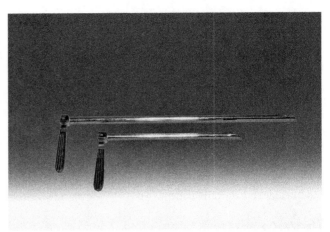

FIGURE 8-16 Rigid esophagoscopes.

light cord or fibers, a light source box, and suction. If tissue or specimens are anticipated, biopsy forceps, graspers, or cup forceps should be available. A mouth guard should be placed over the patient's upper teeth before insertion of the scope to protect the teeth from damage.

Patient positioning varies according to institution or surgeon preference, but generally the patient is placed supine with a shoulder roll or doughnut headrest.

## Rigid Esophagoscopy

Rigid esophagoscopy is used for direct visualization of the esophagus and top of the stomach. Similar to the rigid bronchoscopes, the rigid esophagoscopes are long, hollow, metal tubes that are inserted into the esophagus, usually for one of the following reasons:

■ Visualize masses or lesions.
■ Remove foreign body; this is the most common reason this procedure is done in pediatrics.
■ Inject esophageal varices.
■ Obtain tissue or specimens for biopsy or examination.
■ Dilate strictures or stenosis (narrowing).

The setup for rigid esophagoscopy is similar to that of rigid bronchoscopy except that the scopes are longer (Fig. 8–16). You need the light cord or fibers, a light source box, and suction. If tissue or specimens are anticipated, biopsy forceps, graspers, or cup forceps should be available. A mouth guard should be placed over the patient's upper teeth before insertion of the scope to protect the teeth from damage.

Patient positioning varies according to institution or surgeon preference, but generally the patient is placed supine with a shoulder roll or doughnut headrest.

## Mediastinoscopy

The mediastinoscope is a lighted hollow metal tube with a handle attached at a right angle (Fig. 8–17) used to look inside the space under the sternum between the lungs (the mediastinum). Located in this space are the large vessels, heart, lymph

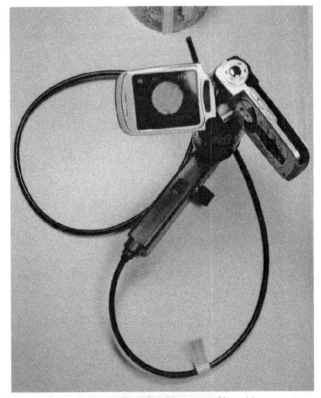

FIGURE 8-17 Mediastinoscope. (Courtesy of http://www.entscope.com/servlet/the-template/about/Page.)

nodes, trachea, and esophagus. A mediastinoscopy is usually done for one of the following reasons:

■ Detect lymphoma (including Hodgkin's disease).
■ Diagnose sarcoidosis.
■ Biopsy masses or tumors.
■ Stage cancer (including obtaining lymph nodes).
■ Diagnose chronic infections.

As with other endoscopes, a light source box is required, and a camera may be attached to allow for viewing of the surgical field on a video monitor. Newer scopes have the camera built into the handle, which is less awkward and provides a better picture quality than a separate attachment.

The patient is placed in a supine position with the head and neck hyperextended. An incision is made into the suprasternal notch for insertion of the scope.

*Note:* The use of an incision requires that the mediastinoscopy be treated as a sterile procedure rather than a surgically clean procedure like other endoscopes. The surgical team must follow strict aseptic techniques when handling supplies and instruments as well as when prepping and draping for this procedure. Failure to do so could result in postoperative infection and possible death of the patient.

## Thoracoscope

The procedure abbreviated VATS (video-assisted thoracoscopic surgery) uses a rigid telescope and three to four ports to perform minimally invasive surgery on the lung (Fig. 8–18). Two 10-mm scopes should be available: a 0-degree and a 30-degree. As with other endoscopic procedures, a light source box, camera, and video monitor are required.

VATS is usually performed for one of the following reasons:

- Biopsy lung, pleura, or diaphragm.
- Resect the lung.
- Decorticate the lung.
- Diagnose cancer or infection.
- Perform wedge resection of the lung.
- Perform pleurodesis for treatment of pneumothorax or pleural effusion.
- Perform sympathectomy or sympathotomy for treatment of hyperhidrosis (excessive sweating).

The patient is placed in a lateral position with the operative side upward. Follow all precautions for lateral positioning, including proper padding of legs, ankles, and arms and placement of an axillary roll and secure fastening of the patient to the bed.

Incisions are used to insert the ports for the camera and instruments; therefore, strict aseptic technique must be followed when handling supplies and instruments as well as prepping and draping for this procedure. Failure to do so could result in postoperative infection and possible death of the patient.

## ARTHROSCOPY EQUIPMENT

The term *arthroscopy* means to look within a joint. Arthroscopes can be used to perform procedures of the shoulder, knee, hip, elbow, wrist, and ankle (Fig. 8–19). It is one of the most common orthopedic procedures performed.

Arthroscopies are performed to diagnose and repair injury to a joint. Some of the most common arthroscopic procedures include ligament, tendon, and cartilage repair; ligament replacement; foreign body removal; chondroplasty; rotator cuff surgery; impingement syndrome treatment; and searching for the cause of chronic pain and swelling.

Equipment setup is much the same as for any other endoscopic procedure. You need an arthroscope, trocars, or cannulas (including an inflow cannula to instill fluid into the joint); one or two video monitors; a light source; arthroscopy pump and tubing; large (3,000 cc) bags of normal saline for irrigation; large-capacity suction device (e.g., Neptune or jug suction); camera; printer with paper; and electrocautery, hooks, probes, shavers, graspers, and other instruments (depending on the procedure). *All* equipment and instruments must be checked before the start of the procedure to ensure that they are working. Make sure to check the printer for an adequate supply of paper.

Arthroscopic surgery requires a large amount of irrigation fluid. The fluid is pumped into the joint using an arthroscopy pump (see Fig. 8–4). There are many models of arthroscopy pumps available; make sure you are familiar with the pump(s) your institution uses. The pump should be set up and tested before the start of the procedure. If the pump is not pumping fluid properly, check the tubing to make sure it is inserted correctly and does not have a kink in it. If the pump still fails to pump properly, get another pump.

It is the responsibility of the circulator to keep an eye on the fluid level in the irrigation bag. Fluid should never be

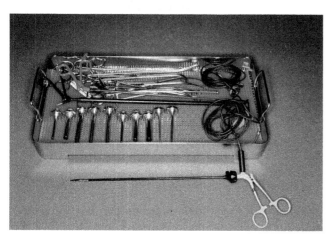

FIGURE 8–18 Thoracoscopy instrument set.

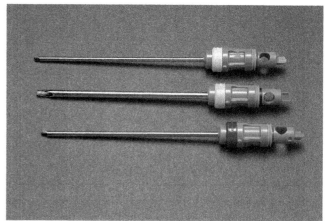

FIGURE 8–19 Shaver and arthroscopic instruments.

allowed to run out. Most pumps have an alarm that signals a low fluid level, but do not rely solely on the alarm. Keep an eye on the fluid level and change the bag before it runs out.

It is the responsibility of the scrub person to check the arthroscope (Fig. 8–20) and camera to make sure the picture is clear and that the lens is not broken or cracked. The scope should be checked to make sure it is not bent or damaged. All cords must be checked to make sure the fibers are not broken or that the casing is not cracked or damaged. Instruments should be checked to make sure they are in good working order (not difficult to open or close, not sticking).

Patient positioning depends on the procedure being performed. Knee arthroscopy usually requires the patient to be in a supine position with the affected knee in a holder that keeps it bent (e.g., knee-crutch stirrup), although some surgeons do not use the holder and just bend the knee with the foot flat on the bed. Depending on the procedure and the surgeon, shoulder arthroscopy can be performed with the patient supine with the affected arm suspended in traction or with the patient positioned sitting using a "beach chair" positioner. Hip arthroscopy can be performed with the patient positioned on a fracture bed, with the affected leg in traction. Make sure you have all the required positioning equipment available before bringing the patient into the OR.

## FLEXIBLE ENDOSCOPES

Flexible endoscopes are available for use in a variety of nonsurgical procedures. Bronchoscopy, esophagoscopy, endoscopic retrograde cholangiopancreatography (ERCP), gastroscopy, colonoscopy, and sigmoidoscopy are the most common, but flexible endoscopes are available to perform hysteroscopy, cystoscopy, and rhinolaryngoscopy as well.

As its name implies, the flexible endoscope is a long, hollow, flexible tube with a light on the end (a light source box is required) and a camera attached that is used to inspect passageways within the body (Fig. 8–21). Located within the scope are channels where biopsy, suction, and irrigation instruments can be inserted. The tip of the scope can be rotated 360 degrees to allow for complete visualization of tissue. The diameter and length of the tube vary depending on the intended use and the size of the patient (pediatric or adult).

Flexible endoscopies are most commonly used to diagnose or treat problems within the digestive tract, including the following:

- Abdominal pain
- Gastric ulcers
- Tumors, masses, and polyps

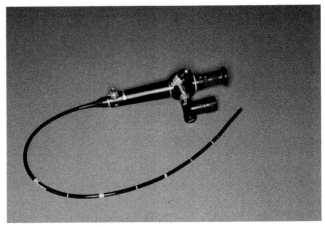

FIGURE 8–21 Flexible scope.

- Intestinal tract bleeding (e.g., vomiting blood or passing blood rectally)
- Gastritis
- Common bile duct stones
- Changes in bowel habits
- Tissue retrieval for examination

The performance of flexible endoscopy alone does not (in most cases) require the use of general anesthesia. Most procedures are performed with sedation and a topical anesthetic. As with any procedure, the scope, light source, video monitor, and other equipment must be checked *before* the start of the procedure to make sure they are working properly.

Patient positioning depends on what procedure is being performed, with supine being the most common position for endoscopy of the upper tract and either side lying (Sims) or lithotomy for endoscopy of the lower tract.

### Care of Flexible Endoscopes

As with any delicate (and expensive!) piece of equipment, care is needed when handling flexible endoscopes. Here are some general rules to follow when handling and cleaning flexible scopes, but be sure you read and are familiar with the manufacturer's instructions before using the scope:

- Flexible endoscopes contain fiberoptic bundles. Coil the scope loosely; coiling scopes too tightly can break the fibers.
- Do not place heavy instruments or equipment on top of the endoscope because it could damage the fiberoptic bundles or make a hole in the outer casing of the scope.
- Lay scopes on a flat surface when not in use to avoid kinking or twisting the shaft of the scope.
- Before use, inspect all scopes for holes or tears on the outer casing. Hook up all equipment to the scope and turn it on to make sure you have a clear picture (dark spots within the picture can indicate broken fiberoptic bundles).
- Before use, inspect all scopes to make sure they are free of bioburden.

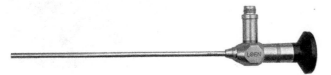

FIGURE 8–20 Arthroscope.

- Clean bioburden (e.g., blood, secretions, and feces) from the scope and instruments as needed during the procedure to ensure adequate visualization of the cavity. Wipe the scope immediately after use to prevent bioburden from drying on the scope.
- Follow the manufacturer's instructions for cleaning the scope. Soak the scope only if it is immersible. Clean all channels within the scope as well as all valves and ports. Long, thin, soft brushes are available for cleaning hard-to-reach areas. Flush all channels, ports, and valves clean after using the brush to loosen debris.
- Test all flexible scopes for leaks according to manufacturer's instructions.
- Rinse the scope with copious amounts of fresh water to remove debris and cleaning solution.
- Dry the scope according to manufacturer's instructions. All channels, ports, and valves must be free of moisture.
- Routinely inspect all scopes for broken fiberoptic bundles, control switches, or deflectors. Inspect lenses for scratches and looseness.
- Lay scopes flat or hang them up with the control handle in the upright position and the tube hanging downward for storage. They should not be stored near the edge of a table or where they could easily be bumped against something hard and damaged.

## NEEDLES, TROCARS, AND INSTRUMENTS

When a procedure of the abdomen or pelvis is going to be performed laparoscopically, the abdominopelvic cavity must first be filled with carbon dioxide, creating a *pneumoperitoneum*. The purpose of the pneumoperitoneum is to help prevent injury to tissue and organs as well as to provide space for the insertion of trocars and instruments.

Carbon dioxide is used to inflate the abdomen because it is readily available, is odorless, does not support combustion, has a lower incidence of embolism than air, and is reabsorbed by the body. Carbon dioxide can have side effects, the most serious being hypercarbia (see warning box later in this section). Additional side effects that could occur are nerve irritation, leading to postoperative pain in the shoulder area, venous embolism, cerebrovascular accident (stroke), or the introduction of infectious germs from the carbon dioxide tanks.

To introduce carbon dioxide into the abdomen, the surgeon will use a *Veress needle* (also known as a *pneumoperitoneum needle*). Veress needles come in various lengths to accommodate patients of differing abdominal girths (Fig. 8–22).

The usual technique for insertion of the Veress needle is for the surgeon to make a small "stab" incision into the upper abdominal tissues; lift up the skin with a Kocher, Backhaus, or other penetrating clamp; and push the distal end of the needle through the tissue at an angle to avoid injuring underlying

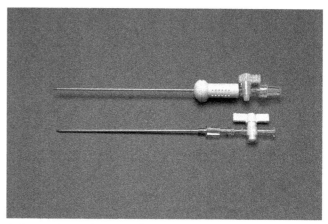

FIGURE 8-22 Veress needles.

structures. The proximal end of the needle is attached to insufflator tubing, which is attached to the insufflating control box (Fig. 8–23). The tubing must have a filter and should be flushed with carbon dioxide (to remove air) before insufflation of the abdomen.

An alternative to using the Veress needle is for the surgeon to insert a *Hasson cannula* (Fig. 8–24). This technique requires the surgeon to make a 1-cm incision in the area of the umbilicus and place a heavy suture into the fascia on each side of

**WARNING! Hypercarbia**

- *Hypercarbia* is defined as excess carbon dioxide in the body.
- Excess carbon dioxide in the body can create metabolic acidosis, leading to cardiac and respiratory abnormalities.
- Despite the potential for hypercarbia, carbon dioxide remains the safest and most commonly used gas to create a pneumoperitoneum.

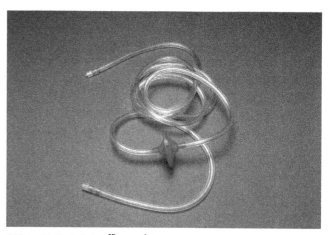

FIGURE 8-23 Insufflator tubing.

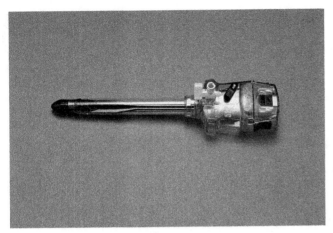

FIGURE 8-24 Hasson cannula.

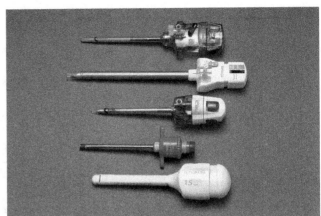

FIGURE 8-25 Trocar/cannula systems.

the incision. The surgeon then bluntly dissects down to the peritoneum, lifts the peritoneum with clamps, and incises it. The Hasson cannula (with a blunt obturator) is inserted into the abdominal cavity, taking care to protect the viscera. The sutures are wrapped around the locking tabs on the cannula to hold it in place. The insufflator tubing is attached to a port on the cannula.

Once the abdomen is inflated, the surgeon makes several more small incisions that allow for the introduction of the trocar-cannula system (Fig. 8–25). The trocar is the part of the device that pierces the tissue, whereas the cannula is the part that is left after the trocar is removed. The tip of the trocar can be blunt or sharp, although blunt or bladeless trocars are now more common because they pose less threat of injury to internal organs. The cannula is used to create a port for introducing the camera or instruments into the internal cavity. The cannulas vary in size from 5 mm to 15 mm; 5 mm and 10 mm are the most commonly used sizes.

There are times when you may have a 10-mm trocar inserted into the abdomen, but the instrument the surgeon wants to use is 5 mm. In that case, you place a *reducer* onto the trocar (Fig. 8–26). This reducer has a soft, pliable opening that closes around the 5-mm instrument so that carbon dioxide is not lost out of the abdomen. If the surgeon were just to insert a 5-mm instrument into a 10-mm trocar, there would be open space around the instrument that would allow the carbon dioxide to escape and decrease your pneumoperitoneum.

## Instruments

If you look at the tips of laparoscopic instruments, they look very similar to the tips of your common surgical instruments: allis, Kocher, hemostat, scissors, Mixters, and so on. The difference lies in the shaft length and handle. Laparoscopic instruments have a long, narrow shaft and a trigger-style handle (Fig. 8–27). The long, narrow shaft allows the instrument to be inserted through the cannula into the abdomen. The trigger-style handle allows for more precise manipulation of the instrument. These instruments tend to be very delicate and

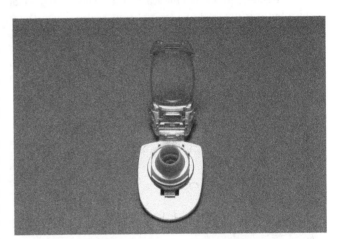

FIGURE 8-26 Reducer cap.

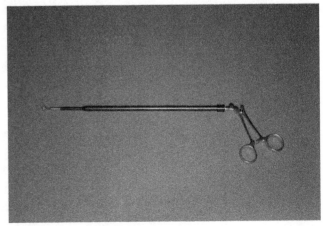

FIGURE 8-27 Laparoscopic instrument.

should be handled with extra care. The length of the shaft makes it more susceptible to bending or breaking; the handle mechanisms can become too stiff or too loose to manipulate precisely; and the tips can become loose, fall off, or become damaged.

Laparoscopic instruments can be disposable or reusable. Some laparoscopic instruments have a place to attach an electrosurgery unit cord, allowing the instrument to be used for cauterization (Fig. 8–28).

Some instruments have a device near the handle that allows for rotation of the tip, making it so the user can manipulate the tip without having to rotate the entire instrument (Fig. 8–29).

Suturing inside the cavity during laparoscopic surgery always presents a challenge. A number of different devices are used for suturing. Each device has its own merits and drawbacks. The device used is generally based on what the surgeon is comfortable with and what tissue he or she is suturing.

Stapling devices are available for laparoscopic use. Similar to standard instruments, some of these devices can either place a single staple (Ligaclip) or a row of staples (Fig. 8–30). The tip of the stapler looks like the tip of a regular clip applier or stapler, but it is attached to a long, narrow shaft.

Laparoscopic irrigation devices consist of a long, thin tube that has multiple holes along the sides of the tip and at the end (Fig. 8–31). Some of these devices are a combination of irrigation and suction with a hand control at the proximal end to allow the operator to switch between the two modes.

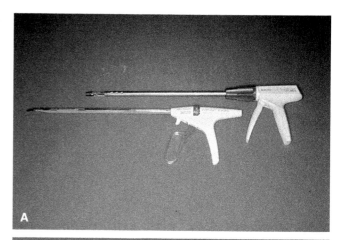

A

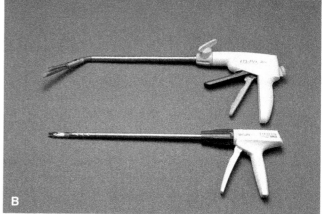

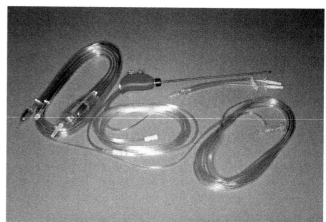

B

FIGURE 8–30 Laparoscopic stapling devices. (A) Single clip applier. (B) Multiple staple appliers.

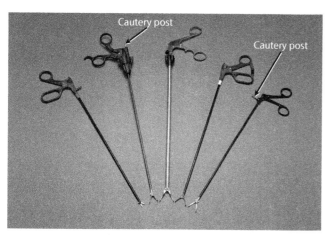

FIGURE 8–28 Laparoscopic instrument with cautery.

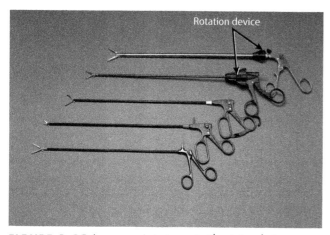

FIGURE 8–29 Laparoscopic instrument with rotation device.

FIGURE 8–31 Laparoscopic irrigation devices.

Generally, 3,000-cc bags of normal saline are attached to the device to use as an irrigating solution.

Suction devices need a power source: nitrogen or batteries. If using nitrogen, be sure to follow the manufacturer's recommendations for pressure setting. If the pressure is too low, the device will not work properly. Too high a setting can cause the spike to come out of the bag, and the whole bag of irrigation fluid will drain onto the floor!

**Surgical Session Review**

1) *Rhinoscopy* refers to viewing inside the
   a. Mouth
   b. Nose
   c. Ear
   d. Throat

2) *Fluoroscopy* uses _____ to view inside tissues or organs.
   a. Ultrasound waves
   b. Laser
   c. X-ray
   d. Electrical current

3) *Gastroscopy* refers to viewing inside the
   a. Small intestine
   b. Large intestine
   c. Esophagus
   d. Stomach

4) Which of the following is *false* concerning a ureteroscope?
   a. The shaft is longer and thinner than a cystoscope.
   b. It can be rigid, semirigid, or flexible.
   c. The shaft is shorter and thinner than a cystoscope.
   d. It is used to view inside the ureter.

5) The most common gas used to create a pneumoperitoneum is
   a. Carbon dioxide
   b. Carbon monoxide
   c. Oxygen
   d. Helium

6) Video towers are not sterile; therefore, you need to make sure they are positioned at least _____ inches from the sterile drapes.
   a. 6 to 10
   b. 12 to 18
   c. 26 to 28
   d. 32 to 40

7) If the monitor video screen is dark, what should you check first?
   a. The fuses
   b. The power box to make sure it is not overloaded
   c. Whether it is plugged in and turned on
   d. Whether it is connected to the printer

8) Your patient is scheduled for a laryngoscopy. The surgeon will be looking inside the patient's _____.
   a. Nose
   b. Throat
   c. Ear
   d. Stomach

9) A mediastinoscopy can be used to aid in diagnosing
   a. Cervical cancer
   b. Hodgkin's disease
   c. AIDS
   d. Paget's disease

10) All of the following structures are located in the mediastinum *except* the
   a. Trachea
   b. Heart
   c. Esophagus
   d. Lungs

11) Thoracoscopy can be performed for all of the following reasons *except*
   a. Lung biopsy
   b. Wedge resection of the lung
   c. Decortication
   d. Pneumonectomy

12) The acronym VATS means:
   a. Video-activated thoracoscopic surgery
   b. Video-assisted thoracoscopic surgery
   c. Video-aided thoracic surgery
   d. Video-aligned thoracic surgery

13) To avoid possible damage, cystoscopes should be handled by the
   a. Middle of the shaft
   b. Tip end of the shaft
   c. Light cable connector
   d. Bridge

14) The patient is undergoing a TURBT that will involve electrocautery of bladder tumors. Which irrigation fluid would you anticipate using?
   a. Normal saline
   b. Dextrose in water
   c. Lactated Ringer's
   d. Glycine

15) _____ is the most common position for a patient undergoing cystoscopy.
   a. Supine
   b. Prone
   c. Kraske
   d. Lithotomy

16) Arthroscopy can be used for all of the following *except*
   a. Ligament damage repair
   b. Tendon damage repair
   c. Bone fractures
   d. Chondroplasty

17) The needle used to insert gas into the abdomen is known as a _____ needle.
   a. Veress
   b. Vegan
   c. Vargan
   d. Verrin

18) Excess carbon dioxide in the body is known as
   a. Hypoxia
   b. Hypocarbia
   c. Hypercarbia
   d. Hypoxemia

19) Enteroscopy is viewing inside the:
   a. Large intestine
   b. Small intestine
   c. Liver
   d. Spleen

20) If a video camera is outside the body and not in use, it should be in _____ mode.
   a. Still picture
   b. Active
   c. Panning
   d. Standby

# 9

# Robotics

Robotic surgery, once considered a technology of the distant future, is now routine in a number of surgical procedures. The robotic equipment is designed to enhance minimally invasive procedures. The instruments and camera are attached to the machine's robotic arms, which are manipulated by a surgeon who is seated at a console. This allows him or her to perform the surgery without standing at the surgical field, thus reducing surgeon fatigue. Furthermore, surgeons in one location can view or perform surgery in another location *(telesurgery)*. Robotics systems are becoming more sophisticated and capable of performing more precise procedures as the technology advances.

Robotic surgery is now an accepted way of performing surgery across a number of specialties. Surgical procedures in which robotics are used include the following:

- Genitourinary: Radical prostatectomy, pyeloplasty, cystectomy, nephrectomy, ureteral reimplantation, donor nephrectomy, adrenalectomy
- General surgery: Single-site cholecystectomy, Nissen fundoplication, gastric bypass, splenectomy, bowel resection, treatment of pancreatic disease, stomach cancer
- Gynecology: Hysterectomy, myomectomy, Bilateral Salpingo-Oophorectomy (BSO), pelvic reconstructive surgery
- Cardiothoracic: Internal mammary artery mobilization and cardiac tissue ablation, mitral valve repair, endoscopic atrial septal defect closure, mammary to left anterior descending coronary artery anastomosis for cardiac revascularization, chest cancer, mediastinal procedures, Coronary Artery Bypass Graft (CABG)
- Ear, Nose, Throat (ENT) surgery (transoral route): Laryngeal cancer, cancer at the base of the tongue, treatment of sleep apnea, laryngeal cleft repair

(Adapted from www.intuitive.com and uclahealth.org)

## ADVANTAGES AND DISADVANTAGES OF ROBOTIC SURGERY

One of the major disadvantages of robotic technology is that it is expensive—a single robot can cost about $2 million. Therefore, the advantages versus the cost need to be considered before investing in this technology. The technological advantages include the following:

- Elimination of hand tremor and cramping
- 3D viewing of the surgical field

- Decrease in the number of surgical assistants needed; some systems have an optional fourth arm that can be used for providing countertraction or aiding in suturing, allowing some procedures to be performed without an assistant
- Increase in dexterity; the arm of the robot that holds the instruments can be rotated 360 degrees with 90 degrees of articulation
- Binocular optics, allowing for better depth perception, aids in nerve sparing
- Less fatigue for the surgeon

The patient advantages include less recovery time, less bleeding, less pain due to decreased tissue trauma/manipulation and quicker recovery, less time missed from work, and other activities. These are the same types of advantages common to other types of endoscopic surgery.

## COMPONENTS OF THE ROBOTIC SYSTEM

There are a few different manufacturers of robotic surgical systems, but their systems all have the same basic components.

The *patient cart* contains the robotic arms and is the "working" part of the system. The instruments are attached into the arms (Figs. 9–1A and 9–1B), and the surgeon can position and manipulate the arms and instruments as needed to perform the surgery. The instruments are designed to work like a human wrist: they can be rotated 360 degrees and have 90 degrees of articulation. This amount of freedom of movement allows for more precision working around delicate structures.

The *console* (Fig. 9–2) where the surgeon sits is designed to allow the surgeon to control the movements of the instruments and robotic arms through the use of hand controls and foot pedals. The surgeon looks into binocular lenses and is able to see a high definition, magnified 3D view of the surgical field.

The third component of the system is the *viewing or image system (cart)*. The image system enables the procedure to be viewed by all personnel in the room (Fig. 9–3). Components of the system include the camera system, endoscope, light source, touch screen, video processing unit, and stereo viewer.

Figures 9–4 and 9–5 show examples of how a robotic surgery suite might be set up.

Configuration will depend on the size of the room. These robotic ORs can be permanent or temporary (as the equipment will be moved in and out).

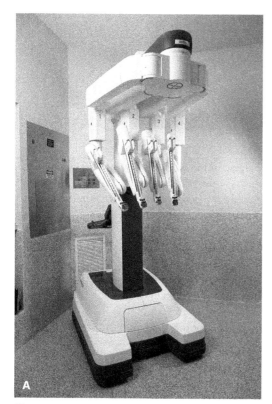

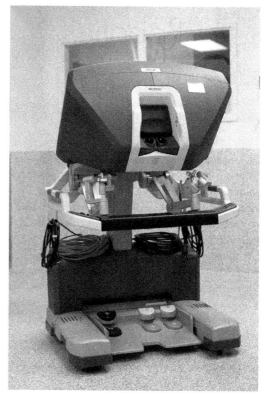

FIGURE 9-2 Surgeon console.

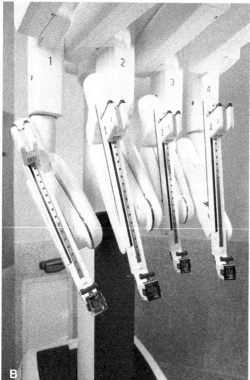

FIGURE 9-1 (A) Patient-side cart. (B) Attachment points on the arms for the customized instruments.

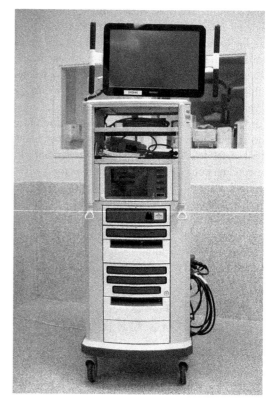

FIGURE 9-3 Image system (viewing cart).

Video monitors
for staff viewing

Surgeon console
room (where surgeon
sits to do the surgery)

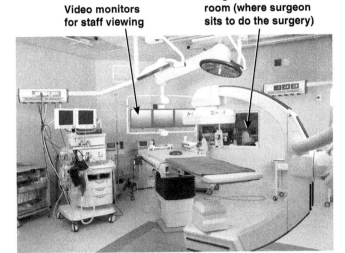

**FIGURE 9-4** One example of a robotic OR (russellglenister/RooM/Getty Images).

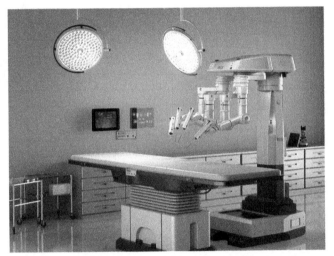

**FIGURE 9-5** Patient side carts (placement around the operating room table will depend on the procedure being performed) (PhonlamaiPhoto/iStock/Getty Images Plus).

## ROLE OF THE PERSONNEL ASSIGNED TO ROBOTIC CASES

Any staff member who is assigned to a room where a robotic surgery is to be performed should meet the following general standards (adapted from AST Recommended Guidelines for Best Practices During Robotic Surgery). Please check your institution's policies and procedures for further guidance.

- Staff members must complete training specific to the robotic device being used; because of the complexity of these devices, staff MUST be properly trained on all of the components of the device use and assembly/setup—including proper draping of the instrument arms (Fig. 9–6), troubleshooting, proper cleaning, and proper transportation of the device if there is not a dedicated room.

- An individual who is properly trained and familiar with the devices can be designated a robotics team leader.
- Policies and procedures should be reviewed annually.
- They should have a thorough understanding of the patient and vision carts and be able to assist in setting up the components, whether they are scrubbed in or acting as a circulator or an assistant circulator.
- They need to have a thorough understanding of the robotic—how they work and how to care for them.

## ADDITIONAL ROLES OF SCRUBBED PERSONNEL

- They must be able to assist in providing for a safe procedure—checking all equipment for proper working order before the procedure, assist when needed to defog the camera lens, remove and exchange instruments from the robotic arms as needed during the procedure, facilitate the removal of tissue or organs from the body cavity, remove instruments then the endoscope at the conclusion of the procedure.
- Be prepared for conversion to an open procedure if needed—have proper instruments available for immediate use, remove the robotic instruments and endoscope from the patient, be familiar with scrubbing the open version of the procedure.
- At the case conclusion they are responsible for breaking down the sterile back table and initial decontamination of the instruments and accessories.

Robotic surgery has become the "cutting edge" of minimally invasive surgery. The increased use of this technology requires scrubbed personnel and circulators to be familiar with the technology, how to set up the equipment and attach the instruments, and how to troubleshoot the equipment. Similar to any technology, there are limitations. As with any minimally invasive procedure, the OR personnel must be able to convert to an "open" procedure if necessary. Personnel must also be ready to take over and finish the procedure manually if the robotics equipment malfunctions.

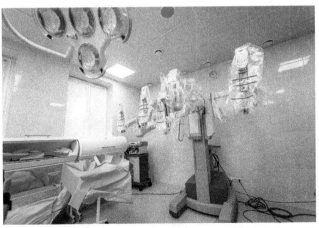

**FIGURE 9-6** Robotic instrument with arms draped (Vadym Terelyuk/iStock/Getty Images Plus).

## Surgical Session Review

1) The viewing system for robotic surgery includes which components?
   a. Touch screen, endoscope, and robotic arms
   b. Endoscope, camera, and surgeon hand controls
   c. Touch screen, endoscope, and camera
   d. Endoscope, camera, and graspers

2) Which of the following is an advantage of robotic surgery?
   a. Two-dimensional viewing of the surgical field
   b. Three-dimensional viewing of the surgical field
   c. Monocular optics
   d. Decreased dexterity

3) One of the major disadvantages of robotic surgery is:
   a. Decreased physician fatigue
   b. Elimination of tremors
   c. Initial cost of the equipment
   d. Binocular optics

4) Which of the following components contain the robotic arms?
   a. Patient cart
   b. Viewing cart
   c. Graspers
   d. Console

5) A Nissen fundoplication falls into which category of robotic surgery?
   a. Genitourinary
   b. Cardiothoracic
   c. Gynecological
   d. General surgery

# Specialty Equipment

## IMAGE GUIDANCE SYSTEM

The image guidance system (also known as the *stealth station system* or the *stealth*) takes computed tomography (CT) scan, ultrasound, magnetic resonance imaging (MRI), or conventional radiograph images and transforms them into three-dimensional (3D) images (Fig. 10–1). The 3D images allow the surgeon to know the exact location of the lesion or tissue to be removed. These images can be rotated and manipulated to give the surgeon the precise view needed. The imaging is done before surgery to aid in preprocedure planning or is used intraoperatively.

Surgeons use the image guidance systems for *neurosurgery* (removal of brain tumors and spinal procedures); ENT procedures (polypectomy, functional endoscopic sinus surgery [FESS]; cholesteatomas); orthopedic procedures (total knee or hip and trauma); and biopsies of the liver, breast, or prostate.

The image is projected on a touch screen monitor. The surgeon uses special instruments that register their location in relation to the location of the lesion. The image on the screen shows where the instrument is situated so that the surgeon can protect surrounding tissue and blood vessels. For example, during polyp surgery, the ENT surgeon can see, within 1 mm, where the instrument is in relation to the brain, thus allowing the surgeon to extract more polyp tissue without fear of inadvertently causing damage or contamination to the brain.

Similar to any technology, the use of an image guidance system requires that OR personnel know how to load images into the machine, set up and position the machine in the room, and troubleshoot the equipment during a procedure. Personnel must make sure that they are knowledgeable about the manufacturer's instructions and recommendations on equipment function before being assigned to a case.

## IMPLANTS

Implants are objects that are placed in a person's body by means of surgery to replace diseased, damaged, or abnormal tissue. They may also be used to strengthen or repair bone, allowing it time to heal or to deliver medication.

Implanting an external product into a patient requires special handling of the implant (see the Guidelines box). It also requires careful documentation of exactly what was implanted into the patient. The documentation should include the device name, type, size, and serial number. Other documentation may be required by your facility; please check the policies regarding implant documentation. Something as small as a screw or as large as a heart valve or spinal rod may be considered an implant and requires the same special considerations.

## NEUROSURGERY EQUIPMENT

Neurosurgery requires specialized equipment, and it is essential for OR personnel to be familiar with it. In Chapter 2, some of the specific positioning devices (e.g., Mayo headrest) and furniture (e.g., large Mayo stand and overhead table) are described. Chapters 3 and 4 include some specific supplies (e.g., neuro patties or cottonoids) and drains (e.g., ventricular drain). In this section, some of the equipment used for surgery on the brain is described.

### Cranial Access Kit

The disposable cranial access kit (Fig. 10–2) is used to perform an emergency or bedside *ventriculostomy* (burr hole access into the cranium). This procedure enables the medical team to monitor intracranial pressure (ICP) or to drain

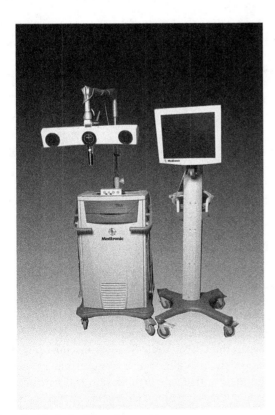

FIGURE 10-1 Stealth station machine.

## Guidelines for Handling of Implants

- Any implant used must be documented in the patient's intra-operative record.
- Implants should be handled as little as possible to avoid possible contamination.
- If an implant must be immediate-use sterilized (not recommended but sometimes necessary), a biological indicator must be flashed along with the implant. A chemical paper indicator is not sufficient.
- The circulator should double-check the implant size and type with the surgeon before opening the package. Implants are very expensive; you must make sure you have the correct one before opening it onto the sterile field.
- Scrub personnel should always measure any screws before handing them to the surgeon. Do not rely on the numbers on the package or on the side of the tray. Mistakes happen, and a screw could end up in the wrong section of the tray.

- Scrub personnel should double-check pin size before handing pins to the surgeon. Trays could have been restocked incorrectly.
- Never reuse an implant. They are single-use devices. Reuse could weaken them.
- Do not use any implant that has been damaged; get a new one. Implants that are dropped, scratched, or dented need to be discarded.
- Bending plates to conform to the bone should be avoided whenever possible. If a plate must be bent, a proper plate-bending instrument should be used, not a pair of pliers.
- Use implants of the same metal or alloy for the surgery. If implants of differing alloys are used, they can corrode and cause implant breakdown.

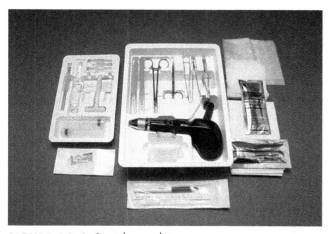

FIGURE 10-2 Cranial access kit.

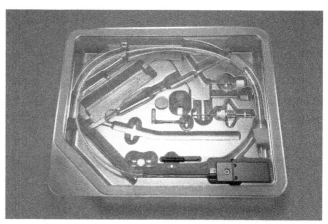

FIGURE 10-3 Intracranial pressure monitor kit.

cerebrospinal fluid or blood from the central nervous system to relieve pressure.

This kit is designed for single-patient use. Although contents of the kits vary, most of them include a hand drill and drill bits, prepping supplies (including razors and prep solution), drapes, scissors, suturing equipment, tubes for collecting cerebrospinal fluid samples, disposable scalpels, needles, syringes, and local anesthetic.

### Intracranial Pressure Monitor

The ICP monitor (Fig. 10–3) is used to continuously monitor the pressure surrounding the brain. Patients requiring ICP monitoring include those who have sustained head trauma or brain hemorrhage, those who have undergone brain surgery, and those who have cranial tumors.

A small plastic tube is inserted into the brain, usually in the left or right ventricle. The tube is connected to a monitor that continuously displays ICP. Normal ICP in an adult

is 5 to 15 mm Hg. An increased pressure reading could be indicative of brain swelling, which could lead to herniation or permanent neurological damage if uncorrected. Complications of ICP monitor insertion include infection or hemorrhage.

### Cavitron Ultrasonic Surgical Aspirator/Sonopet

The Cavitron Ultrasonic Surgical Aspirator (CUSA) enables a surgeon to break up and remove tumors, tissue, and bone requiring fragmentation, emulsification, and aspiration. The device uses ultrasonic waves to fragment the tumor and then removes it by irrigation and suction.

Similar to the CUSA is the Sonopet machine (Fig. 10–4). The Sonopet also uses ultrasonic waves to fragment tissue and bone and remove them through suction and irrigation. It is also a bone-cutting aspirator. Unlike conventional cranial sawing devices, there is minimal heat generation at the tip when cutting bone.

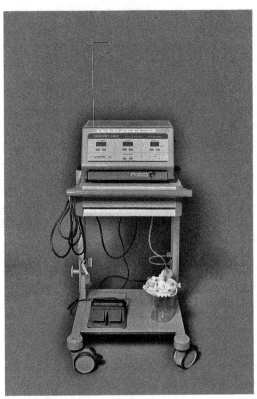

FIGURE 10-4 Sonopet machine.

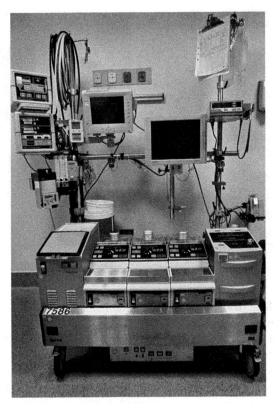

FIGURE 10-5 Heart-lung machine.

There are many tips available for the handpieces of both devices to allow for use on a variety of tumor types and locations. The Sonopet machine also has a variety of bone-cutting tips available. Although both machines mainly started out being used in neurosurgical procedures, they are now used in most surgical specialties.

## CARDIAC SURGERY EQUIPMENT AND SUPPLIES

### Cardiopulmonary Bypass Machine

The cardiopulmonary bypass machine, also known as the *heart-lung machine* or *pump oxygenator,* is used to replace the heart and lungs during some cardiac surgery procedures (Fig. 10–5). The machine gathers the blood, removes excess carbon dioxide, oxygenates it, and returns it to the body. In addition, it filters the blood and controls its temperature. The machine is used during many cardiac procedures, including the following:

- Coronary artery bypass graft (CABG)
- Heart or heart-lung transplant
- Heart valve replacement or repair
- Birth defect repair (e.g., septal defects, tetralogy of Fallot, transposition of great vessels)
- Pulmonary thrombolectomy
- Large aortic aneurysm repair
- Rewarming of severe hypothermia victims

The cardiopulmonary bypass machine is operated by a perfusionist. He or she is specially educated, having 2 to 4 years of undergraduate training before enrolling in a 2-year perfusion training program. The perfusionist is responsible for supporting the metabolic and physiological needs of the patient while he or she is on the bypass machine, for monitoring physiological parameters (e.g., blood gases, acid base balance, electrolytes, and anticoagulation), for adjusting machine parameters as needed, and for collecting autologous blood. Perfusionists monitor the pump lines for the presence of air. Any air must be removed immediately to prevent possible air embolus or stroke. All lines must be monitored to make sure none becomes disconnected from the machine as a patient could quickly exsanguinate from a disconnected line.

Special cannulae (Fig. 10–6) are inserted into the vena cava and the ascending aorta, and the pump tubing is attached to the cannulae. The blood is taken out of the body via the cannula in the vena cava (or right atrium), which is called the *venous cannula.* This cannula is straight ended with multiple holes in the tip. The blood is returned to the body through the aortic cannula. The aortic cannula may have a straight or angled tip. The femoral artery and femoral vein occasionally are used to collect and return the blood, generally when the great vessels cannot be used. The femoral artery catheter is tapered and has a beveled end for ease of insertion.

Cardiopulmonary bypass can be total or partial. *Total cardiopulmonary bypass* means that all the blood returning to the heart is forced into the venous cannula and out to the heart-lung

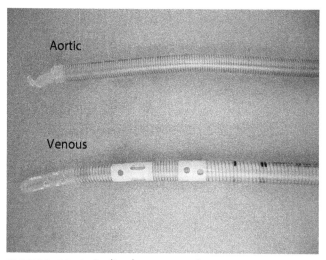

FIGURE 10-6 Cardiopulmonary cannulae.

machine (see Fig. 10–5). Total cardiopulmonary bypass is used for many cardiac surgeries: CABG, transplants, repair of most cardiac birth defects, and valve replacements.

*Partial cardiopulmonary bypass* means that some blood is allowed to flow into the heart and "normal" circulation while the rest of the blood is diverted into the machine. Partial cardiopulmonary bypass can be used during some types of cardiothoracic surgery (e.g., repairs of some aortic anomalies) and as a temporary measure after coronary bypass grafting to wean the patient from the bypass machine.

## Additional Cardiac Surgery Supplies

### Vessel and Patch Grafts

Synthetic grafts are used to replace diseased, injured, or abnormal segments of blood vessels (veins or arteries). To accommodate the shape of the vessels they are replacing, grafts can be straight or bifurcated (Fig. 10–7). They are made of knitted or woven Dacron or Teflon. Grafts are very expensive; therefore, graft sizers should be used to determine the correct size before the package is opened.

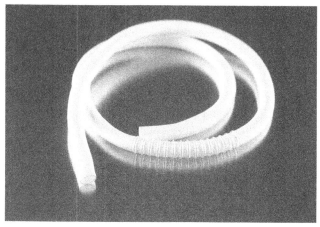

FIGURE 10-7 Vascular graft.

Grafts are considered implants, necessitating the documentation in the medical record of the type, size, and serial number of the graft. Check your institutional policy for any further documentation that may be required relating to implants.

### Prosthetic Heart Valves

Replacement of the heart valve occurs when the valve is too diseased or damaged to repair. Valve replacement requires a full set of sizers, handlers, and holders. OR personnel assigned to these cases must be familiar with this type of equipment and its use.

Two common types of prosthetic heart valves are mechanical (e.g., St. Jude Medical) and biological (porcine, bovine, or human tissue). The surgeon's choice of valve depends on a thorough assessment of each patient's needs. Biological valves may come stored in gluteraldehyde solution that must be rinsed off in three separate basins of normal saline, 2 minutes in each basin (a total of 6 minutes of rinsing).

Bioprinting, using a 3D printer to create tissue or organs, is currently being used to create heart valves. Using a computer-assisted design, the bioprinter deposits ultrathin layers of living cells upon each other, following a precise geometric pattern that matches the heart valve dimensions.

Prosthetic valve replacement is the standard procedure for adults but has proved inadequate for younger adults and growing children, because as the child grows, the prosthesis does not grow, necessitating another surgical procedure to replace it. Tissue engineering has the potential to address this by providing living tissues that can grow, remodel, and integrate with the patient.

Valve replacements are considered implants, necessitating the documentation in the medical record of the type, size, and serial number of the valve. Check your institutional policy for any further documentation that may be required relating to implants.

### Internal (Permanent) Pacemakers and AICDs

Pacemakers and AICDs (automatic implantable cardioverter defibrillator) are implanted when the heart is too diseased or damaged to function properly on its own long term (Fig. 10–8). Insertion of a permanent pacemaker or AICD necessitates a skin incision; therefore, it should be done under sterile conditions, either in the OR or a cardiac catheterization laboratory.

A pacemaker produces electrical impulses that stimulate the heart muscle to beat. There are four basic types of pacemakers. The type of pacemakers inserted depends on the needs of the patient.

- Single-chamber pacemakers—In a single-chamber pacemaker, only one wire (pacing lead) is placed into the heart. The wire is either placed into one of the upper chambers or atrium or in one of the lower chambers or ventricles, depending on the needs of the patient.
- Dual-chamber pacemakers—In dual-chamber pacemakers, wires are placed in two chambers of the heart. One lead paces the atria (upper chambers), and one paces the ventricles (lower chambers). This type of pacemaker

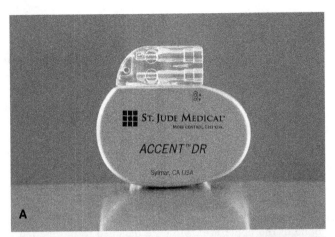

A

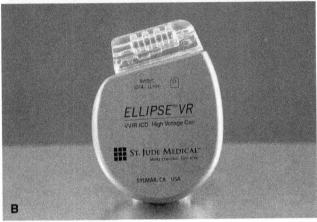

B

FIGURE 10-8 (A) Dual-chamber pacemaker. (B) Defibrillator AICD.

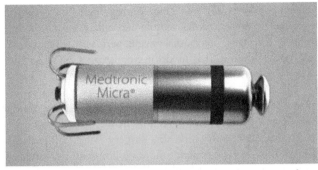

FIGURE 10-9 Micra pacemaker. Reproduced with permission from Medtronic.

monitors the patient's heart rate and rhythm and automatically gives the heart a shock if the rate is too irregular or very rapid. In some cases, an AICD can act as a pacemaker and stimulate the heart to beat faster if the heart rate drops too low.

Permanent pacemakers and AICDs require documentation in the medical record of the type, size, and serial number of the device. Check your institutional policy for any further documentation that may be required relating to implants.

### Intra-Aortic Balloon Pump

The intra-aortic balloon pump (IABP) is an external machine attached to a sheath and balloon that is inserted through the femoral artery (Fig. 10-10). The balloon is placed in the

can coordinate function between the atria and ventricles and more closely matches the heart's natural pacing mechanism.
- Rate-responsive pacemakers—These types of pacemakers have sensors that automatically adjust to changes in the person's heart rate and activate only when needed.
- Leadless pacemakers are a more recent option. They are small (about 90% smaller than a regular pacemaker), self-contained, and are inserted through a catheter in the femoral vein (Fig. 10-9). They are implanted directly into the right ventricle to treat certain symptomatic bradycardias (slow heart rate) that require single-chamber pacing. They DO NOT contain a defibrillator component and are therefore not used in patients with a history of ventricular fibrillation nor are they used for those who require dual-chamber pacing. The advantages to this type of pacemaker are that there are no chest incisions and no exposure of the heart, lessening the chance of infection. There are no wires (leads) implanted into the heart so there is less chance of reoperation to fix dislodged or broken wires. Generally patients do not have the arm restrictions postprocedure that they do with a pacemaker.

An AICD is implanted in a patient at risk of sudden cardiac death caused by a very rapid or irregular heartbeat. The AICD

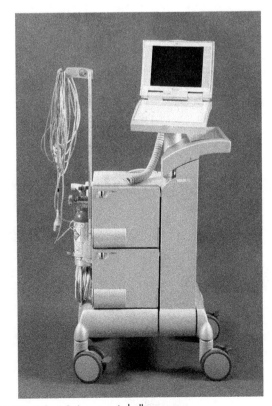

FIGURE 10-10 Intra-aortic balloon pump.

descending aorta. The machine controls the balloon, causing it to deflate during cardiac systole and inflate during diastole, thereby increasing myocardial oxygen perfusion while increasing cardiac output. It is used for circulatory support in cases when the heart is severely damaged.

The IABP can be used in patients waiting for a heart transplant, for treatment of cardiogenic shock after myocardial infarction, or in patients who cannot be weaned off the cardiopulmonary bypass machine after surgery. The IABP is a temporary measure; the patient cannot go home on this device. It provides support and allows more time until a more permanent solution to the patient's cardiac dysfunction can be found.

## ORTHOPEDIC SUPPLIES

### Repair and Fixation Implants

The screws, plates, nails, rods, and pins used in orthopedic surgery are considered implants because they are inserted into the bone or tissue and left inside the patient. Most of the time these implants are permanent, although some can be removed after the fracture heals if they are bothersome to the patient (e.g., causing pain or discomfort). This section covers the use of these devices.

### Staples

The primary use of fixation staples is to reconnect soft tissue to bone, including anterior cruciate ligament repair. Other uses include tendon and ligament repair, bone fragment fixation, and bone growth control.

Staples come in a variety of sizes and types (two, three, or four prongs) to accommodate surgery on all types and sizes of bone and tissue (Fig. 10–11). Most staples are straight, but some have an offset to allow for stable fixation of an osteotomy that has steps. There are specific staples available for use in open procedures and for use in arthroscopic procedures.

Staples are commonly made of stainless steel, but some are made from chromium-cobalt and nitinol alloy or titanium.

Staples are inserted with a staple driver and a mallet.

### Nails and Rods

Nails and rods are used to fix fractures of long bones (i.e., femur, tibia, and humerus) (Fig. 10–12). They are driven into the medullary canal to span the fracture sites. There are several manufacturers of these devices; make sure you are familiar with both the implant and the insertion instrument system being used by your institution.

Tibial nails are used to fix fractures of the large bone of the lower leg. The nails are designed to be used reamed or unreamed. Locking screws hold them in place. They vary in diameter from 8 mm to 14 mm and are available in 26-cm through 42-cm lengths. They are made of stainless steel or a titanium alloy.

Humeral nails are used to repair fractures of the long bone of the upper arm. Most are designed to be inserted at either the elbow or the shoulder. There are two main styles of humeral nails: one style has a bend at the proximal end and is used to repair fractures of the proximal third of the humerus, whereas the other style is straight and is used to repair fractures of the shaft of the humerus. Some humeral nails have a flexible head and could be used to repair fractures anywhere in the humerus. The nails are held in place with a locking screw system. Humeral nails are available in 6-mm to 13-mm diameters and 18-cm to 30-cm lengths.

The femoral intramedullary (IM) rod or nail is used to repair and align fractures of the femur. The rod is inserted into the bone marrow canal (IM canal). This allows the rod to share the weight-bearing load with the bone, making it possible for the patient to be mobile sooner. Femoral nails are available as antegrade, retrograde, natural, uniflex, or distal, depending on the type of fracture in need of repair. Most femoral nails are 10 to 16 mm in diameter with lengths that range from 16 cm to 44 cm. Distal femoral nails are available in 9-mm to 13-mm diameters and 160-mm to 460-mm lengths. Rods and nails are generally made of titanium or a titanium alloy.

### Bone Plates

Plates, along with screws, are used to traverse the surfaces of two bone fragments to repair fractures or stabilize bones. Plates

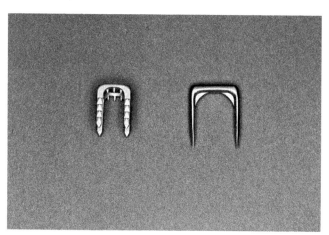

FIGURE 10–11 Fixation staples.

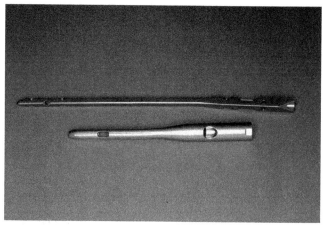

FIGURE 10–12 Nails.

come in a variety of sizes and shapes to accommodate a variety of bone surfaces and sizes (Fig. 10–13). Plates are used in cranial surgery (e.g., holding craniotomy bone flap in place), maxillofacial surgery (e.g., repair fractures of the jaw, facial bones, and zygoma), orthopedic surgery (e.g., repair of fractures), and spinal surgery (e.g., stabilization of vertebrae). Plates generally are made of titanium, titanium/nickel alloy, or stainless steel. As a general rule, it is best to avoid bending plates because this can weaken the metal, but if a plate must be bent to fit the fracture site, a plate bender made specifically for that purpose must be used. Plates come with anywhere from 2 to 12 holes, depending on the length, and in a variety of shapes.

### Bone Screws

Bone screws can be used to attach a plate or soft tissue to bone, or they can be placed directly across the fracture ends of small bone fractures to repair them. There are three types of bone screw: *cancellous, locking head,* and *cortical* (Fig. 10–14). It is very important that OR personnel be able to differentiate between the types of screws so that the correct screw is available to the surgeon.

The cancellous screw has threads that reach about one-half to two-thirds of the way up the *shank* of the screw. Cortical

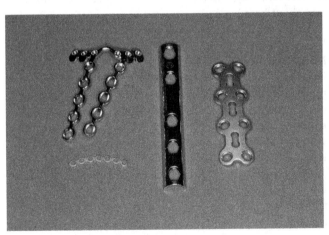

**FIGURE 10-13** Bone plates.

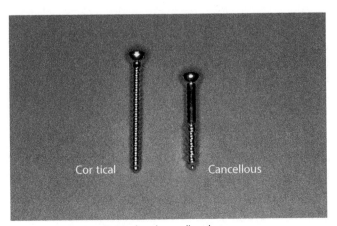

**FIGURE 10-14** Cortical and cancellous bone screws.

screws have threads all the way up the shank to the head of the screw. Locking head screws have a larger core diameter and a shallow, blunt thread.

Screws can be self-tapping, self-tapping/self-drilling, or they may require the use of a "tap" (non-self-tapping) to make ridges in the bone for the screw to follow. There are four steps for screw insertion with which scrub personnel should be familiar in order to anticipate what will be needed next:

1. *Drill:* Make a hole with a drill bit that is a smaller diameter than the screw being used.
2. *Measure:* Use a depth gauge to determine the length of the screw needed.
3. *Tap:* Use a bone tap to create ridges for the screw to follow (not necessary if self-tapping screws are used).
4. *Screw:* Set the screw in place using a screwdriver.

To remember the steps for screw insertion I once heard someone use the pneumonic "**D**on't **M**arry **T**oo **S**oon" to stand for *drill, measure, tap, screw.*

Screws are commonly made from titanium, stainless steel, or cobalt-chromium alloy. Cortical screws are available in 1.5-mm to 5.0-mm diameters and 6-mm to 110-mm lengths. Cancellous screws are available in 3.5-mm to 6.5-mm diameters and 10-mm to 110-mm lengths (thread length, 5 mm to 32 mm). Locking head screws are available in 2.4 mm to 7.3 mm diameters.

## Joint Replacement Implants

Joint implants can be used to totally or partially replace diseased or damaged joints. They are generally made from one of three materials: metal, polyethylene (plastic), or ceramic. Metal alloy implants are very strong, and some manufacturers are returning to metal-on-metal joint replacement systems instead of the plastic and metal hybrid systems. Polyethylene plastic is low friction and highly durable. It is used to make components for the hybrid systems. Ceramic is hard and found to resist wear and scratching. The primary disadvantage of ceramic is that it is brittle and can shatter or break. Ceramic prostheses are generally only used in hip replacements.

The type of implant used depends on the patient's condition, including his or her activity level, the condition of the bone, the patient's age, and whether it is a total or partial joint replacement. Figure 10–15A shows one example of the components of a total knee implant. Figure 10–15B shows an example of a total hip implant. No matter which implant you are using, they all need the same handling precautions and documentation standards that are stated in the "Implants" section at the beginning of this chapter.

## BONE GRAFTS

Bone grafts are one of two types: autograft (using the patient's own bone) or allograft (using cadaver bone). These grafts are used to repair or reconstruct bone.

Bone graft tissue should be kept on the back table in a basin covered with sponges that are moistened with saline. *Do not*

**A** 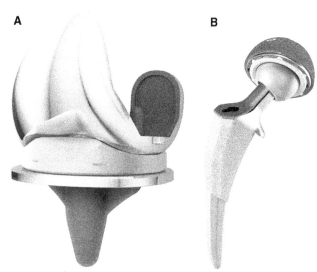 **B**

FIGURE 10-15 (A) ATTUNE™ Knee, Cruciate Retaining (CR) Rotating Platform (RP); (B) ACTIS™ Hip Stem, Standard Offset Stem Ceramic on Poly Side V. Photos courtesy of DePuy Synthes.

use water to moisten bone grafts as it can cause cellular damage. *Do not* soak the grafts in a basin of saline unless directed to by the surgeon.

Bone graft substitutes can be used in place of an autograft or allograft. The substitutes are made of ceramic or polymer and available in a number of forms: chips, putty, blocks, paste, and granules. Figure 10–16 shows cancellous chips that can be used for a bone graft.

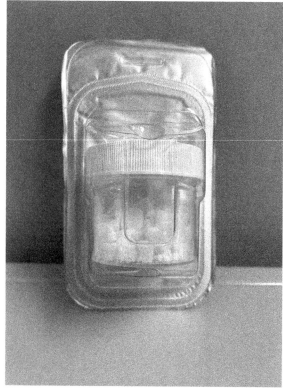

FIGURE 10-16 Cancellous chips.

# OPHTHALMIC SURGERY EQUIPMENT

## Vitrectomy and Cataract Removal Machines

A vitrectomy is an ophthalmic operation to remove the vitreous humor. Surgeons evacuate the vitreous to remove scar tissue, repair retinal damage or detachment, clear blood and debris from the eye, repair a macular hole, or repair injury to the eye resulting from previous surgery.

During surgery for retinal detachment, the surgeon uses either *diathermy* (heat) or *cryothermy* (cold) to create adhesions (scar tissue) between the layers of tissue and repair the detachment. The detached area adheres to the scar tissue as it heals, with the goal being for the damaged tissue to return to its normal position. A scleral buckle (small silicone or foam band) is attached to the sclera, causing it to indent and come in close contact with the retina during healing. The vitreous of the eye is replaced with a gas bubble or silicone oil. The oil or gas holds the retina in place and prevents traction or pulling on the newly repaired retina.

OR personnel must be familiar with a few pieces of important ophthalmic surgery machinery: the vitrectomy machine, the cryotherapy machine, the phacoemulsifier (for cataract removal), and the laser (see Chapter 7 for information about lasers).

### Vitrectomy Machine

Many vitrectomy machines (Fig. 10–17) are capable of allowing the surgeon to perform procedures in the anterior or posterior chamber as well as to perform "combined" procedures involving cataract excision and vitreoretinal surgery. The machines are capable of phacoemulsification, diathermy, and vitreous removal. They offer cutting, irrigation, aspiration, vacuum, and viscous fluid control mode options.

Any vitrectomy machine requires setup time. It is the responsibility of the OR personnel assigned to the room to be familiar with the setup for the machine—and its probes, tubing, and irrigation—used at their institution. Be sure you are familiar with manufacturer's guidelines for priming the tubing and probe or instrument attachment as well as the various modes at which the machine can be set.

## Cryotherapy Machine

*Cryotherapy* is the use of extreme cold to freeze tissue. This therapy is used to treat retinal detachment by freezing the scleral tissue at the area(s) where the retina is detached, thereby avoiding damage to adjacent tissue. It can also be used for some forms of cataract extraction.

An insulated probe is attached to the machine (Fig. 10–18) and the cold is delivered to the tissue. The type of probe used depends on the surgical procedure. Probes are available for the following:

- Retinal surgery (treatment of detachment)
- Cataract surgery
- Trichiasis (ingrown eyelashes) treatment

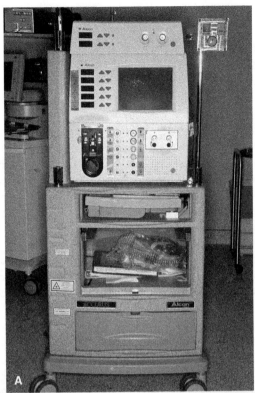

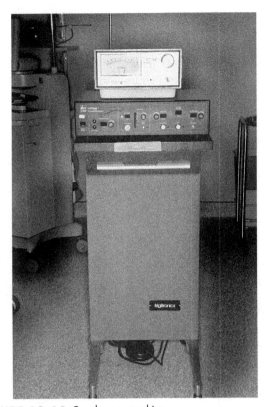

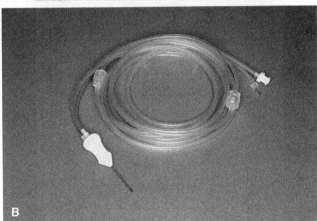

FIGURE 10-17 (A) Vitrectomy machine. (B) Probe.

- Endocryocoagulation
- Dislocated lens removal or repositioning
- Intravitreal foreign body removal

## Phacoemulsifier

The phacoemulsifier (also referred to as the *phaco*) is used during cataract extraction (Fig. 10–19). This machine uses ultrasonic energy to fragment the affected lens into tiny pieces while irrigating and suctioning to remove the pieces. This allows the lens to be removed using a very tiny incision, which in most cases does not require suturing. The tiny incision causes less trauma to the eye than open surgery and allows the procedure to be performed in about 15 minutes.

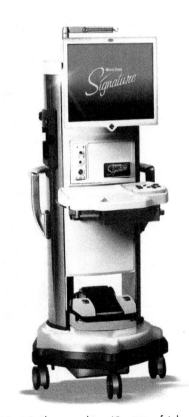

FIGURE 10-19 Phaco machine. (Courtesy of Advanced Medical Optics, Inc.)

Operating room personnel are responsible for setting up and running the phacoemulsifier. There are several models of machines available; before the procedure make sure you are familiar with the machine in your institution. All phacoemulsifiers require the use of irrigating solution, usually balanced saline solution (BSS). In addition to irrigating lens fragments, the BSS helps to maintain intraocular tissue fluid levels. Verify that the BSS is hooked up to the tubing correctly and that the tubing is primed before the procedure. The level of BSS in the bottle needs to be monitored to ensure it does not run out during the procedure.

There are several types of handpieces available, which allow the surgeon to customize the surgery to the needs of the patient.

## EAR, NOSE, AND THROAT EQUIPMENT

### Coblator

Surgeons use the Coblator (Fig. 10–20) for tissue destruction and coagulation during ENT procedures, most notably tonsillectomy and adenoidectomy. The tissue is removed by molecular disintegration, and the tissue bed is coagulated using bipolar energy.

Most of the handpieces used with the machine have built-in suction and irrigation (saline delivery). The different handpieces (also called *wands*) allow the machine to be used for the following:

- Tonsillectomy
- Adenoidectomy
- Uvulopalatoplasty
- Submucosal tissue shrinkage in the oral and nasal cavities

### Powered ENT Instruments

The powered microdissector (also known as a *straight shot*) is used for sinus surgery (Fig. 10–21). The available handpieces allow the machine to be used for medial and lateral cutting in the frontal sinuses as well as polyp removal in the maxillary sinus. The cutting is done by a rotating blade at the tip of the handpiece.

Another version of this type of system offers the option of running a high-speed otologic drill for treatment of acoustic neuroma or performance of a cochleostomy. The drill burr rotates in both forward and reverse and has a built-in water-cooling system.

## GYNECOLOGICAL SURGERY MACHINES

There are very few machines specific to OB-GYN surgeries except for the vacuum curettage. The other machines, most notably the robotics machine and the laser, are discussed

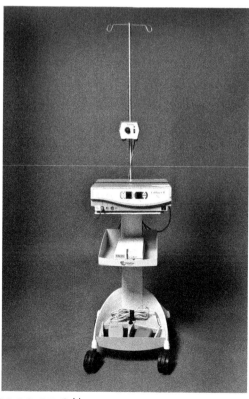

FIGURE 10–20 Coblator.

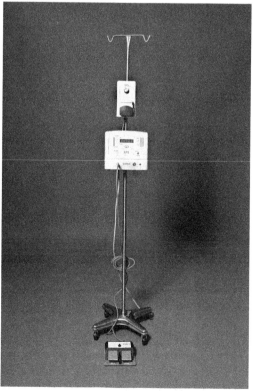

FIGURE 10–21 Powered ENT instrument.

elsewhere in this book because they are used in many types of surgery.

The electric vacuum curettage (Fig. 10–22) is used during dilation and evacuation (D&E) to remove endometrial tissue or products of conception. The D&E can be performed electively or to treat conditions such as a miscarriage, missed or incomplete abortion, or retained placental tissue. This procedure is used most commonly to treat conditions occurring in the first trimester of pregnancy.

A dilation and curettage (D&C) is performed once the cervix is dilated. A disposable curette is attached to the vacuum aspirator suction tubing, the vacuum is activated, and the uterine contents are evacuated. The machine has two collection bottles where the specimen is collected for later retrieval.

The vacuum power on the machine is adjustable. Curettes are available in a variety of diameters from 6 mm to 14 mm.

## LIPOSUCTION

Liposuction is the surgical aspiration of excess fat for the purpose of improving body contours. The excess fat is suctioned out through the use of specially designed suction cannulas and an aspiration machine. Liposuction can be performed on almost any part of the body and has become one of the most commonly performed aesthetic surgeries.

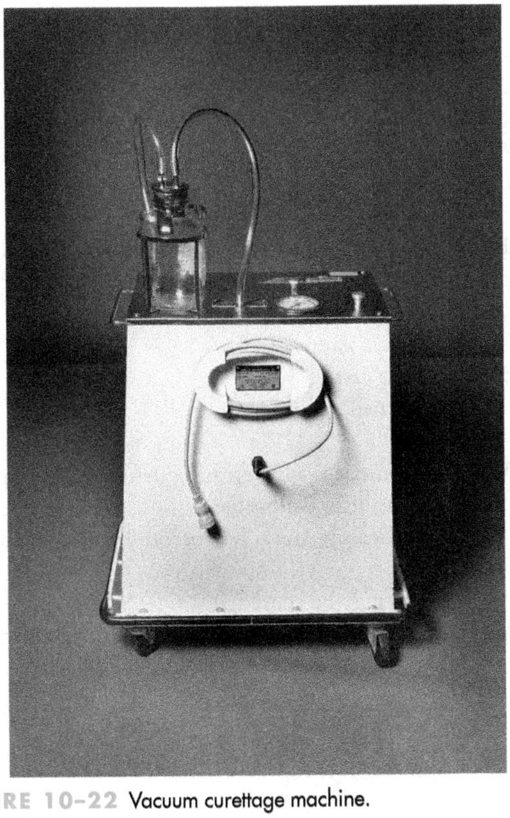

There are many types of liposuction machines in use today. The type of machine being used depends on the setting it is being used in and what procedures it is being used for. Some are larger machines, used for a variety of procedures, and some are smaller machines, used in clinics or doctor's offices for specific procedures.

The aspiration machine (Fig. 10–23) is a high-vacuum machine because fat is thick and cannot be removed from the body using regular suction. The manufacturer will give guidelines for the amount of suction that is safe to use with their machines. Make sure you follow the manufacturer's instructions and guidelines for the specific machine your institution uses.

Before skin incision, the tissue is injected with a mixture of lidocaine, epinephrine, and Ringer's lactate or 0.9% saline intravenous solution. The purpose of the injection is to expand the tissue for easier insertion of the cannula, to provide hemostasis (epinephrine), and to provide local anesthesia (lidocaine). Small incisions are made, the cannula is passed under the skin, and the excess fat is suctioned out.

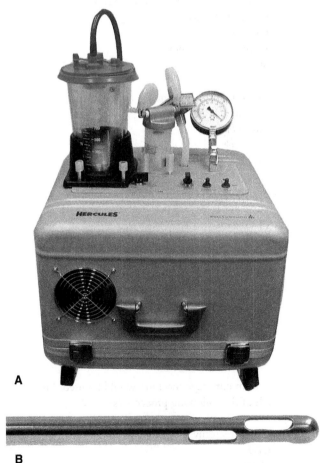

**A**

**B**

FIGURE 10–23 (A) HERCULES 230 VAC aspirator. (B) 3-Port Radial Plus liposuction cannulae. With permission from Wells Johnson Company, Tucson, AZ.

FIGURE 10–22 Vacuum curettage machine.

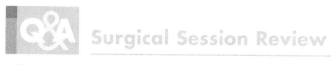 **Surgical Session Review**

1) An ICP monitor measures pressure within the
   a. Chest
   b. Cranium
   c. Carpals
   d. Coronaries

2) Phacoemulsification is used to remove
   a. Cataracts
   b. Wrinkles
   c. Chalazions
   d. Vitreous humor

3) A micropacemaker is appropriate for patients requiring:
   a. Dual-chamber pacing
   b. Support after open heart surgery
   c. Single-chamber pacing
   d. Defibrillation

4) A scleral buckle procedure is used to treat
   a. Corneal abrasion
   b. Glaucoma
   c. Retinal detachment
   d. Sties

5) Trichiasis is another name for an ingrown
   a. Toenail
   b. Fingernail
   c. Abscess
   d. Eyelash

6) Cryotherapy uses _____ to destroy tissue.
   a. Heat
   b. Electricity
   c. Cold
   d. Ultrasound

7) Diathermy uses _____ to destroy tissue.
   a. Heat
   b. Electricity
   c. Cold
   d. Ultrasound

8) A vacuum curettage machine would be used during which of the following procedures?
   a. Hysterectomy
   b. Oophorectomy
   c. D&E
   d. Cerclage

9) The cardiopulmonary bypass machine is operated by a
   a. Surgeon
   b. Nurse
   c. Surgical technologist
   d. Perfusionist

10) In which of the following procedures would cardiopulmonary bypass definitely *not* be used?
   a. Repair of tetralogy of Fallot
   b. Heart transplant
   c. Aortofemoral bypass graft
   d. CABG

11) The straight shot device is used for surgery of the
   a. Hand
   b. Foot
   c. Back
   d. Sinuses

12) A Coblator is used most commonly for a
   a. Coronary bypass graft
   b. Cerclage
   c. Tonsillectomy
   d. Adenoma removal

13) All of the following are types of cardiac valve implants *except:*
   a. Biological
   b. Mechanical
   c. Bioprinted
   d. Metabolic

14) Examples of bone implants include all of the following *except:*
   a. Staple
   b. Cancellous screw
   c. Fiberglass cast
   d. Femoral nail

15) Which statement is *false* regarding handling of implants:
   a. Handle as little as possible
   b. Always measure any screw before handing it to the surgeon
   c. Implants may be reused
   d. Do not use any implant that has been damaged

16) The proper order for the steps for screw insertion is
   a. Measure, drill, tap, screw
   b. Tap, measure, drill, screw
   c. Drill, measure, tap, screw
   d. Drill, tap, measure, screw

17) A bone tap is used to
   a. Create ridges for the screw to follow
   b. Determine the length of screw needed
   c. Screw the plate to the bone
   d. Drill the hole for the screw

18) Which of the following is NOT generally found in the solution used in liposuction?
   a. 0.9% Saline
   b. Gentamycin
   c. Epinephrine
   d. Lidocaine

19) The initials IM in IM nailing or rodding refers to:
   a. Intermedullary
   b. Intramaxillary
   c. Intramandibular
   d. Intramedullary

## TYPES OF ANESTHESIA

The word *anesthesia* comes from the Greek *anaisthesis*, meaning "without sensation." Anesthesia allows us to perform surgery on patients without them feeling pain and, in most cases, recalling the events of the operating room (OR).

Several types of anesthesia are available: general, regional blocks (i.e., spinal, epidural and nerve blocks), monitored anesthesia care (MAC), and local. Depending on what type of surgery is being performed, the patient may have a choice of the type of anesthetic.

This chapter contains a brief description of each type of anesthesia, the surgery for which it is usually used, and common side effects, as well as Watch Out! boxes. Pay particular attention to the Watch Out! boxes because they describe what you need to look for or report if you are the person assisting the anesthesia care provider during the administration of the anesthetic.

### General Anesthesia

#### Description

Commonly described by patients as "going off to sleep," general anesthesia consists of four components: heavy sedation (alteration of consciousness), muscle relaxation, loss of response to pain, and lack of recall of events while under anesthesia. There is not one single medication that produces an adequate level of all four of these components; therefore, the anesthesia provider must use a combination of medications (usually given by the inhalation or intravenous [IV] routes) to achieve optimum results.

#### Stages of General Anesthesia

There are four stages to general anesthesia: induction, maintenance, emergence, and recovery.

**Induction Phase.** During the induction phase, the patient goes from a state of consciousness to a state of unconsciousness. His or her reflexes are also depressed. Respiratory depression may occur. **Maintenance of airway is crucial during this phase!**

Cricoid pressure (also known as *Sellick's maneuver*) is performed to reduce the risk of aspiration or help the anesthesia provider visualize the vocal cords. Firm pressure is applied to the cricoid cartilage using the thumb and index finger in a V formation (Fig. 11–1). This causes the esophagus to be occluded between the cricoid cartilage and the lower cervical vertebrae, thus decreasing the chance of aspiration. Applying pressure to the cartilage can also help to visualize the cords, especially if the patient's anatomy is less than optimal, thus making intubation

easier. When applying cricoid pressure, *do not release the pressure until instructed to do so by the anesthesia care provider.*

**Maintenance.** The second phase of anesthesia is maintenance of the anesthetic. It is during this phase that the surgical procedure takes place. The patient is constantly monitored for homeostasis of all vital functions, and the anesthesia care provider adjusts the anesthetic levels accordingly.

> **WATCH OUT!** | **Induction Phase**
>
> - During induction, another trained person, other than the anesthesia provider, should be positioned by the patient's side near the head of the bed to help, as needed.
> - Personnel helping with anesthesia should have the skill and knowledge to maintain the patient's airway if need be.
> - If the anesthesia provider is using an endotracheal tube, the person assisting should hold the tube and be ready to hand it to the anesthesia provider as soon as he or she visualizes the vocal cords.
> - If the provider is using a stylet to intubate, pull the stylet when asked; be careful not to pull too hard or you might dislodge the tube.
> - If you are providing cricoid pressure (see text for description), do not release pressure until instructed to do so by the anesthesia provider.
> - Hearing is the last sense that leaves the patient during induction. *Talking and noise should be kept to an absolute minimum; be careful what you say!*

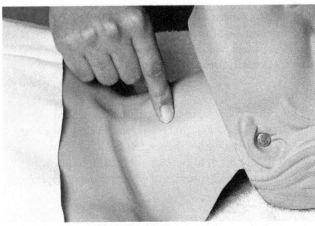

**FIGURE 11–1** Cricoid pressure being held on a mannequin's neck.

**WATCH OUT! Maintenance Phase**

- The circulator needs to be aware of what is going on with the anesthesia care provider. Increased activity "behind the screen" could indicate a change in patient condition. Always keep an eye and ear out and be ready to respond if help is needed.
- Scrubbed personnel need to keep track of the amount of irrigating fluid used and report that number to the anesthesia provider. This is an important step in estimating blood loss.
- Scrubbed personnel need to tell the anesthesia provider when they are about to irrigate with large amounts of fluid. The anesthesia provider needs to be aware of this extensive irrigation so that he or she will not think a large amount of bleeding has suddenly occurred.
- When local anesthetic is used during a procedure, scrubbed personnel need to keep track of the amount injected. The amount, type, and strength of local anesthetic used needs to be reported to the anesthesia care provider.

**WATCH OUT! Emergence Phase**

- During emergence, another trained person, other than the anesthesia provider, should be positioned by the patient's side near the head of the bed to help as needed.
- Personnel helping with anesthesia should have the skill and knowledge to maintain the patient's airway if need be.
- Hearing is often the first sense to return during emergence. *Keep noise to an absolute minimum and be careful what is said!*
- Be prepared to assist if needed after extubation. In rare cases, the patient may need to be reintubated.
- Have oxygen ready for transport to the PACU. (Make sure you have checked the amount of oxygen in the tank before the end of the case!)

**Emergence.** Emergence is the third phase of general anesthesia. This phase occurs as the surgical procedure is finishing. The goal is to have the patient as awake as possible at the end of the procedure. The focus during emergence is on monitoring the patient's ability to resume breathing on his or her own and restoring a gag reflex. The patient is usually extubated, if necessary. A major concern during this phase is the risk of laryngospasm or bronchospasm, which can lead to airway obstruction. The airway must be monitored closely.

**Recovery.** The last phase of general anesthesia is recovery. In this phase, the patient returns to his or her optimal level of consciousness. This phase begins in the OR, continues in the postanesthesia care unit (PACU), and may continue through discharge. Patients are closely monitored in the OR and PACU for signs of increasing levels of consciousness and function.

## Procedures Performed Under General Anesthesia

Any surgical procedure can be performed while the patient is under general anesthesia. The anesthesia care provider, along with the patient and surgeon, decide if the patient is a candidate for general anesthesia.

## Advantages

- Medication dosages can be adjusted as needed.
- Muscle relaxation can be achieved, making for easier visualization within the surgical field.
- Rate and depth of respiration can be controlled.
- Patient is usually unaware of what goes on intraoperatively.

## Disadvantages

- A small percentage of patients are aware of intraoperative events.

- General anesthesia is not for everyone. If the patient has many comorbidities, then he or she may not be a good candidate to undergo general anesthesia.
- Risk of aspiration is greatest during the induction and emergence phases.
- Risk of laryngospasm or bronchospasm is real.
- Risk of malignant hyperthermia is real, although rare, because anesthesia personnel screen patients preoperatively for risk of malignant hyperthermia.
- The chance of postoperative nausea and vomiting is increased.
- The chance of postoperative pain compared with regional anesthesia is increased.

## Regional Anesthesia

### Spinal Anesthesia

To perform a spinal block, the anesthesia care provider injects an anesthetic agent into the subarachnoid space using a spinal needle inserted into an intervertebral space in the lower lumbar area. The patient experiences loss of sensation below the diaphragm.

### Procedures Performed Under Spinal Anesthesia

Spinal anesthesia can be used for procedures below the waist. It is commonly used for orthopedic procedures on the lower limbs (e.g., total knee arthroplasty, total hip arthroplasty), genitourinary procedures, and gynecological procedures.

### Advantages

- Patients remain conscious and in control of their own airways.
- Patients can receive sedation that is titrated to their desired levels of consciousness during the procedure.
- Patients have fewer systemic effects with spinal anesthesia than with general anesthesia; therefore, spinal anesthesia may be a less risky choice of anesthetic for those with multiple comorbidities.

- Patients do not experience the sore throat or hoarseness postoperatively that an endotracheal tube (ETT) can cause.
- Produces bowel contraction, which can facilitate exposure during surgery of the abdomen or pelvis.
- Produces muscle relaxation, making retraction easier.

### Disadvantages

- Hypotension is a major risk!
- The spinal block could travel upward and block the muscles necessary for respiration.
- In a small percentage of cases, the spinal anesthetic is not effective, and the patient must be given a general anesthetic.
- The dosage of medication cannot be titrated. Once it is given, it cannot be adjusted.
- The patient could experience a spinal headache postoperatively.
- The patient could possibly develop temporary or permanent paresthesia or paralysis (very rare).
- Spinal anesthesia cannot be used for procedures of long duration. The length of time depends on the anesthetic agent that is used.

### Epidural Anesthesia

Epidural anesthesia is accomplished by the anesthesia care provider injecting an anesthetic agent into the epidural space that surrounds the dural sac. The anesthetic agent is absorbed slowly through the dura mater into the cerebrospinal fluid.

---

**WATCH OUT!** Spinal Anesthesia

- Hypotension (sudden drop in blood pressure) is a major risk with spinal anesthesia. The person assisting the anesthesia care provider must keep an eye on the blood pressure monitor and report a drop of more than 20 mm Hg systolic to the anesthesia provider immediately. Often, the anesthesia provider's back is to the monitors while inserting the spinal needle; therefore, it is up to the person assisting to watch for hypotension. Continuous monitoring of vital signs is necessary.
- There is a small chance that the spinal block could move upward, thereby blocking the diaphragm and accessory respiratory muscles. The person assisting the anesthesia care provider needs to monitor the patient for signs of difficulty breathing or respiratory distress.
- Proper positioning of the patient before needle insertion is important. A spinal anesthetic can be administered with the patient either lying on his or her side or sitting up and leaning forward (this is usually the anesthesia provider's preference). The person assisting needs to help the patient into the proper position and help the patient maintain that position throughout the procedure; this may require holding the patient in position, especially if he or she has been sedated.
- *Remember:* Watch what is said in the room. The patient is awake!

---

Epidural anesthesia can be a single shot of anesthetic agent or, more commonly, a small catheter is inserted into the back and an intermittent or continuous drip of medication is administered through the catheter to provide ongoing pain control.

### Procedures Performed Under Epidural Anesthesia

Epidural anesthesia is commonly used for procedures of the rectum and pelvis (e.g., obstetrical, gynecological, and urological). It can be used for intraoperative and postoperative pain control or, in some cases, control of intractable pain.

### Advantages

- The agent is more slowly absorbed; therefore, hypotension develops more slowly than with a spinal block, making it easier to treat.
- Medication dosage can be titrated.
- When the need is no longer there, the catheter can be removed.
- Postoperative pain control can be achieved, yet the patient is able to walk and move about.
- The medication pump delivering the agent can be programmed to allow the patient to deliver supplemental doses of medication, as needed.
- The patient remains conscious and cooperative (important during labor).
- The patient remains in control of his or her own airway.

### Disadvantages

- Hypotension can result, although more slowly than with a spinal block.
- In rare cases, the epidural may not be effective, necessitating a switch to another type of anesthetic.
- Accidental puncture of the dura during the insertion could result in total spinal anesthesia, leading to respiratory paralysis and bradycardia.

## Combined Spinal-Epidural Anesthesia
### Description

An epidural needle is passed into the epidural space in the usual manner. A spinal needle is passed through the epidural needle until the dura is pierced. Medication is injected into the subarachnoid space. The spinal needle is removed, and an epidural catheter is placed into the epidural space.

---

**WATCH OUT!** Epidural Anesthesia

- Accidental puncture of the dura during needle insertion could result in total spinal anesthesia. Signs of total spinal anesthesia include bradycardia, respiratory paralysis, and vasodilation.
- Continuous monitoring of vital signs is necessary during insertion of an epidural.
- *Remember:* Watch what is said in the room; the patient is awake!

**WATCH OUT!** Combined Spinal-Epidural Anesthesia

- Same as for epidural and spinal anesthesia.
- Some patients experience pruritus (itching) after injection of the narcotic.
- *Remember:* Watch what is said in the room; the patient is awake!

## Procedures Performed Under Spinal-Epidural Anesthesia

Combined spinal/epidural anesthesia is commonly used for obstetrical procedures or labor pain relief. This technique can also be used for surgical procedures that have extended surgery times.

### Advantages

- Spinal-epidural anesthesia provides immediate benefits from the spinal injection, and the epidural catheter allows for continued anesthesia.
- This type of anesthesia offers less motor block than spinal anesthesia alone.
- The patient remains conscious and cooperative, which is important during labor.
- The patient remains in control of his or her own airway.

### Disadvantages

- Hypotension is a major risk! Monitor the patient for signs of decreased blood pressure.
- The patient could experience a spinal headache postoperatively.
- The patient could potentially develop temporary or permanent paresthesia or paralysis (very rare).

## Nerve Block

Nerve blocks are another option for regional anesthesia. The anesthesia care provider injects an anesthetic agent into either a large peripheral nerve or the area of a *major nerve plexus* (a large bundle or group of nerves). This type of anesthesia allows for temporary loss of sensation to the area innervated by the nerve or plexus.

### Procedures Performed Under Nerve Block

Nerve blocks are commonly used for procedures on the arm or leg. In addition to intraoperative anesthesia, nerve blocks help control postoperative pain (many agents last 18 to 24 hours). In selected cases, a nerve block can be used to control intractable pain (e.g., injection of the intercostal nerves to control rib pain).

### Advantages

- Nerve blocks can be given to a specific area only, without the systemic impact of a general or spinal anesthetic.
- Nerve blocks allow analgesia to continue into the postoperative period.

**WATCH OUT!** Nerve Blocks

- Most of the major nerves run near major arteries. If the medication is accidently injected into the artery, anesthetic overdose could occur. The patient's vital signs should be monitored closely throughout the procedure.
- The anesthesia care provider may ask the person assisting him or her to inject the medication once the correct spot is found. The assistant should aspirate (pull back slightly on the plunger) and then inject 5 to 10 cc of the medication slowly. The assistant should aspirate every 5 to 10 cc until the anesthetic is injected.
- *Remember:* Watch what is said in the room; the patient is awake!

- The duration of the block is medication specific, allowing it to be tailored to the specific needs of the patient or procedure.
- The patient is conscious and in control of his or her own airway.
- Nerve blocks can be combined with other types of anesthesia (e.g., general).

### Disadvantages

- Anesthetic overdose could occur if a major artery is accidently injected, causing seizures or cardiac arrest.

## Bier Block

A Bier block is a regional block of the distal end of an upper extremity. A tourniquet is placed on the upper arm, and the anesthetic is injected intravenously at an area close to the surgical site. The limb is exsanguinated using an Esmarch bandage, and the proximal tourniquet is inflated to about 100 mm Hg above the patient's systolic blood pressure. The tourniquet remains inflated throughout the procedure to prevent the anesthetic agent from being redistributed from the area.

### Procedures Performed Under Bier Blocks

Bier blocks are used for procedures of the distal upper extremity that are less than 1 hour in duration (e.g., closed reduction of a Colles fracture).

### Advantages

- Bier block is a short-acting, localized anesthesia without systemic impact.
- It has a short recovery time after the procedure.
- The patient is conscious and in control of his or her own airway.

### Disadvantages

- It has limited uses (distal upper extremity procedures of short duration).
- The patient could experience adverse cardiovascular effects due to systemic administration of the medication.

> ### WATCH OUT! Bier Block
>
> - If the tourniquet fails or the tourniquet is released too rapidly at the end of the procedure, the patient may experience systemic administration of the medication. Systemic administration can adversely affect the cardiovascular system, causing sudden changes in heart rate and blood pressure. The patient's vital signs should be closely monitored throughout the injection, surgical procedure, and release of the tourniquet.
> - *Remember:* Watch what is said in the room; the patient is awake!

> ### WATCH OUT! Monitored Anesthesia Care
>
> - Supplemental oxygen should be available.
> - The patient's vital signs (especially respiratory status) and level of consciousness need to be closely monitored; usually this is done by the anesthesia care provider, but the circulator must be aware of what is happening.
> - Scrubbed personnel need to keep track of the amount of local anesthetic injected at the surgical site. They need to report to the anesthesia care provider the type, strength, and amount of local used.
> - *Remember:* Watch what is said in the room; the patient is awake!

## Monitored Anesthesia Care

The patient receives sedatives, analgesics, or amnesics to make him or her less aware of intraoperative events. This is done in conjunction with a local anesthetic at the surgical site.

### Procedures Performed Under Monitored Anesthesia Care

Monitored anesthesia care (MAC) can be used for procedures that can be done using local anesthesia when the patient wants some sedation.

### Advantages

- MAC can be used for patients with complex medical problems who are undergoing procedures requiring only local anesthesia.
- It has fewer systemic effects than other types of anesthesia.
- Medication dosages can be titrated.
- The recovery time is shorter after the procedure.
- The patient is conscious and in control of his or her own airway.

### Disadvantages

- MAC cannot be used for complex procedures.
- The patient must be capable of cooperation (e.g., not moving the area the surgeon is working on).

## Local Anesthesia

Local anesthesia is produced when the surgeon injects an anesthetic agent into the tissue surrounding the operative site. This produces a small, localized area of anesthesia/analgesia at the operative site. The length of the anesthesia/analgesia depends on the agent.

### Procedures Performed Under Local Anesthesia

Local anesthesia can be used for simple or short procedures (e.g., wound suturing, pacemaker insertion, chest tube insertion, and removal of small skin lesions). Some surgeons perform breast biopsy and hernia repairs using local anesthesia.

> ### WATCH OUT! Local Anesthesia: Topical Anesthesia
>
> - Depending on institution policy, if the patient is undergoing only local anesthesia, a registered nurse (RN) may be monitoring the patient's vital signs intraoperatively. The RN should NOT be the same nurse who is performing the circulating duties; a dedicated nurse should be assigned to monitor the patient.
> - Supplemental oxygen should be available.
> - If sedation (e.g., Versed) is used, the institution's policy for conscious sedation must be followed.
> - Scrubbed personnel need to keep track of the amount of local anesthetic injected at the surgical site and report to the person monitoring the patient the type, strength, and amount of local used.
> - *Remember:* Watch what is said in the room; the patient is awake!

### Advantages

- Local anesthesia can be used for patients with complex medical problems who are undergoing simple or short procedures.
- Local anesthesia has fewer systemic effects than other types of anesthesia.
- The recovery time is shorter after the procedure.
- The patient is conscious and in control of his or her own airway.
- The surgeon can regulate the amount of medication that the patient receives based on the patient's needs.

### Disadvantages

- Cannot be used for complex procedures.
- The patient must be capable of cooperation (e.g., not moving the area the surgeon is working on).
- May require another RN to be assigned to monitor the patient, depending on institution policy.

## Topical Anesthesia

Topical anesthesia is produced by instilling or swabbing a local anesthetic agent onto mucous membranes or tissue.

### Procedures Performed Under Topical Anesthesia

Topical anesthesia can be used for minor, short-duration procedures of the mucous membranes or skin (e.g., skin tag removal, throat endoscopy, and IV insertion) or as a supplement to other anesthesia (e.g., cocaine in nasal procedures). Topical anesthesia is often used for cataract surgery.

### Advantages

- Topical anesthesia requires a very short recovery time.
- There are fewer systemic effects following topical than other types of anesthesia.
- The patient is conscious and in control of his or her own airway.

### Disadvantages

- Topical anesthesia cannot be used for complex procedures.
- The patient must be capable of cooperation (e.g., not moving the area the surgeon is working on).

## AIRWAYS

When a patient can no longer adequately maintain a patent airway independently, several types of adjuncts can be used. The type of airway chosen depends on the situation: why the person can no longer maintain his or her own airway, how long the surgical procedure is expected to last, or if the person is expected to need ventilatory support postoperatively. This section covers oral and nasal airways, laryngeal mask airways (LMAs), and several types of ETTs.

## Oral Airways

An oral airway is a curved piece of rigid plastic with an opening through the middle or along the sides (Fig. 11–2). It can help to establish or maintain a patent airway in an unconscious patient, or it can be inserted in the mouth to keep the patient from biting down on the endotracheal tubes (EETs).

The oral airway works by lifting the tongue forward to keep it from obstructing the pharynx. This type of airway is to be used only in an unconscious patient without a gag reflex. If

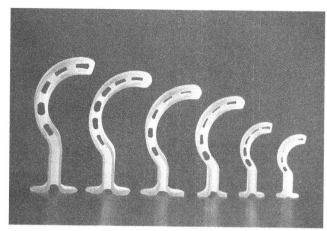

FIGURE 11–2 Oral airway.

the patient has a gag reflex, insertion of an oral airway could lead to gagging, vomiting, or laryngospasm.

Oral airways do not require any special equipment to insert. The airway is inserted into the mouth with the curve facing the roof of the mouth, and then the airway is rotated 180 degrees as you move it toward the back of the oral cavity. The airway tip should come to rest at the front of the pharynx, just behind the back of the tongue, with the phalange of the airway between the patient's lips. The curve of the airway is resting on the tongue, holding it down and keeping the passage to the pharynx open. An alternative method of inserting an oral airway is to depress the tongue with a tongue blade and insert the airway with the tip facing the floor of the mouth.

Oral airways are available in a variety of sizes from newborn (size 000 or 30-mm long) to large adult (size 6 or 120-mm long). To approximate the correct size for your patient, place the phalange of the airway at the base of the patient's ear lobe and lay the airway diagonally across the cheek to the corner of the patient's mouth (on the same side of the face). The tip of the airway should reach the corner of the mouth without overlap (Fig. 11–3). If the airway overlaps

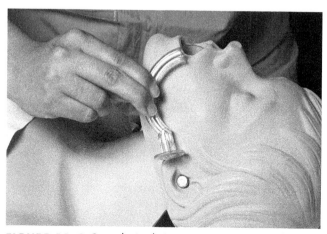

FIGURE 11–3 Correctly sized airway next to mannequin's face.

the lips, the airway is too large; if it doesn't reach the corner of the mouth, the airway is too small.

## Nasal Airways

Unlike the oral airway, nasal airways can be used to help maintain an airway in a patient who still has a gag reflex (Fig. 11–4). The nasal airway is a soft hollow tube with a phalange at one end to prevent it from slipping all the way into the nasal cavity. It rests in the nasopharynx and does not go down far enough into the throat to trigger the gag reflex.

To insert the airway, lubricate it with water-soluble lubricant and insert it into the nares, advancing along the floor of the nasal passage and into the nasopharynx. Nasal airways come in a variety of diameters ranging from 12 Fr to 36 Fr.

Nasal airways can cause *epistaxis* (nasal bleeding) and should not be used in a patient who is on anticoagulants. They should also not be used in children with prominent adenoids or in a patient with a basilar skull fracture.

## Laryngeal Mask Airway

The LMA consists of a wide tube with a 15-mm connector at one end that connects to an anesthesia breathing circuit and an elliptical inflatable cuff at the other end that, when inflated, sits in the laryngopharynx. Three fenestrations in the cuff allow for ventilation of the patient (Fig. 11–5). The cuff is inflated through a pilot tube.

The LMA is becoming increasingly popular as a device to deliver anesthetics for general anesthesia. The LMA does not go through or below the vocal cords and, when properly used, can have less complications than an endotracheal tube.

Not all general anesthesia patients are candidates for the use of an LMA. The LMA should not be used in patients with a full stomach or hiatal hernia, patients with pharyngeal pathology (e.g., abscess, tumor, or obstruction), patients undergoing lengthy procedures, or patients requiring high peak inspiratory pressures.

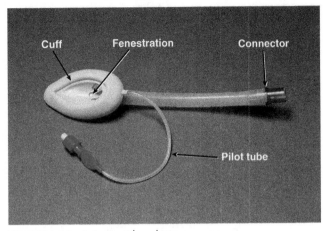

FIGURE 11–5 Laryngeal mask airway.

The LMA comes in both resterilizable and disposable types. Sizes range from size 2 (infant) to size 6 (large adult).

In addition to providing a patent airway, facilitating ventilation, and providing a conduit to deliver anesthetic gases, a special type of LMA can be used to help facilitate placement of an ETT in a patient with a difficult airway. This type of LMA is known as a *Fastrach LMA* (Fig. 11–6).

## Endotracheal Tubes

The ETT (also known as an ET or a TT) is a tube used to provide a patent airway, deliver anesthetic gases, control ventilation, and prevent aspiration during general anesthesia. When you hear about a patient "being intubated," it is generally a reference to the placement of an ETT.

ETTs come either *cuffed,* meaning that they have an inflatable balloon on one end that holds them in place in the trachea, or *uncuffed,* which means there is no inflatable balloon (Fig. 11–7). Although there are exceptions, generally uncuffed tubes are used in small children (to avoid pressure injury to the trachea from the balloon), and cuffed tubes are used in older children and adults.

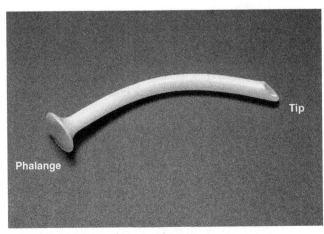

FIGURE 11–4 Nasal airway.

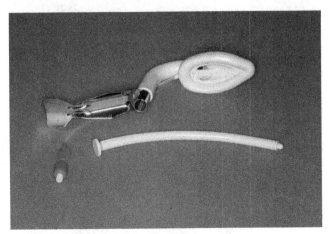

FIGURE 11–6 Fastrach laryngeal mask airway.

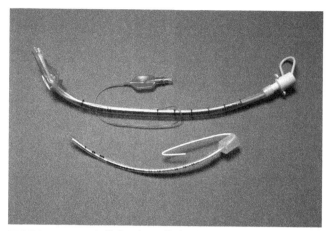

FIGURE 11-7 Cuffed and uncuffed endotracheal tube.

ETTs come in sizes ranging from 2.5 (infant) though 9.0 (large adult). ETTs are single-patient use and cannot be resterilized.

To insert an ETT, the anesthesia care provider uses a laryngoscope. The laryngoscope consists of a handle with an electrical contact onto which a blade with a light bulb is attached. The lighted blade is inserted into the larynx, allowing the anesthesia care provider to examine the larynx and visualize the vocal cords.

Two different types of blades can be attached to the laryngoscope. The Macintosh (or Mac) blade is curved, and the Miller is straight (Fig. 11–8A). Which type of blade the anesthesia care provider uses depends on patient anatomy and, to some degree, personal preference.

As with the ETTs, laryngoscope blades come in a range of sizes from infant/small child (size 0) to large adult (size 4). Laryngoscope handles come in pediatric and adult sizes.

The video laryngoscope gives the anesthesia care provider the ability to view the patient's airway on a video screen in real time, allowing for a well-lit, clearer view of the airway (Fig. 11–8B). The provider intubates the patient while looking

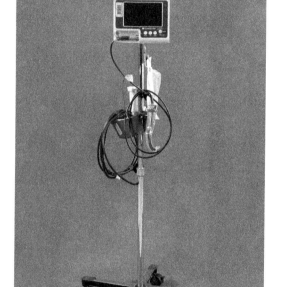

FIGURE 11-8 (A) Laryngoscope handle along with a Miller and a Mac blade. (B) Video laryngoscope.

## Troubleshooting the Laryngoscope

If the light on the laryngoscope is dim or doesn't work, consider the following:
- Does the handle need new batteries?
- If it is a rechargeable handle, does it need to be plugged into a socket to recharge? In this case, you need to get another handle to use.
- Is the electrical contact on the top of the handle tight? If it has come loose, you will not get good contact between the blade and the handle. You can turn this to hand-tighten it.
- Is the light bulb on the blade screwed into the socket tightly?
- Does the light bulb on the blade need to be replaced?

at the video screen, using the special laryngoscope blades and stylets that are part of the system.

The reusable blades come in three sizes, for small to morbidly obese patients. These blades must be resterilized between uses according to the manufacturer's instructions and institutional policy.

### Specialty Endotracheal Tubes

In addition to regular ETTs, there are several tubes designed for specific purposes.

**Right-Angle Endotracheal Tubes.** The right-angle ETT (Fig. 11–9) is specially designed for use in ear, nose, throat, and ophthalmic surgery. This tube has a preformed right-angle bend at the

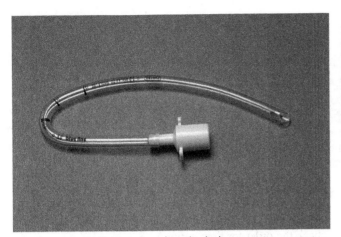

FIGURE 11-9 Right-angle endotracheal tube.

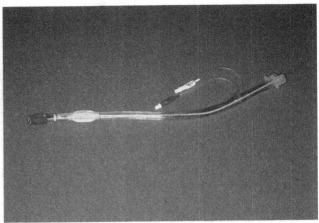

FIGURE 11-11 Double-lumen endotracheal tube.

level of the teeth that allows it to exit the mouth away from the surgical field.

**Laser Surgery Endotracheal Tubes.** Because of the possible danger of fire if a conventional ETT is used during laser surgery of the face and neck, a specially designed laser surgery ETT may be necessary. These tubes are made to resist laser strikes. The cuff of the tube should be inflated with saline mixed with methylene blue to signal if the cuff is hit with the laser and ruptured (Fig. 11–10).

**Double-Lumen Bronchial Tubes.** The double-lumen bronchial tube (Fig. 11–11) is used for thoracic surgery. The advantage to this tube is that it allows the anesthesia care provider to ventilate one lung at a time or both together and allows suctioning of either lung.

## Tracheotomy Tubes

Tracheotomy tubes are airways that are specially designed to fit inside a tracheostomy stoma to keep the stoma open and provide a patent airway. A tracheostomy (also called a *tracheotomy*) can be temporary or permanent, depending on the need

of the patient. It can be done as an emergency procedure or as an elective procedure. Acute upper airway obstruction is the most common reason for an emergency tracheostomy. Conditions causing upper airway obstruction include tumor, infection, foreign body, congenital, or neurological conditions and trauma. Electively, a tracheostomy is often performed for patients who require long-term ventilator support or have a condition causing chronic upper airway obstruction.

Tracheotomy tubes are available cuffed (with a balloon) or uncuffed (Fig. 11–12). Cuffed tracheotomy tubes are used for adults, especially those on ventilators. When the patient is on a ventilator, the cuff must be inflated to prevent air from leaking out around the tube. The cuff may also help prevent saliva or other secretions from entering the lungs. Similar to ETTs, the uncuffed tracheotomy tubes are generally used on children. Uncuffed tracheotomy tubes also can be used in adults who do not require ventilatory support.

Tracheotomy tubes consist of an outer tube and an obturator (introducer). Many tracheotomy tubes also have a removable inner cannula (Fig. 11–13). The inner cannula slides inside the outer tube and can be removed for ease of cleaning or to unblock the tube if it becomes plugged with mucus.

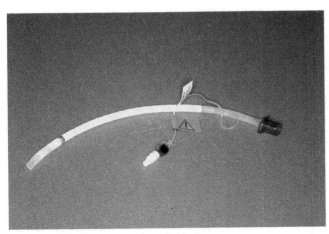

FIGURE 11-10 Laser endotracheal tube.

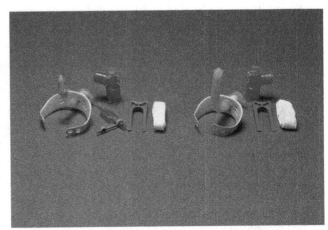

FIGURE 11-12 Cuffed and uncuffed tracheotomy tubes.

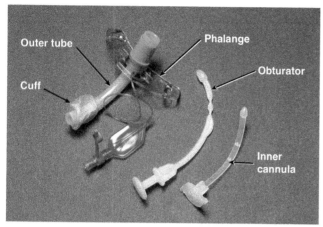

FIGURE 11-13 Parts of a tracheotomy tube.

Tracheotomy tubes are available in a variety of styles, are usually made of plastic, and come with outer diameter sizes ranging from 4 mm (infant) to 13 mm (large adult).

## SUPPLEMENTAL OXYGEN

Oxygen is one of the most important gases in our environment. Without it, our cells could not function, and we would die. We need a constant supply of oxygen, usually from the air we breathe. There are people whose bodies cannot supply their cells with adequate oxygen from breathing, commonly due to lung or heart disease. They need an additional oxygen source, usually a portable or fixed oxygen tank.

Even if we are breathing adequately, there are times that additional oxygen is needed. Preoperatively or intraoperatively, regional or MAC, medication may be given to help patients relax, but it can make them drowsy, less apt to take deep breaths, and in need of an additional source of oxygen. Before induction of general anesthetic, patients are asked to breathe oxygen to fill their lungs and give them an oxygen reserve. Oxygen is given (along with the gases) during general anesthetic to keep the body cells functioning properly. Postoperatively, oxygen is given to help the patient wake up from anesthesia as well as to help combat the effects of the anesthetics and narcotics.

Several devices can be used to deliver supplemental oxygen: nasal cannulas, reservoir and nonreservoir masks, bag-valve-mask devices, and nebulizers. These devices and their use are covered in this section.

### TIP Oxygen Is a Medication

Because oxygen is used so commonly in the OR environment, we tend to forget that it is a *medication,* requiring a doctor's (or certified registered nurse anesthetist's) order for its use. Many institutions have standing orders for the use of oxygen. Be sure to check your institution's policies and procedures.

## Nasal Cannula

A nasal cannula, also called *nasal prongs,* consists of two soft plastic tubes that are inserted into the patient's nostrils (Fig. 11–14). These tubes are attached to a narrow plastic hose that is looped around the patient's ears and under his or her chin to keep the prongs in place. The hose is attached to an oxygen supply (tank or wall source). Nasal cannulas are available in several styles and in adult and pediatric sizes.

A nasal cannula delivers a lower concentration of oxygen (23% to 35%) than an oxygen mask. It is used for those patients requiring smaller amounts of supplemental oxygen (e.g., patients who have been medicated and are drowsy). The oxygen flow is generally set at 1 to 4 L/min. (*Note:* Be sure to check the order for flow setting.)

Most patients tolerate a nasal cannula well, even those who are claustrophobic, because it does not cover the mouth and nose like an oxygen mask does. The nasal prongs can be irritating, mostly because the oxygen is not humidified, and it dries out the mucous membranes of the nostrils.

## Nonreservoir Mask

The nonreservoir or "simple" oxygen mask is a lightweight, plastic, somewhat triangle-shaped device designed to cover the patient's mouth and nose (Fig. 11–15). The mask is placed on the patient's face with the pointed end over the top of the patient's nose and the rounded end below the patient's mouth. It is attached to the patient's head using an elastic strap to secure it in place. The hose is attached to an oxygen supply (tank or wall source). Nonreservoir masks are available in adult and pediatric sizes.

Simple masks can deliver oxygen concentrations of 30% to 45% with a flow rate of 5 to 6 L/min and 40% to 60% with a flow rate of 7 to 8 L/min. These masks should be used for patients requiring higher oxygen concentrations than can be delivered by nasal cannulas but who are expected to need the oxygen for short-term use (e.g., patients in the PACU waking up from anesthesia). These devices are not for use in patients who are profoundly hypoxic or tachypneic.

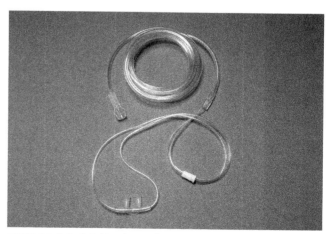

FIGURE 11-14 Nasal cannula.

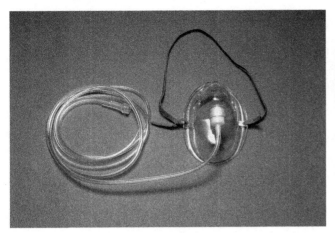

FIGURE 11-15 Nonreservoir mask.

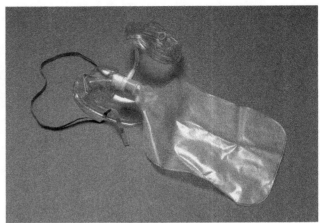

FIGURE 11-16 Partial rebreather mask.

## Reservoir Mask

The reservoir mask is an oxygen mask with a built-in gas reservoir. Reservoir masks are the delivery device of choice for patients needing high concentrations of oxygen for short periods of time—that is, those who may have significant hypoxemia but are breathing relatively normally (e.g., myocardial infarction or trauma patients). There are two types: partial rebreathing mask and nonrebreathing mask. The differences are in the valves in the mask and between the mask and bag.

The partial rebreathing mask has a reservoir where "part" (thus the phrase *partial rebreathing*) of the patient's expired gas volume fills the reservoir bag (Fig. 11–16). The expired gas mixes with the fresh gas (oxygen). Usually, this expired gas is mostly dead space and does not result in the patient rebreathing a significant amount of carbon dioxide. The mixing of the fresh and expired gases can potentially conserve oxygen use. The partial rebreathing mask can deliver oxygen concentrations of 35% to 60% with a flow rate of 7 to 10 L/min.

The nonrebreathing mask has a flap-type valve between the mask and bag (reservoir) and over at least one of the mask's side ports (exhalation port). The valve between the bag and reservoir prevents expired air from entering the mask (and being rebreathed) whereas the valve over the side port limits the amount of room air that can enter the mask. Oxygen concentrations of 100% can be obtained with a flow rate of 15 L/min.

### Guidelines for the Simple Oxygen Mask

- The body of the mask acts as a reservoir for oxygen and expired carbon dioxide. In order for the patient to avoid rebreathing his or her own carbon dioxide, a *minimum* flow rate of 5 L/min is required when using a simple mask.
- One important factor in determining the oxygen concentration of any mask is that it fits the face properly. The mask should completely cover the mouth and nose and fit snugly against the face without large gaps.

Reservoir masks are available in adult and pediatric sizes. To work properly, these types of masks must be used with a flow rate of at least 7 L/min. Fill the reservoir (bag) with oxygen before placing on the patient's face.

## Bag-Valve-Mask Device

Commonly referred to as a *BVM device,* the bag-valve-mask is used to provide ventilation to the patient who is unable to breathe (or breathe adequately) on his or her own. There are two types of devices: the anesthesia bag (Fig 11–17A) and the disposable self-inflating "Ambu"-type bag (Fig. 11–17B).

The anesthesia bag is a non–self-inflating bag that requires a continuous oxygen source to keep the reservoir (bag) inflated. These systems have adjustable valves to allow for the regulation of oxygen flow in response to changing breathing patterns or demands. The bags on these systems should not be allowed to deflate substantially; therefore, oxygen flow to the system should be kept relatively high (although the bag should not be allowed to overinflate either).

The self-inflating bags are used most often when a patient is in respiratory arrest or when a patient who cannot adequately breathe is being transported to another area such as a PACU or intensive care unit. In order to ventilate the patient, the bag is attached to a mask or ETT and the bag is repeatedly squeezed (just hard enough to make the chest rise) and released.

*Caution:* Unlike the anesthesia bag that deflates if the flow of oxygen is inadequate (a visual sign that something is wrong), these bags do not look any different. The equipment needs to be checked to make sure that the hose is attached to the oxygen source, that the oxygen source is turned on, and that there is an adequate flow rate (15 L/min).

## Nebulizers

Nebulizers can be used to deliver moistened (mist) oxygen therapy or medications to patients. These devices are adjustable to allow for the delivery of a variety of oxygen concentrations, depending on patient need. One common use for these devices in the surgical setting is postintubation in the

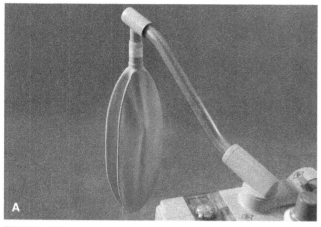

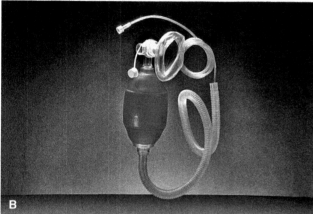

FIGURE 11-17 (A) Anesthesia bag valve mask. (B) Self-inflating bag.

PACU; the aerosol (mist) properties help moisten the airway (Fig. 11–18).

Nebulizers used for mist therapy come in a variety of devices, including face tents, tracheostomy collars, or T pieces (that fit on ETTs). Depending on the liter flow of gas and the valve adjustment, these devices can deliver oxygen concentrations of 24% to 100%.

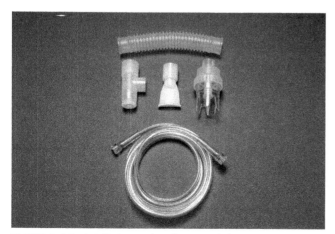

FIGURE 11-18 T-piece and medication nebulizer.

## Guidelines for Nebulizer Treatments

When nebulizers are used for mist, there are several things to look for:
- Observe the mist. If it disappears during inspiration, the oxygen flow to the system is inadequate.
- Some patients may have bronchospasm due to irritation from the aerosol. In this case, a heated, nonaerosol humidification system can be substituted.
- Check the tubing frequently for water collection. Excess water in the tubing can obstruct gas flow.

Nebulizers that are used for medication administration are handheld. The medication and a small amount of saline are added to the chamber of the nebulizer, and oxygen flow is turned on. The medication is converted to an aerosol form that the patient can inhale. The medication nebulizer is used to administer bronchodilators either preoperatively or postoperatively.

## SUCTION

In the OR, suction is used to clear blood, mucus, and other secretions from the patient's airway or the surgical site (Fig. 11–19). Suction also can be used to remove smoke plume from the surgical field. There should always be at least two suction devices available: one for the surgical field and one to help with airway maintenance.

Suction systems consist of several parts. A suction tip or catheter is attached to sterile tubing. The tubing is attached to a vacuum source that is attached to a collection device for the secretions. When activated, the system uses a vacuum power unit to suck the secretions up through the tip/tubing and into the collection device. The vacuum unit can be fixed (e.g., wall suction) or portable. The collection device can be disposable (e.g., rigid plastic container) or reusable or have a disposable liner (e.g., suction carousel).

Suction devices have regulators at the vacuum source so that the strength of the vacuum power can be adjusted. The suction power is expressed in millimeters of mercury (mm Hg). The maximum suction strength depends on the unit, generally varying from −550 mm Hg to −700 mm Hg. The amount of suction used depends on what it is being used for. For wound suction, it is generally set in the high medium range; for suctioning airway secretions, it is generally in the high range (airway secretions are thicker and therefore require a higher vacuum setting).

Several types of suction tips are available, but the two most commonly used to maintain the airway are the Yankauer (tonsil) and the flexible suction catheter (Fig. 11–20). The Yankauer or tonsil suction is a long, semirigid tip that is curved toward the end to allow for suctioning the back of the throat. It has a

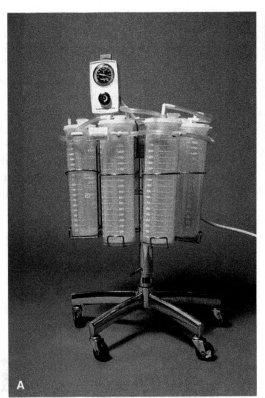
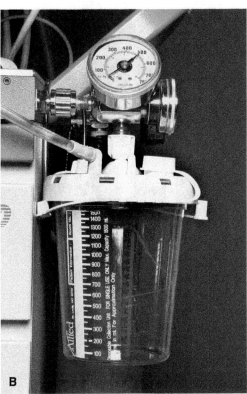

FIGURE 11-19 (A) Suction carousel. (B) Rigid collection canister.

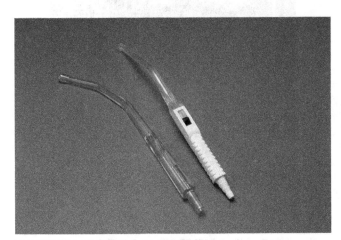

FIGURE 11-20 Yankauer suction tips.

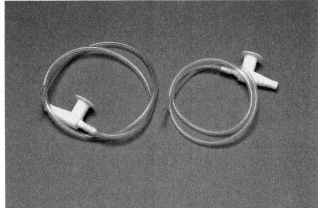

FIGURE 11-21 Small and large suction catheters.

rounded tip with several holes and can suction large amounts of secretions. This tip is used to suction the mouth and pharynx. It is available in a reusable (metal) or disposable (plastic) models.

The soft suction catheter is a flexible tube with holes at the end. It has a thumb control at the proximal end that you occlude with your thumb when you want to apply suction (Fig. 11–21). This tip is used to suction the nasopharynx, the oropharynx, or inside the ETT. To accommodate suctioning varying sizes of ETTs and patients, the flexible suction catheter is available in sizes 5 Fr to 24 Fr.

## ANESTHESIA MACHINERY

Walk into any OR and look toward the head of the bed. What do you see? Usually the answer is the anesthesia machine and a variety of other machines used by anesthesia personnel to provide patient care. This section provides a brief description of the commonly used machines, their use, and the precautions that OR staff need take.

### Anesthesia Machine

The largest and most noticeable machine at the head of the OR bed is the anesthesia machine (Fig. 11–22), which is needed to

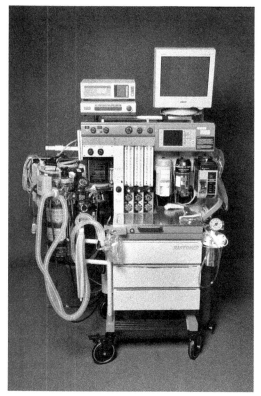

FIGURE 11-22 Anesthesia machine.

administer general anesthesia. There are many different models of anesthesia machines, but most can be divided into its two parts: the anesthetic delivery system and the monitoring system. The monitors usually are positioned on the top of the machine. They allow the anesthesia care provider to monitor the patient's cardiac rhythm (electrocardiogram [ECG]), blood pressure, pulse, end-tidal carbon dioxide (end-tidal $CO_2$), and oxygen saturation. In most cases, the monitoring system is configured to allow blood pressure monitoring through the use of a cuff (noninvasive) or an arterial line (invasive).

The anesthetic delivery portion of the machine delivers air, oxygen, and nitrous oxide to the patient (either from tanks or wall outlets) and converts the volatile anesthetics to gas vapors that the patient can breathe. After general anesthetics have been administered to the patient, this machine allows for manual or mechanical ventilation.

The anesthetic gases are delivered to the patient through a series of hoses that are configured to create a circular flow. This is known as a *circuit*. There are three types of circuit configurations: *open (semiopen), closed,* and *semiclosed.*

As the name implies, the *open* system allows atmospheric gases to enter the system; it is "open" to the outside atmosphere. In this system, almost all the exhaled gases are vented out of the system instead of being rebreathed. An open system can be more expensive to use because of the increased amount of anesthetic required by the patient. This system is used mostly for pediatric patients.

In contrast to the open system, the *closed* system enables the patient to rebreathe exhaled anesthetic. The exhaled anesthetic

is captured and recycled through the circuit. This system uses less anesthetic gases, which means that it can be less expensive to use, and it helps to maintain respiratory humidity and core body temperature.

In a *semiclosed* system, some anesthetic gases are allowed to escape whereas some are recycled through the system. In both the open and semiclosed systems, a gas salvaging system captures the exhaled gases. To prevent the patient from rebreathing his or her own carbon dioxide, a soda lime reservoir is part of the circuit (Fig. 11–23). The soda lime absorbs the carbon dioxide.

Another part of the anesthesia machine is the vaporizer (Fig. 11–24). The vaporizer converts volatile liquid anesthetics

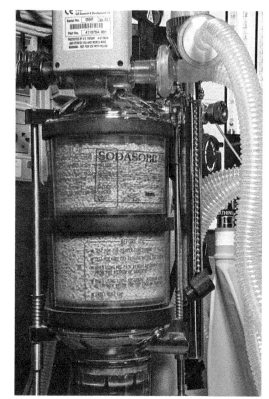

FIGURE 11-23 Soda lime canister.

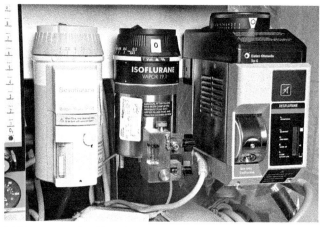

FIGURE 11-24 Vaporizer.

such as desflurane, sevoflurane, and isoflurane to a gaseous state so they can be inhaled by the patient through the circuit. Each liquid anesthetic has different characteristics; therefore, the machine contains a separate vaporizer for each.

The last part of the machine controls the patient's ventilation. The anesthesia care provider can deliver gases and control the patient's ventilatory rate and volume either manually (by squeezing the bag) or automatically (by switching on the ventilator) (Fig. 11–25).

## Bispectral Index Monitor

The bispectral index (BIS) monitor allows the anesthesia care provider to monitor the patient's level of consciousness under general anesthesia (Fig. 11–26). The machine takes electroencephalogram (EEG) data from the patient's brain and processes it to come up with a single number that corresponds to the patient's depth of anesthesia. The use of this device may reduce the incidence of patient awareness during anesthesia, and it may reduce the amount of drug needed to ensure amnesia, thus leading to faster wake-up times. Numeric values of 40 to 60 have been recommended for ensuring adequate levels of general anesthesia (and patient amnesia).

The monitor is attached to the patient by use of a special sensor strip attached to the patient's forehead. The sensor strip is then attached to a cord coming from the machine.

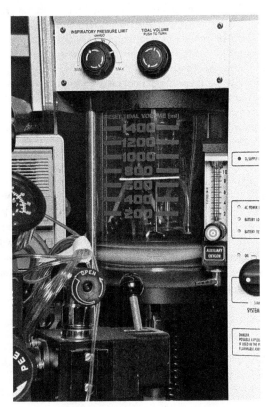

FIGURE 11-25 Ventilator.

### Guidelines for Cleaning the Anesthesia Machine Between Patients

Decontamination and cleaning of the anesthesia machine between patients may be the responsibility of an anesthesia tech, an anesthesia care provider, or the OR staff, depending on the institution. Institutional policies for cleaning and decontamination may vary (be sure to check your institution's policies), but there are some general rules:

- Follow standard precautions when handling any contaminated equipment or supplies.
- Change all equipment that comes in contact with the patient (single-use items such as masks, hoses, ventilation bag, ECG leads) or decontaminate it (blood pressure cuffs, nondisposable pulse oximeter probes, ECG lead wires).
- Change soda lime canisters between patients or when they are used up, depending on institutional policy. The soda lime granules turn purple when they are used; too much purple is an indication that they need to be changed.
- Remove used laryngoscope blades from the room and clean or sterilize them according to your institution's policies.
- Check all hoses to make sure they are connected and snug, not loose.

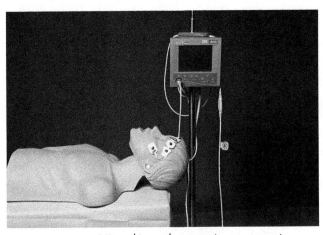

FIGURE 11-26 BIS machine and sensor strip on mannequin.

## Syringe Infusion Pump

Syringe infusion pumps are designed so that anesthesia or other care providers can insert a syringe of medication (e.g., propofol) and infuse the medication into the patient's IV at a set rate. Infusion rates can be adjusted using dials on the face of the machine. For the model shown in Fig. 11–27, a library of SMART LABELS is available for various commonly used medications. The SMART LABELS are magnetically coded and drug specific. The provider changes the SMART LABEL when he or she inserts a syringe of new medication into the machine. The dosages are already figured on the label, thus saving calculation time and decreasing chance of calculation errors.

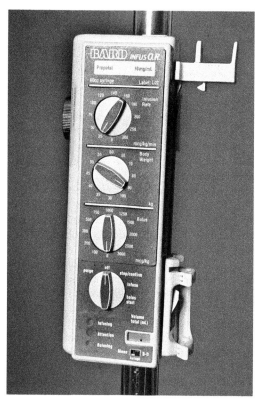

FIGURE 11–27 Syringe infusion pump.

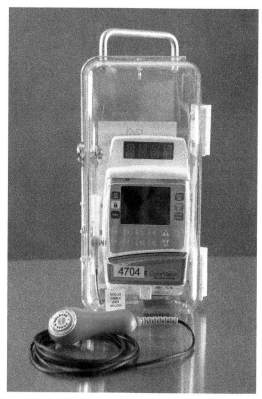

FIGURE 11–28 Patient-controlled anesthesia and epidural pump.

The newer models of syringe infusion pumps have fully programmable screens that are used to set the medication infusion rates.

## Patient-Controlled Anesthesia and Epidural Pump

Patient-controlled anesthesia and epidural pumps are programmable, allowing the care provider to set the machine to deliver a preset amount of medication to the patient at given intervals (Fig. 11–28). These pumps can be used to deliver medication through an epidural catheter or an IV line. The pump can be programmed to deliver the medication continuously, intermittently (by having the patient push a button), or both. These pumps require special tubing.

## PATIENT WARMING EQUIPMENT

Intraoperative and postoperative *hypothermia* (lower than normal body temperature) can lead to a multitude of complications: increased risk of surgical site infection, coagulation problems, increased risk of morbid cardiac events, and delayed drug absorption. To help combat hypothermia, devices exist to help regulate body temperature, both interoperatively and postoperatively.

## Forced-Air Warming Blankets

Forced-air warming blankets blow forced hot air into a special blanket that is used to continuously warm the patient. The Bair

**WATCH OUT!** **Bair Hugger**

- Bair Hugger devices should be used only with the special blanket attached. The unattached hose should NEVER be placed next to the patient's skin or under the regular blankets. Patient skin burns have occurred when the hose was used without the blanket!
- Bair Hugger hoses should not be used to warm the sheets before the patient's arrival in the OR; heating the sheets could cause a burn or fire. The air from the hose also causes the sheets to flap around and increases the amount of air current, which spreads contamination in the OR.

Hugger is one such device (Fig. 11–29). The temperature can be adjusted to low, medium, or high (depending on the patient, length of surgery, type of procedure, and temperature of the OR). Approximately 25 different blankets are available for use with the Bair Hugger; many are designed to allow access for specialized procedures (e.g., cardiac surgery, cath laboratory, outpatient) whereas other modules are specifically for the upper, lower, or full body.

## Liquid Circulating Heating and Cooling Devices

Liquid-filled devices, such as the Blanketrol, circulates heated or cooled water through coils in a special blanket, allowing for control of patient body temperature (Fig. 11–30). Many machines can be operated in one of three modes: *automatic* (controls patient temperature), *manual* (controls water temperature), and *monitor* (monitors the patient's temperature through use of a probe). The devices have a warming mode to help prevent intraoperative hypothermia and a cooling mode to help decrease patient body temperature (e.g., in patients with high fevers). Blankets are available in single-patient use or reusable styles, although most institutions now use the single-use style.

## Fluid Warmer

Fluid/blood warmers heat IV solutions or blood before infusion into the patient. The model shown in Fig. 11–31 uses a warm water bath to heat the fluid to between 95°F and 105°F in about 4 minutes. Special tubing is required for use with this machine.

# DEFIBRILLATOR

The purpose of a defibrillator is to allow for monitoring, defibrillating, cardioversion, or pacing during an untoward cardiac event. Most models use pads for "hands-off" delivery of electricity. The defibrillator pictured in Fig. 11–32A and B allows for use of pads or "paddles" (hands-on delivery). Paddles cannot be used for pacing; therefore, most practitioners prefer to apply the pads because they can be used for any mode.

The electricity delivered to the heart can be either a monophasic or biphasic configuration. Biphasic technology is the newer technology. A biphasic defibrillator requires a lower setting of electricity (200 joules maximum), whereas a monophasic defibrillator requires a setting of 360 joules maximum. Make sure you know which type (monophasic or biphasic) of defibrillator your department has; its recommended settings; how to operate it safely; and how to attach the pads, paddles, and internal paddles. Pads, paddles, and internal paddles are available in adult and pediatric sizes.

The internal paddles require far less energy (10 to 40 joules for an adult) and are applied directly to the heart. They can

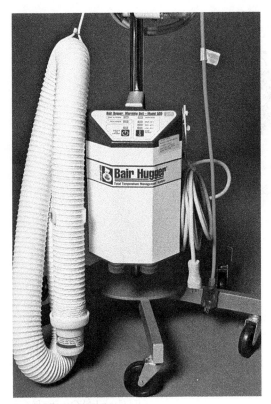

FIGURE 11–29 Bair Hugger.

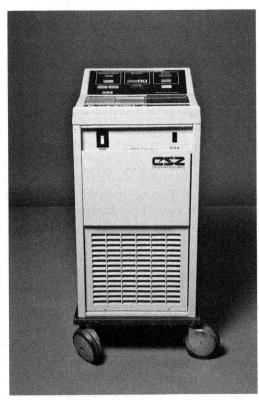

FIGURE 11–30 Blanketrol device.

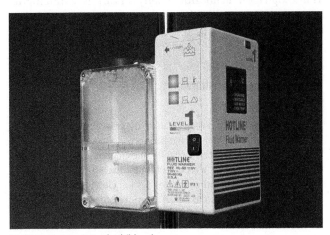

FIGURE 11–31 Fluid/blood warmer.

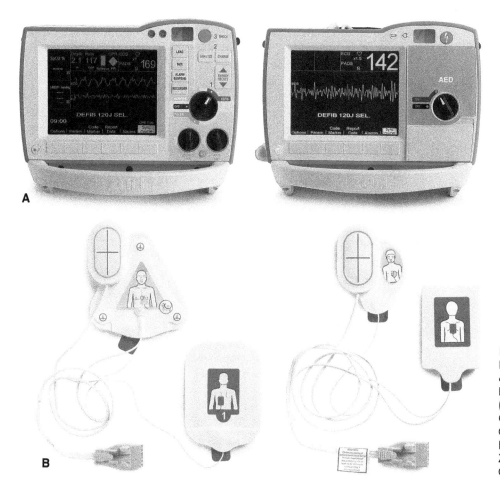

FIGURE 11-32 (A) (From left) R Series® Monitor/Defibrillator and R Series Plus Monitor/Defibrillator in AED Mode. (B) (From left) OneStep™ CPR Complete Electrode (adult) and OneStep™ Pediatric CPR Electrode (pediatric). Courtesy of Zoll Medical Corporation, Chelmsford, MA.

only be used if the chest cavity is opened up (e.g., thoracic surgeries, open heart procedures).

## SCOPES

### Transesophageal Echocardiography Scope

Transesophageal echocardiography (TEE) is a fiberoptic scope with an ultrasound transducer connected to the distal end (Fig. 11–33). The scope and transducer are threaded through the patient's mouth and into the esophagus. The esophagus sits directly behind the heart; therefore, the ultrasound beam has less obstructions to travel through than a standard external ultrasound in which the transducer is placed on the outside of the chest and the beam has to travel through skin, tissue, muscles, and ribs. The TEE gives a much clearer picture of the heart. Most modern TEE machines have features that allow for color Doppler imaging of blood flow through the cardiac valves. These types of images are most often done in patients undergoing cardiac surgery, but they could be done for any patient with suspected cardiac disease (especially valve, atrial, or ventricular abnormalities). In the OR setting, TEE should be performed by anesthesia providers who are familiar with its use and interpretation.

### Fiberoptic Bronchoscopes

Fiberoptic bronchoscopes are used for direct visualization of the respiratory tract and lungs (Fig. 11–34). These scopes are most often used in the OR for placement of an ETT into a patient who is difficult to intubate using a conventional laryngoscope. They can also be used to place a "double"

---

### Guidelines for Defibrillators

- Defibrillators should only be used by personnel who know how to operate the machine properly. Injury to the patient or other personnel can occur if used improperly.
- Before pushing the "shock" button to discharge the electrical shock, give a verbal cue (e.g., "I'm clear, you're clear, everyone is clear") and LOOK to make sure no one is touching the patient or the stretcher or bed.

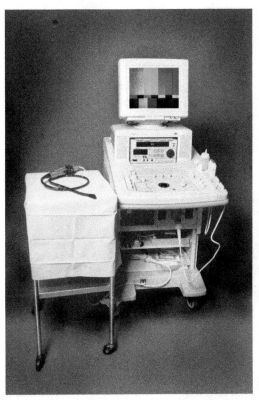

FIGURE 11-33 Transesophageal echocardiography scope and machine.

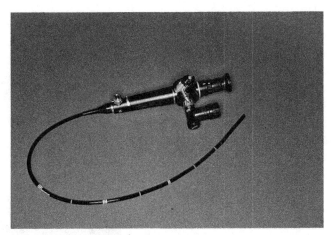

FIGURE 11-34 Bronchoscope.

ETT in a patient who is undergoing lung surgery. Bronchoscopes are available in various sizes, including adult and pediatric.

In this section are pictures and brief descriptions of some of the other equipment and medications that anesthesia care providers use when providing patient care in the OR.

## GENERAL EQUIPMENT

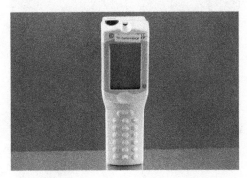

**Name:** POC (point-of-care) blood analyzer
**Alias:** none
**Use:** allows bedside testing of the patient's blood chemistries
**Features:** quick, accurate test; allows for easy testing intraoperatively
**Additional Information:** should be used only by those who have been trained in its proper use; test strips should be checked periodically for outdating

**Name:** glucometer

**Alias:** glucose testing machine

**Use:** allows bedside testing of the patient's blood sugar level

**Features:** quick, accurate test; allows for easy testing intraoperatively

**Additional Information:** should be used only by those who have been trained in its proper use; test strips should be checked periodically for outdating

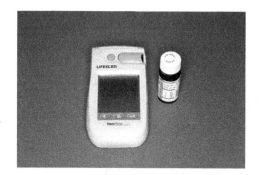

**Name:** transport monitor

**Alias:** none

**Use:** monitors cardiac rhythm and vital signs during transport

**Features:** small, compact size makes for easy portability

**Additional Information:** able to monitor ECG, oxygen saturation, pulse, and blood pressure

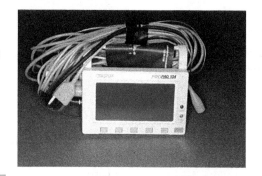

**Name:** temperature monitoring disc

**Alias:** none

**Use:** placed on patient's forehead to monitor skin surface temperature during surgery

**Features:** peel-off backing allows for adhesion to the patient's skin

**Additional Information:** single-patient use

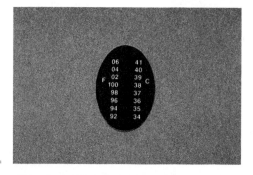

**Name:** Broselow tape

**Alias:** none

**Use:** estimates weight of pediatric patients for medication dosage calculation

**Features:** color-coded by weight; provides common emergency medication calculations estimated on it by weight; provides the size of tubes, etc., to use by weight; weight is estimated according to child's height: lay the marked end of the tape at the child's head and where the bottom of his or her feet fall is the estimated weight

**Additional Information:** laminated for easy cleaning between patients; has calculations up to 34 kg

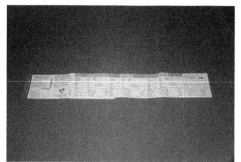

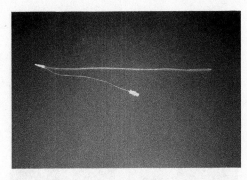

**Name:** esophageal stethoscope

**Alias:** none

**Use:** monitors heart and breath sounds during surgery

**Features:** hooked up to a fitted earpiece to allow the anesthesia care provider to monitor heart and breath sounds while listening to other OR sounds and communication

**Additional Information:** inserted by anesthesia care provider after patient is asleep and intubated

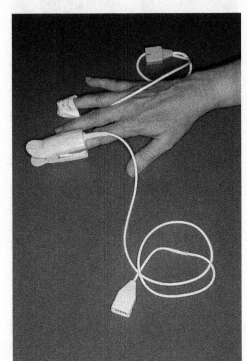

**Name:** oxygen saturation probe

**Alias:** none

**Use:** measures the oxygen saturation present in the patient's hemoglobin

**Features:** noninvasive; probe clips or tapes onto finger or toe

**Additional Information:** available with reusable or disposable probes

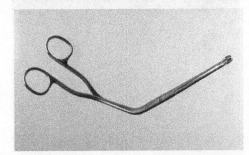

**Name:** Magill catheter introducing forceps

**Alias:** intubating forceps

**Use:** grasping ETT during intubation; grasping and removing foreign bodies from the airway

**Additional Information:** can be used to grasp other types of catheters during insertion

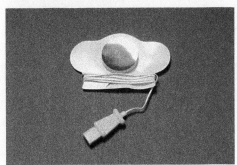

**Name:** skin temperature sensor

**Alias:** none

**Use:** enables intraoperative skin temperature monitoring

**Features:** adhesive side has a tiny probe embedded that is touching the skin to monitor the skin temperature

**Additional Information:** plug end is attached to the temperature monitor

**Name:** tracheal tube introducer

**Alias:** Bougie

**Use:** aids with insertion of ETT

**Features:** flexible; atraumatic Coude type tip

**Additional Information:** available in 6-Fr, 10-Fr, and 15-Fr sizes

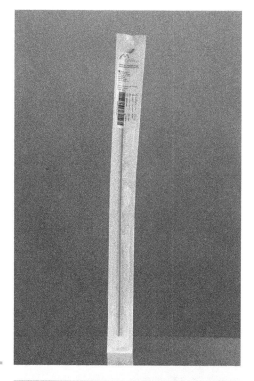

**Name:** ECG leads

**Alias:** monitor electrodes

**Use:** placed on the chest to allow for attachment of ECG monitoring electrodes

**Features:** self-adhesive

**Additional Information:** available in adult and pediatric sizes; single use only

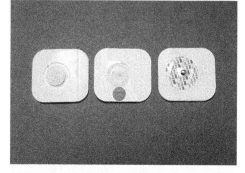

**Name:** Bullard laryngoscope

**Alias:** none

**Use:** aids in visualizing the airway when there is an inability to align the axes of the airway, such as in patients with upper body burns, unstable cervical fractures, anterior larynx, or temporomandibular joint immobility

**Features:** rigid; needs a fiberoptic light source; can be used in a patient whose mouth opening is as little as 6 mm; can be used to aid in nasal and oral intubations

**Additional Information:** available in pediatric and adult sizes

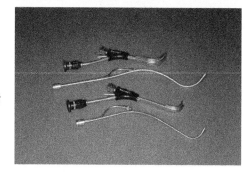

# BLOCK NEEDLES AND SUPPLIES

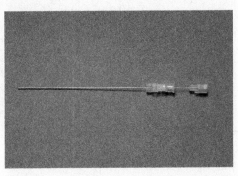

**Name:** Sprotte spinal needle

**Alias:** none

**Use:** creates a pathway for the introduction of regional anesthetics into the spinal canal for spinal analgesia/anesthesia; can be used to inject medication into deep or hard-to-reach areas (e.g., cervix)

**Features:** 3.5 to 5 inches long; pencil tip point; designed for atraumatic dural puncture; "noncutting point"

**Additional Information:** available in 22-gauge to 29-gauge sizes; available with or without an introducer

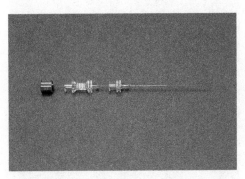

**Name:** Quincke spinal needle

**Alias:** none

**Use:** creates a pathway for the introduction of regional anesthetics into the spinal canal for spinal analgesia/anesthesia; can be used to inject medication into deep or hard-to-reach areas (e.g., cervix)

**Features:** 90-mm long; sharp, cutting point

**Additional Information:** available in 18-gauge to 29-gauge sizes; available with or without an introducer

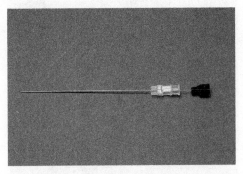

**Name:** Whitacre spinal needle

**Alias:** none

**Use:** creates a pathway for the introduction of regional anesthetics into the spinal canal for spinal analgesia/anesthesia; can be used to inject medication into deep or hard-to-reach areas (e.g., cervix)

**Features:** pencil point tip; 3.5- to 5.5-inches long

**Additional Information:** available in 18-gauge to 27-gauge sizes; available in regular or high-flow style

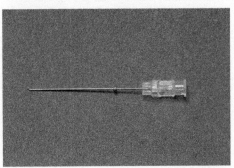

**Name:** regional block needle

**Alias:** security bead needle

**Use:** administers medication for regional nerve blocks

**Features:** 1.5-inch-long security bead on the shaft of the needle to prevent overinsertion

**Additional Information:** available in 20- and 22-gauge sizes

**Name:** spinal block kit

**Alias:** none

**Use:** used to insert needle for administration of spinal anesthesia

**Features:** contains all needed supplies and equipment to administer spinal anesthesia

**Additional Information:** practitioner may choose to add additional supplies per personal preference; inside of the kit is considered sterile

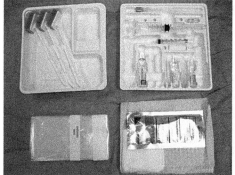
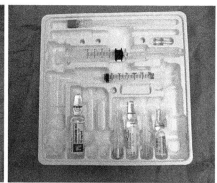

**Name:** epidural kit

**Alias:** none

**Use:** used to insert epidural catheter for administration of epidural anesthesia

**Features:** contains all needed supplies and equipment to administer epidural anesthesia

**Additional Information:** practitioner may choose to add additional supplies per personal preference; inside of the kit is considered sterile

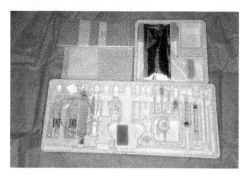

**Name:** epidural catheter

**Alias:** none

**Use:** used to administer medication into the epidural space for regional anesthesia or analgesia

**Features:** can stay in the patient's back for several days postoperatively to provide analgesic medication

**Additional Information:** comes in a variety of sizes and lengths

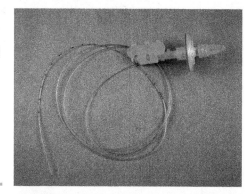

**Name:** peripheral nerve stimulator

**Alias:** none

**Use:** stimulates nerves; used for insertion of regional nerve blocks

**Features:** output control can be adjusted for higher or lower stimulation

**Additional Information:** use with disposable nerve stimulator needle

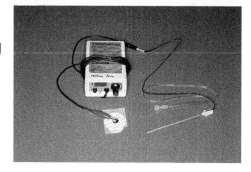

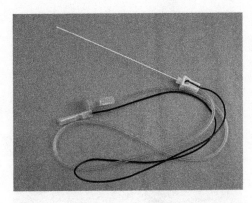

**Name:** nerve stimulator needle

**Alias:** nerve block needle

**Use:** inserts into the nerve plexus to allow for injection of regional anesthetic

**Features:** attaches to peripheral nerve stimulator machine; single-patient use

**Additional Information:** needs to be irrigated before insertion into patient; available in 4- and 1.5-inch lengths

# IV SUPPLIES AND SOLUTIONS

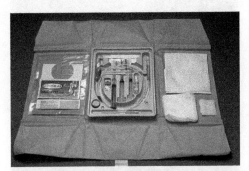

**Name:** central venous pressure monitoring kit

**Alias:** central venous pressure (CVP) line kit

**Use:** used to monitor the patient's fluid status by monitoring the pressure in the vena cava and right atrium

**Features:** kit comes with everything needed to insert the line

**Additional Information:** none

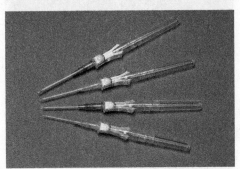

**Name:** IV catheters

**Alias:** IV needles

**Use:** starts an IV infusion on a patient

**Features:** safety needle; once the catheter is in place, the white button is pushed and the needle retracts into the plastic sheath

**Additional Information:** come in a variety of gauges (16, 18, 20, 22, and 24 gauge are the most common sizes); the larger the gauge number, the smaller the catheter diameter (e.g., a size-16 catheter has a much larger diameter than a size-24)

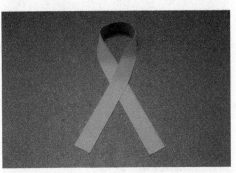

**Name:** tourniquet

**Alias:** none

**Use:** starts IV infusions; may be used in a dire emergency to control bleeding from limbs

**Features:** some have Velcro closures; most are latex free

**Additional Information:** comes in a variety of sizes and styles

**Name:** Walrus tubing

**Alias:** anesthesia IV tubing

**Use:** connects IV solution to IV catheter

**Features:** multiple stopcocks for injection of medications during induction and intraoperatively

**Additional Information:** latex free

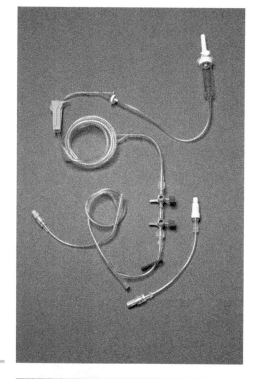

**Name:** extension set

**Alias:** none

**Use:** extends the length of IV tubing; attach to IV catheter to extend saline lock site

**Features:** comes in a variety of lengths

**Additional Information:** single use

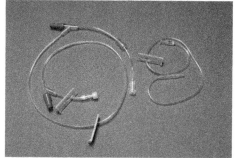

**Name:** sodium chloride 0.9%

**Alias:** normal saline

**Use:** provides fluid replacement or volume expansion

**Features:** isotonic solution; does not contain potassium

**Additional Information:** available in several sizes of bags (50 mL, 100 mL, 250 mL, 500 mL, 1,000 mL)

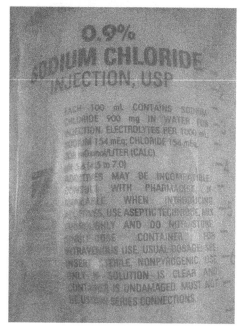

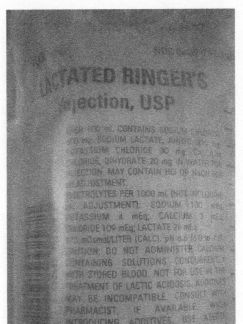

**Name:** lactated Ringer's solution

**Alias:** LR

**Use:** provides fluid replacement or volume expansion

**Features:** electrolyte solution; contains sodium, potassium, calcium, and chloride

**Additional Information:** available in several sizes of bags (250 mL, 500 mL, 1,000 mL)

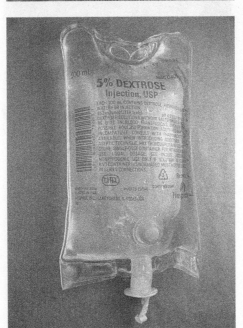

**Name:** dextrose 5%

**Alias:** D5W

**Use:** acts as a glucose and fluid replacement

**Features:** contains glucose for sugar replacement

**Additional Information:** provides calories to patient

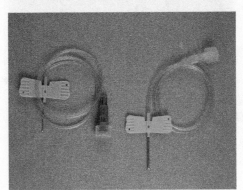

**Name:** butterfly infusion set

**Alias:** none

**Use:** used to draw blood in people with difficult veins

**Features:** uses a metal needle rather than a plastic catheter that stays in the patient's vein; needle tends to be shorter than an IV catheter, sometimes making it easier to dislodge

**Additional Information:** available in a variety of gauges (19, 21, 23, and 25 gauge are the most common)

**Name:** three-way stopcock

**Alias:** none

**Use:** allows more than one medication or fluid to be administered in rapid succession, such as a medication that needs to be followed with a saline flush

**Features:** lever turns to allow opening and closing of each port

**Additional Information:** available in plastic (disposable) or metal (resterilizable)

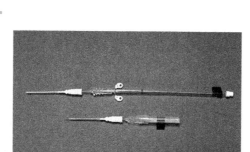

**Name:** arterial line needles

**Alias:** none

**Use:** inserted into an artery, it allows access for monitoring, blood drawing, or administration of fluids and medications

**Features:** has slider to allow for easier insertion once the artery is cannulated

**Additional Information:** available in short or long sizes

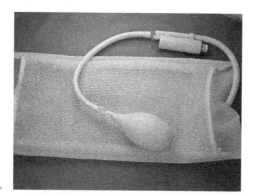

**Name:** IV pressure bag

**Alias:** none

**Use:** exerts pressure on IV solution bags to increase flow rate

**Additional Information:** available in several styles

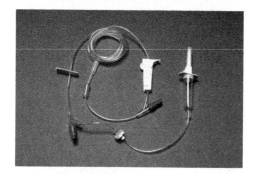

**Name:** microdrip tubing

**Alias:** none

**Use:** administers small amounts of IV solution or medication to a patient; used when patient fluid intake needs to be limited or on pediatric patients

**Features:** small drip size: 60 drops equals 1 mL

**Additional Information:** none

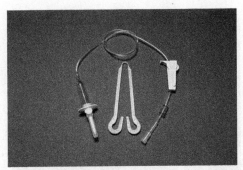

**Name:** secondary IV tubing

**Alias:** piggyback tubing

**Use:** piggyback medication drips into main IV line

**Features:** comes with plastic hanger for main IV bag and a blunt needle to use for insertion into the main IV line

**Additional Information:** main IV should be hung below the piggyback IV bag using the plastic hanger

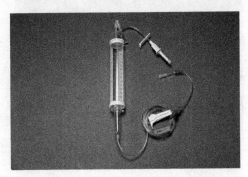

**Name:** burette

**Alias:** none

**Use:** measures and administers small amounts of IV medication or fluid; used most commonly with pediatric patients; microdrip administration system

**Features:** chamber allows for the measuring out and administration of restricted amounts of fluid; IV bag can be shut off after the fluid is measured into the chamber so that only the fluid in the chamber is given

**Additional Information:** 150-mL capacity chamber

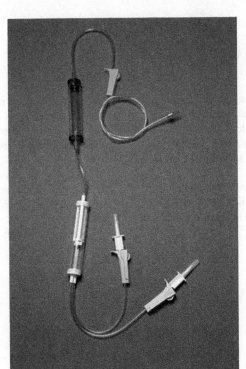

**Name:** blood administration set

**Alias:** Y-tubing

**Use:** used to administer blood

**Features:** double spikes allow blood bag and saline IV bag to be hung together; filter built into the tubing

**Additional Information:** none

**Name:** arterial line setup

**Alias:** none

**Use:** allows for pressure measurements directly from the artery as well as blood drawing

**Features:** IV bag is heparinized saline to keep the line from clotting off; can be set up for one, two, or three transducers (to allow for CVP monitoring as well)

**Additional Information:** setup may vary by institution or equipment

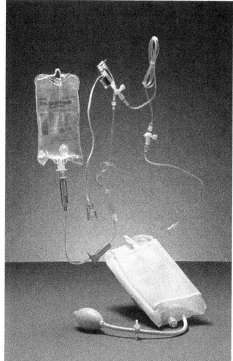
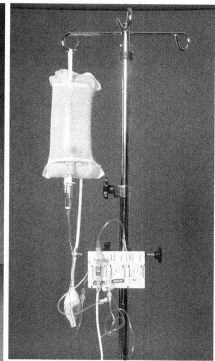

## Guidelines for Needle Safety

When handling injectable, IV, or regional block needles, there are several safety precautions that you should take to minimize the risk of needle-stick injury to yourself or others.

- Use IV or injectable needles that have safety sheaths on them whenever possible. Activate the safety sheath as soon as you are finished with the needle.
- Use a "needleless" system to inject medications into IV tubing whenever available. If your institution does not have a needleless IV tubing system, use blunt needles to inject medication into the ports.
- When possible, load needles onto syringes just before use. Do not leave syringes and needles lying around unattended.
- Know where your needles are at all times. Keep track of where you or the person you are assisting is placing the sharps.
- Place all used needles in a puncture-proof disposal container.
- Never recap used needles with your hands. If you must recap a needle, use the "scoop" method or a recapping device.
- Never use your hands to bend or break needles.

# MEDICATIONS

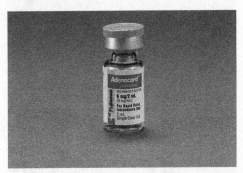

**Name:** adenosine

**Alias:** Adenocard, Adenoscan

**Medication Class:** antiarrhythmic

**Use:** treats narrow, complex tachycardias

**Features:** each vial contains 6 mg; very short half-life, must be given via IV push over 1 to 2 seconds and followed by a 20-cc saline bolus

**Additional Information:** initial dose is 6 mg; up to two more doses of 12 mg each may be given if needed

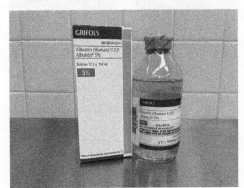

**Name:** albumin

**Alias:** albumin 5%; albumin 25%

**Medication Class:** volume expander

**Use:** restores plasma volume during cardiac bypass procedures or during treatment of burns or shock

**Features:** acts by expanding the volume of circulating blood and maintaining cardiac output

**Additional Information:** 5% albumin is generally used initially to treat shock; 25% may be used after 24 hours

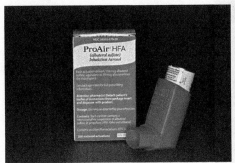
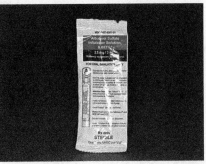

**Name:** albuterol

**Alias:** Proventil, Ventolin, Volmax

**Medication Class:** bronchodilator

**Use:** prevents or treats wheezing, bronchospasm

**Features:** medication can be used with the inhaler or can be squirted down the ETT

**Additional Information:** usual dose is one to two puffs

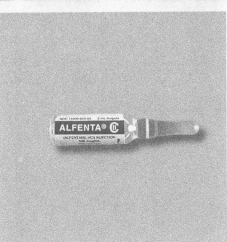

**Name:** alfentanil hydrochloride

**Alias:** Alfenta; Rapifen

**Medication Class:** opioid; narcotic analgesic

**Use:** relieves pain (analgesic)

**Features:** makes the patient drowsy; alters pain perception and response; can cause respiratory depression

**Additional Information:** usual dose depends on length of anesthesia required

**Name:** amiodarone

**Alias:** Cordarone

**Medication Class:** antiarrhythmic

**Use:** treats wide complex tachycardias; also may be used to treat cardiac arrest

**Features:** must be diluted in D5W before infusion

**Additional Information:** usual dose for cardiac arrest is 300 mg given IV via push; usual dose for treatment of tachycardia is 150 mg (diluted in 100 cc of D5W) given via IV drip

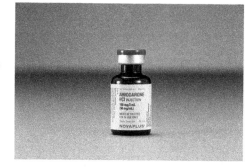

**Name:** ampicillin

**Alias:** Omnipen; Polycillin

**Medication Class:** broad-spectrum antibiotic

**Use:** helps prevent postoperative infection

**Features:** can be given orally (PO), intramuscularly (IM), IV; reconstituted and given preoperatively via IV piggyback; cannot be used for patients with penicillin allergies

**Additional Information:** usual IV dose is 1 g to 2 g

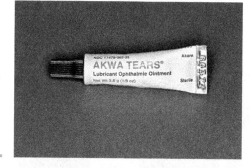

**Name:** artificial tears

**Alias:** Akwa Tears

**Medication Class:** eye lubricant

**Use:** prevents corneal drying during anesthesia

**Features:** comes in ointment form; some brands of artificial tears come as drops

**Additional Information:** apply to each eye as needed during general anesthesia

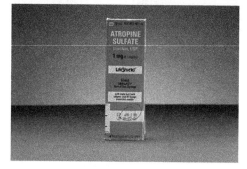

**Name:** atropine

**Alias:** none

**Medication Class:** anticholinergic; antiarrhythmic

**Use:** increases heart rate in symptomatic bradycardic arrhythmias; can be used preoperatively to decrease secretions

**Features:** each bristojet contains 1 mg; also comes in vials; can cause dryness of mouth and mucous membranes

**Additional Information:** dose is 0.5 to 1.0 mg; given via IV push for arrhythmias; preoperative dosage is 0.4 mg to 0.6 mg (adult) and 0.1 mg to 0.4 mg (pediatric)

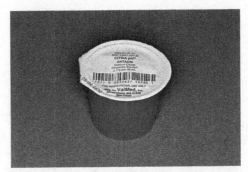

**Name:** Bicitra

**Alias:** citra pH

**Medication Class:** antacid

**Use:** reduces gastric pH

**Features:** given PO

**Additional Information:** usual dose is 15 to 30 cc (may be diluted with water in a 50:50 mixture)

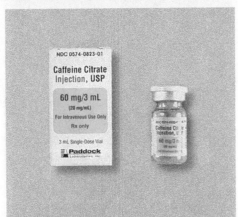

**Name:** caffeine

**Alias:** none

**Medication Class:** stimulant

**Use:** treats migraine headaches; prevents caffeine-induced headaches

**Features:** given via IV drip-mix with D5W or normal saline

**Additional Information:** none

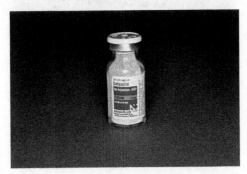

**Name:** cefazolin

**Alias:** Ancef; Kefzol

**Medication Class:** antibiotic (cephalosporin)

**Use:** helps prevent postoperative infection

**Features:** diluted and given via IV piggyback or push; can be given preoperatively, intraoperatively, or postoperatively

**Additional Information:** usual dose is 1 to 2 g; use with caution in patients with penicillin allergies

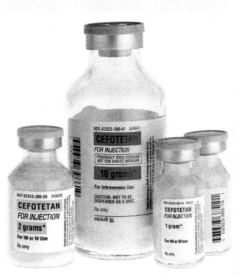

**Name:** cefotetan

**Alias:** Cefotan

**Medication Class:** second generation cephalosporin antibiotic

**Use:** helps prevent postoperative infection

**Features:** diluted and given via IV piggyback or push; can be given preoperatively, intraoperatively, or postoperatively

**Additional Information:** usual dose is 500 mg to 1 g

**Name:** clindamycin

**Alias:** Cleocin

**Medication Class:** antibiotic

**Use:** helps prevent postoperative infection

**Features:** diluted in NS or D5W and given via IV infusion

**Additional Information:** usual dose is 400-mg to 600-mg infusion

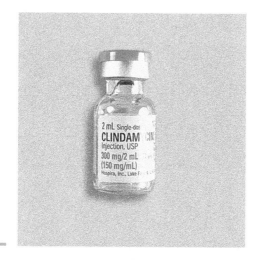

**Name:** clopidogrel

**Alias:** Plavix

**Medication Class:** platelet inhibitor

**Use:** reduces the risk of stroke in high-risk patients

**Features:** do not give to patients with active bleeding; puts patients at risk for increased bleeding; given PO

**Additional Information:** usual dosage is 75 mg/day

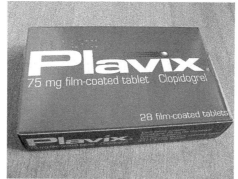

**Name:** cocaine

**Alias:** none

**Medication Class:** topical anesthetic

**Use:** used in nasal procedures as a vasoconstrictor to reduce nasal bleeding

**Features:** can be swabbed on the nasal mucosa, or cocaine-soaked cottonoids can be inserted into the nares

**Additional Information:** for topical use only

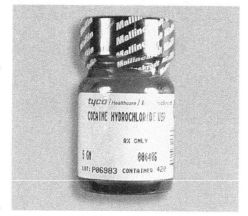

**Name:** Coumadin

**Alias:** warfarin

**Medication Class:** anticoagulant

**Use:** treats deep venous thrombosis, pulmonary embolus, acute myocardial infarction, and postcardiac valve replacement

**Features:** given PO

**Additional Information:** usual dosage is 10 to 15 mg/day, titrated to coagulation studies

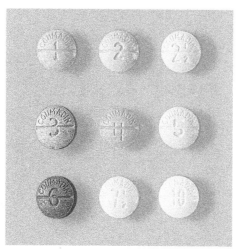

**Name:** dantrolene

**Alias:** Dantrium

**Medication Class:** skeletal muscle relaxant

**Use:** treats malignant hyperthermia

**Features:** comes in a powder form; must be diluted with sterile water

**Additional Information:** loading dose is 2.5 mg/kg mixed with injectable sterile water; using teams of two people to mix it makes for easier and faster mixing

---

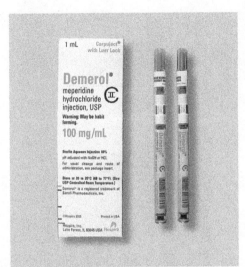

**Name:** Demerol

**Alias:** meperidine

**Medication Class:** opioid; narcotic analgesic

**Use:** relieves pain (analgesic)

**Features:** can be given IV or IM; may make patient nauseated; makes patient drowsy

**Additional Information:** dosages range from 25 mg to 100 mg IM or 25 to 50 mg IV

---

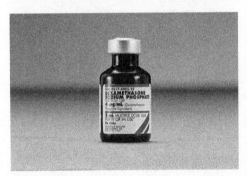

**Name:** dexamethasone

**Alias:** Decadron; Hexadrol; Mymethasone

**Medication Class:** corticosteroid (anti-inflammatory)

**Use:** prevents/reduces inflammation and edema

**Features:** can be given PO, IM, or IV; may be used topically during surgery (e.g., spine surgery); can be injected directly into a joint

**Additional Information:** dose varies depending on route and use

---

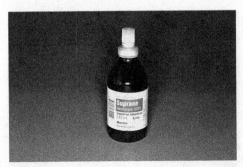

**Name:** desflurane

**Alias:** Suprane

**Medication Class:** inhalation anesthetic

**Use:** induces and maintains anesthesia

**Features:** more rapid onset and recovery than some other gases; strong odor

**Additional Information:** requires the use of a heated vaporizer for administration

**Name:** Dextrose 50%

**Alias:** none

**Medication Class:** carbohydrate

**Use:** increases blood sugar in severe hypoglycemia

**Features:** each bristojet contains 25 g of dextrose

**Additional Information:** average adult dose is 25 to 50 g IV push

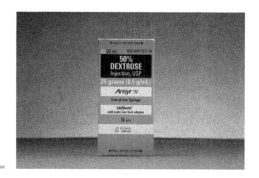

**Name:** diazepam

**Alias:** Valium

**Medication Class:** benzodiazepine

**Use:** reduces anxiety; provides musculoskeletal relaxation; controls acute seizures

**Features:** can be given PO, IM, or IV; short acting; will make patient drowsy

**Additional Information:** usual dose is 2 mg to 10 mg PO; lesser amounts IV

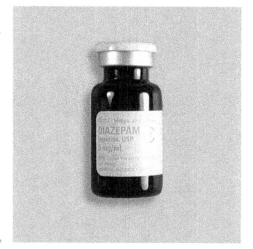

**Name:** Dilaudid

**Alias:** hydromorphone

**Medication Class:** opioid; narcotic analgesic

**Use:** pain reliever (analgesic)

**Features:** makes patient drowsy; can cause respiratory depression; can be given PO, IM, IV, or rectally

**Additional Information:** usual IM or IV dose is 1 mg to 4 mg every 4 to 6 hours

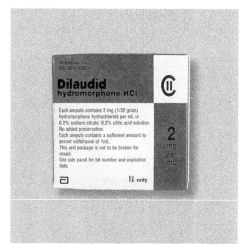

**Name:** diphenhydramine

**Alias:** Benadryl

**Medication Class:** antihistamine

**Use:** treats allergic reactions, motion sickness, insomnia, and cough

**Features:** can be given PO, IM, or IV; may cause drowsiness

**Additional Information:** common ingredient in most over-the-counter allergy medications

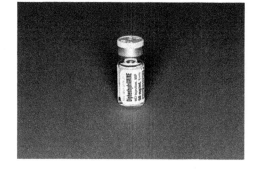

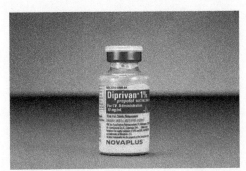

**Name:** Diprivan

**Alias:** propofol

**Medication Class:** general anesthetic

**Use:** induces or maintains anesthesia; sedates patients on ventilators

**Features:** given IV; do not mix with other agents in the same syringe

**Additional Information:** to be used only by personnel trained in anesthesia administration

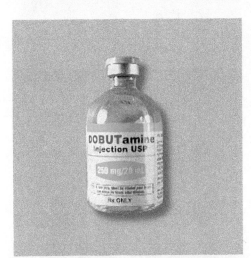

**Name:** dobutamine

**Alias:** Dobutrex

**Medication Class:** catecholamine

**Use:** can be used during cardiac surgery; used to treat shock or refractory heart failure

**Features:** increases cardiac contractility and coronary blood flow; increases heart rate

**Additional Information:** given IV infusion at a rate of 2.5 to 10 mcg/kg/min

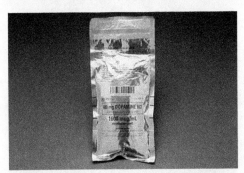

**Name:** dopamine

**Alias:** Intropin

**Medication Class:** catecholamine

**Use:** treats shock and hypotension

**Features:** comes as a premixed drip

**Additional Information:** dose is 2 to 5 mcg/kg/min (not to exceed 50 mcg/kg/min); given as an IV drip; requires careful monitoring of blood pressure

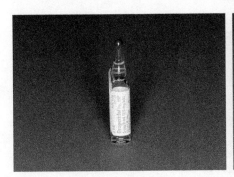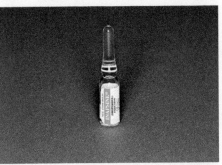

**Name:** droperidol

**Alias:** Inapsine

**Medication Class:** neuroleptic

**Use:** antiemetic; used as premedication for surgery; induces and maintains general anesthesia

**Features:** produces sedation and sleep; can be given IM or IV

**Additional Information:** dose depends on intended use

**Name:** ephedrine

**Alias:** ephedrine sulfate

**Medication Class:** bronchodilator; adrenergic

**Use:** treats hypotension and shock; increases perfusion; bronchodilation

**Features:** causes increased heart rate and cardiac contractility; vasoconstricts blood vessels; given IM, subcutaneously (SC), or IV to treat shock; may also be given PO if used as a bronchodilation

**Additional Information:** usual adult dose to treat hypotension is 10 to 25 mg IV (not to exceed 150 mg/day); usual pediatric dose is 3 mg/kg/day

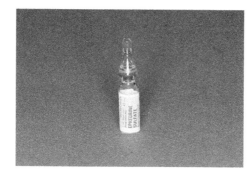

**Name:** epinephrine 1:1000

**Alias:** adrenaline

**Medication Class:** bronchodilator; catecholamine

**Use:** counteracts allergic reactions; treats bronchospasm and asthma

**Features:** 10 times stronger than the cardiac epinephrine: DO NOT confuse the two medications; each ampoule contains 1 mL; can be given IM, subcutaneously (SC), or IV

**Additional Information:** dose is 0.1 to 0.5 cc SC

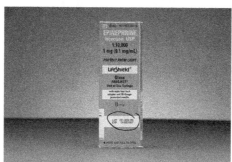

**Name:** epinephrine 1:10,000

**Alias:** adrenaline

**Medication Class:** bronchodilator; catecholamine

**Use:** used during cardiac arrest

**Features:** each bristojet equals 1 mg

**Additional Information:** dosage is 1 mg every 3 to 5 minutes during cardiac arrest; given via IV push

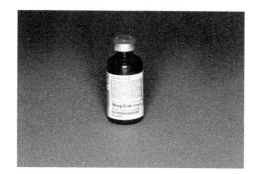

**Name:** esmolol

**Alias:** Brevibloc

**Medication Class:** antiarrhythmic

**Use:** treats hypertension and tachycardia

**Features:** slows heart rate, decreases myocardial oxygen consumption; should not be used in patients with second- or third-degree heart block, congestive heart failure (CHF), or cardiogenic shock

**Additional Information:** adult loading dose is 500 mcg/kg over 1 minute; usual pediatric dose is 50 mcg/kg/min

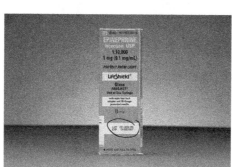

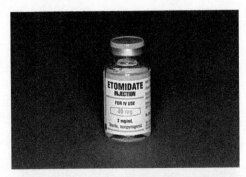

**Name:** etomidate
**Alias:** Amidate
**Medication Class:** general anesthetic
**Use:** induces general anesthesia
**Features:** given IV
**Additional Information:** usual dose is 0.2 to 0.6 mg/kg over 30 to 60 seconds

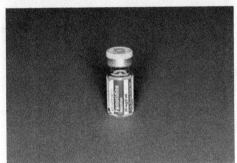

**Name:** famotidine
**Alias:** Pepcid
**Medication Class:** $H_2$ antagonist
**Use:** decreases gastric secretions
**Features:** can be given PO or IV; onset immediate if given IV
**Additional Information:** should be used with caution in children younger than 12 years; usual IV dose is 20 mg

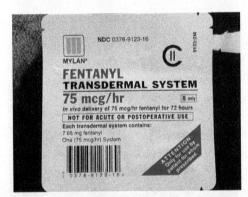

**Name:** fentanyl citrate
**Alias:** Sublimaze
**Medication Class:** opioid; narcotic analgesic
**Use:** relieves pain (analgesic)
**Features:** alters pain perception and increases the pain threshold; makes the patient drowsy; 100 mcg of fentanyl is the analgesic equivalent of 10 mg of morphine or 75 mg of Demerol
**Additional Information:** usual dose is 25 mcg to 50 mcg IV; also available in patch form

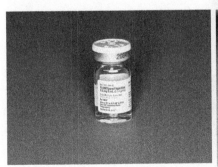 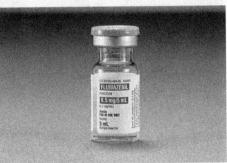

**Name:** flumazenil
**Alias:** Romazicon
**Medication Class:** benzodiazepine antagonist
**Use:** reverses benzodiazepines; commonly given to reverse the effects of midazolam (Versed)
**Features:** given IV only; compatible with normal saline, lactated Ringer's solution, or dextrose in water IV solutions
**Additional Information:** 0.2 mg IV over 15 seconds; may be repeated in 0.2-mg doses every 60 seconds up to a maximum of four doses

**Name:** furosemide
**Alias:** Lasix
**Medication Class:** diuretic
**Use:** used to remove excess fluid from the body
**Features:** comes 10 mg/mL
**Additional Information:** usual dose is 20 to 80 mg IV push

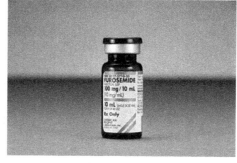

**Name:** gentamicin
**Alias:** none
**Medication Class:** antibiotic
**Use:** helps prevent postoperative infection; used frequently in patients undergoing genitourinary procedures
**Features:** diluted and given via IV piggyback; if the patient is on the medication for several days, he or she should have blood drawn to check medication levels; overdosage can cause ototoxicity or nephrotoxicity
**Additional Information:** usual dose is 60 to 80 mg IV

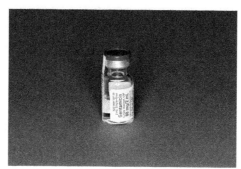

**Name:** glycopyrrolate
**Alias:** Robinul
**Medication Class:** cholinergic blocker
**Use:** decreases gastric secretions preoperatively; reverses neuromuscular blockade
**Features:** may be given PO, IM, or IV (route depends on intended use)
**Additional Information:** usual preoperative dose is 0.002 mg/kg IM; neuromuscular reversal dose is 0.2 mg for each 1 mg of neostigmine (given via IV)

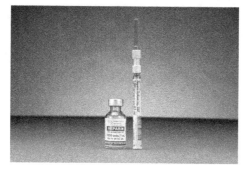

**Name:** heparin
**Alias:** none
**Medication Class:** anticoagulant
**Use:** prevents embolus or thrombus formation; treats deep venous thrombosis (DVT)
**Features:** available in several concentrations — be sure to read label to know how many units/mL it contains; can be given via IV, SC, or IV infusion; during vascular surgery, heparinized saline may be injected directly into the vessels
**Additional Information:** watch for signs of increased bleeding or hemorrhage; peak IV onset is 5 minutes; dosage depends on use

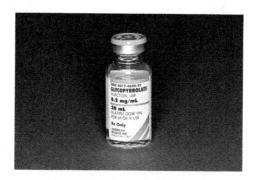

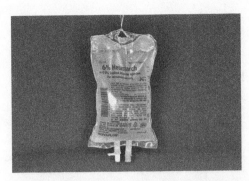

**Name:** Hespan
**Alias:** hetastarch
**Medication Class:** plasma expander
**Use:** expands circulatory volume
**Features:** expands the blood volume one to two times the amount infused
**Additional Information:** usual dose is 30 to 60 g (500 to 1000 mL); should not exceed 20 mg/kg/hr

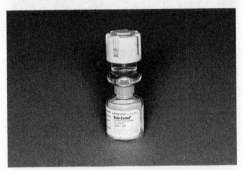

**Name:** hydrocortisone
**Alias:** Cortef; Solu-Cortef
**Medication Class:** corticosteroid
**Use:** prevents or decreases inflammation
**Features:** can be given PO, IM, or IV; drug can mask signs of infection
**Additional Information:** usual IM or IV dose is 100 mg to 250 mg

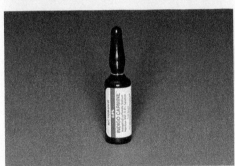

**Name:** Indigo Carmine
**Alias:** none
**Medication Class:** dye
**Use:** used to check for unintentional surgical holes in the urinary system
**Features:** given via IV and excreted by the renal system
**Additional Information:** none

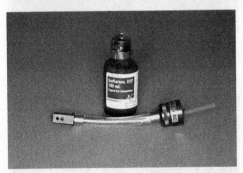

**Name:** isoflurane
**Alias:** Forane
**Medication Class:** inhalation anesthetic
**Use:** induces and maintains general anesthesia
**Features:** rapid induction and recovery
**Additional Information:** causes profound respiratory depression

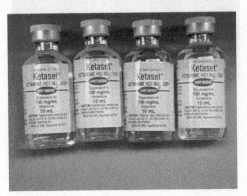

**Name:** ketamine
**Alias:** Ketalar, Ketanest, Ketaset
**Medication Class:** general anesthetic; dissociative agent
**Use:** helps to produce a rapid anesthetic induction
**Features:** can be given IM or IV
**Additional Information:** does not provide relaxation (needs to be used with other medications); can produce vivid imagery and hallucinations

**Name:** ketorolac

**Alias:** Toradol

**Medication Class:** nonsteroidal anti-inflammatory

**Use:** control of mild to moderate pain

**Features:** can be given PO, IM, or IV

**Additional Information:** should not be used in patients with asthma or allergies to NSAIDs; usual IM/IV dosage is 30 mg every 6 hours

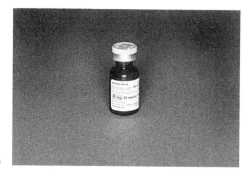

**Name:** labetalol

**Alias:** Normodyne

**Medication Class:** antihypertensive

**Use:** treats hypertension

**Features:** can be given PO or IV; should not be used in patients with cardiogenic shock, heart block, bradycardia, CHF, or asthma

**Additional Information:** onset of action is 5 minutes if given IV; usual IV dose is 20 mg given over 2 minutes; may repeat 40 to 80 mg every 10 minutes; do not exceed 300 mg total

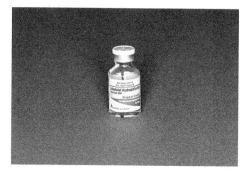

**Name:** lidocaine

**Alias:** Xylocaine

**Medication Class:** local anesthetic

**Use:** used as local and regional anesthesia

**Features:** can be given PO (viscous Xylocaine), local injection around the site, IV (e.g., Bair block), or topically (Xylocaine ointment or cream)

**Additional Information:** comes with and without epinephrine added; red lettering is present on the packaging of bottles that contain epinephrine; usual concentrations are 1%, 2%, and 4%

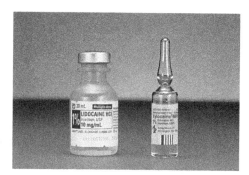

**Name:** LMD 10%

**Alias:** low molecular weight dextrose; dextran 40

**Medication Class:** volume expander

**Use:** used for plasma volume expansion

**Features:** given via IV infusion; expands blood volume one to two times the amount infused

**Additional Information:** usual dose is 500 mL over 15 to 30 minutes

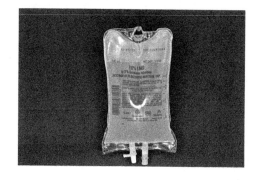

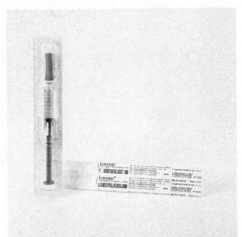

**Name:** Lovenox

**Alias:** enoxaparin

**Medication Class:** anticoagulant

**Use:** prevents pulmonary embolus or DVT in patients undergoing hip or knee replacement surgery or abdominal surgery

**Features:** given SC for 7 to 10 days postoperatively

**Additional Information:** should not be given to patients with pork allergies; should not be used in patients with bleeding disorders or history of bleeding problems; usual dose is 30 mg SC twice a day

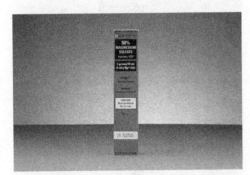

**Name:** magnesium sulfate

**Alias:** none

**Medication Class:** electrolyte

**Use:** treats low serum magnesium, torsades de pointes, and pre-eclampsia or eclampsia

**Features:** can be given PO, IM, or IV

**Additional Information:** dosage depends on condition being treated

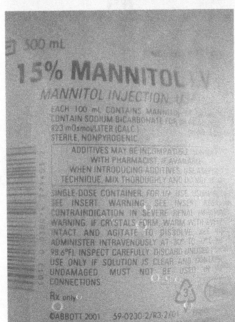

**Name:** mannitol

**Alias:** none

**Medication Class:** osmotic diuretic

**Use:** decreases cerebral edema; decreases intraocular pressure; improves renal function for patients in acute renal failure

**Features:** increases urinary output and sodium excretion; can cause dehydration; needs to be administered with a filter in the IV line

**Additional Information:** usual IV dose is 1 to 2 g/kg of a 15% or 25% solution over 0.5 hour to 1 hour; Foley catheter should be in place when this medication is being used

**Name:** Marcaine

**Alias:** Sensorcaine; bupivacaine

**Medication Class:** local anesthetic

**Use:** used as local and regional anesthesia

**Features:** four times more potent than lidocaine

**Additional Information:** available with or without epinephrine added—red lettering is present on the packaging of bottles containing epinephrine; available in various strengths (e.g., 0.25%, 0.5%, 0.75%)

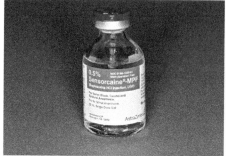

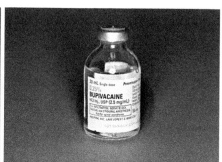

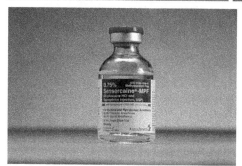

**Name:** methylene blue

**Alias:** none

**Medication Class:** staining agent; dye

**Use:** stains surgical site; checks patency of fallopian tubes during tuboplasty

**Features:** injected into intended site, it creates a blue stain

**Additional Information:** none

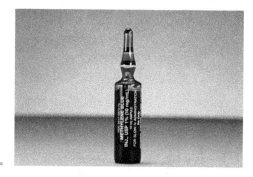

**Name:** methylprednisolone

**Alias:** Medrol; Depo-Medrol; Solu-Medrol

**Medication Class:** corticosteroid

**Use:** treats severe inflammation, adrenal insufficiency, shock

**Features:** can be given PO, IM, or IV; should not be given to patients younger than 2 years or those with tuberculosis or AIDS

**Additional Information:** usual dose for treatment of shock is 100 to 250 mg IV every 2 to 6 hours; usual adult dose for treatment of inflammation is 10 to 250 mg IV

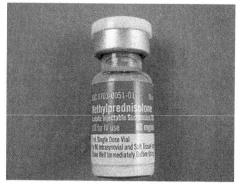

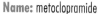

**Name:** metoclopramide

**Alias:** Reglan

**Medication Class:** cholinergic

**Use:** prevents nausea and vomiting; increases gastric emptying

**Features:** can be given PO or IV; should not be given to patients who are sensitive to procaine or procainamide

**Additional Information:** usual dose is 10 mg

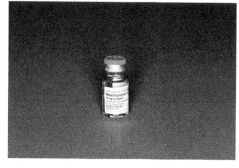

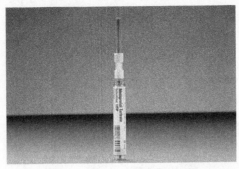

**Name:** metoprolol

**Alias:** Betaloc, Lopressor, Toprol

**Medication Class:** antihypertensive; antianginal

**Use:** treats mild-to-moderate hypertension; controls angina pectoris; used in the setting of acute myocardial infarction to reduce cardiovascular mortality

**Features:** can be given PO or IV; should not be used in patients with heart block, cardiogenic shock, bradycardia, or bronchial asthma

**Additional Information:** usual IV dose is 5 mg every 2 minutes for three doses

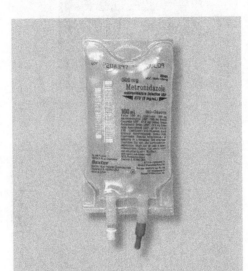

**Name:** metronidazole

**Alias:** Flagyl

**Medication Class:** anti-infective

**Use:** treats or prevents infection

**Features:** can be given PO or IV; has an immediate onset if given IV; may cause vision problems

**Additional Information:** usual IV dose is 15 mg/kg infused over 1 hour

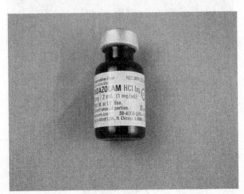

**Name:** midazolam

**Alias:** Versed

**Medication Class:** benzodiazepine

**Use:** reduces anxiety preoperatively; induces conscious sedation; reduces amount needed of more potent anesthetics

**Features:** short acting; will make patient drowsy; twice as potent as diazepam (Valium)

**Additional Information:** 1 to 2 mg IV push; patient's oxygen saturation and respiratory rate must be monitored postadministration (can cause respiratory depression)

**Name:** milrinone

**Alias:** Primacor

**Medication Class:** inotropic; vasodilator

**Use:** treats CHF that does not respond to other medications

**Features:** given IV; contraindicated in the setting of acute myocardial infarction

**Additional Information:** usual adult dosage is 50 mcg/kg given as a bolus over 10 minutes followed by an infusion of 0.375 to 0.75 mcg/kg/min

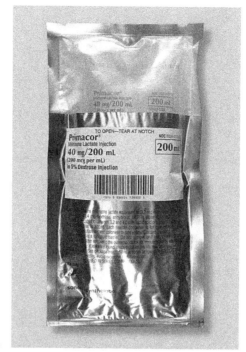

**Name:** mivacurium

**Alias:** Mivacron

**Medication Class:** nondepolarizing neuromuscular blocker

**Use:** causes skeletal muscle relaxation; facilitates intubation

**Features:** given via IV; peak onset is 2 to 3 minutes with reversal in 15 to 30 minutes

**Additional Information:** usual adult dose is 0.15 mg/kg

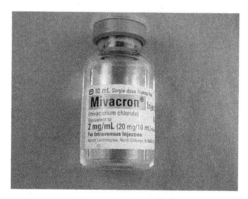

**Name:** morphine sulfate

**Alias:** morphine

**Medication Class:** opioid; narcotic analgesic

**Use:** relieves pain (analgesic)

**Features:** can be given IV or IM; may make patient nauseated; makes patient drowsy

**Additional Information:** usual dose is 1 mg to 10 mg IV push

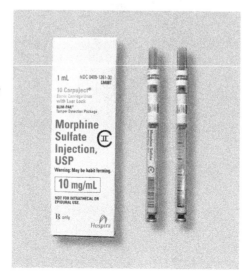

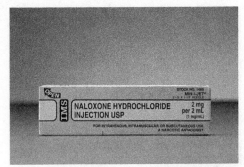

**Name:** naloxone

**Alias:** Narcan

**Medication Class:** narcotic antagonist

**Use:** acts as a reversal agent for narcotics

**Features:** may lead to sudden onset of pain (due to reversal of narcotic effect), which may lead to hypertension and tachycardia

**Additional Information:** usual dose is 0.4 mg to 2.0 mg

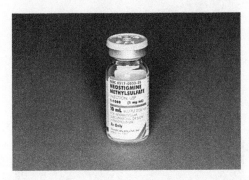

**Name:** neostigmine methylsulfate

**Alias:** Prostigmin

**Medication Class:** anticholinesterase

**Use:** reverses nondepolarizing muscle relaxants (vecuronium, rocuronium); treats myasthenia gravis

**Features:** slows heart rate, so atropine or glycopyrrolate may be given at the same time (using separate syringes)

**Additional Information:** usual reversal dose is 0.5 mg to 2.0 mg IV; can be repeated as needed up to a maximum of 5 mg

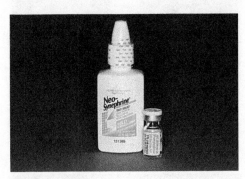

**Name:** Neo-Synephrine

**Alias:** phenylephrine

**Medication Class:** adrenergic

**Use:** treats hypotension and shock; maintains blood pressure during spinal anesthesia; decreases bleeding during nasal surgery

**Features:** causes vasoconstriction; can be given SC, IM, IV, or nasal spray

**Additional Information:** usual adult IV dose to treat hypotension is 0.1 mg to 0.5 mg; may repeat every 10 to 15 minutes as needed

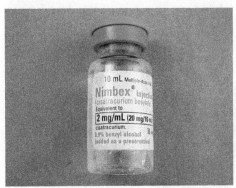

**Name:** Nimbex

**Alias:** cisatracurium

**Medication Class:** nondepolarizing neuromuscular blocker

**Use:** causes skeletal muscle relaxation; facilitates intubation

**Features:** given IV; duration of action is 30 to 40 minutes

**Additional Information:** usual adult dose is 0.15 to 0.2 mg/kg

**Name:** nitroglycerin

**Alias:** Nitro-Bid; Nitrol, NitroQuick

**Medication Class:** antianginal

**Use:** treats pain associated with angina pectoris; can be used to decrease preload and afterload in congestive heart failure (CHF), can be used to create controlled hypotension in surgical procedures

**Features:** causes coronary vessel vasodilation; can be given sublingual (SL), IV, topically (paste), or transdermally (patch)

**Additional Information:** dosage depends on the form of medication being used; IV infusion comes in glass bottles (medication is absorbed into the polyvinyl of infusion bags); usual adult IV infusion dose is 5 mcg/min to start and then increase by 5 mcg every 3 to 5 minutes until desired effect is reached

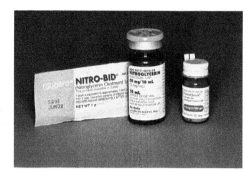

**Name:** nitroprusside

**Alias:** Nitropress

**Medication Class:** antihypertensive

**Use:** treats hypertensive crisis; induces controlled hypotension to decrease bleeding during surgery; treats CHF and cardiogenic shock

**Features:** onset of action is 1 to 2 minutes; given IV infusion; wrap infusion bottle in aluminum foil to protect from light exposure; infuse using an infusion pump

**Additional Information:** usual adult dose is 0.5 mcg to 8 mcg/kg/min; dilute medication in 250 to 1,000 mL of D5W

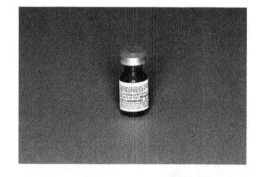

**Name:** nitrous oxide

**Alias:** none

**Medication Class:** inhalation anesthetic

**Use:** used in conjunction with other agents to provide balanced anesthesia

**Features:** has little effect on heart rate or blood pressure; not potent enough to be used alone for general anesthesia

**Additional Information:** gas diffuses into closed spaces thus making it contraindicated for some surgeries (e.g., tympanoplasty)

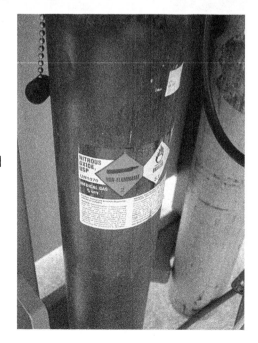

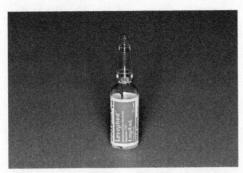

**Name:** norepinephrine

**Alias:** Levophed

**Medication Class:** catecholamine

**Use:** treats acute hypotension and shock

**Features:** onset of action is 1 to 2 minutes; causes increased contractility of the heart, peripheral vasoconstriction, and improved coronary blood flow

**Additional Information:** usual adult dose is 8 to 12 mcg/min; titrate to desired blood pressure

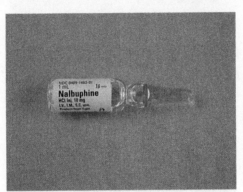

**Name:** Nubain

**Alias:** nalbuphine

**Medication Class:** opiate analgesic

**Use:** controls moderate to severe pain; supplements balanced anesthesia

**Features:** can be given SC, IM, or IV; may cause drowsiness or respiratory depression

**Additional Information:** usual adult dosage is 10 to 20 mg every 3 to 6 hours as needed

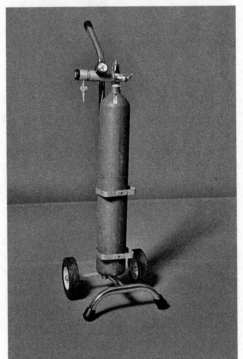

**Name:** oxygen

**Alias:** none

**Medication Class:** essential gas

**Use:** provides supplemental oxygen to organs and tissue

**Features:** can be given via cannula, mask, or Ambu bag; flow rate for cannula should be 1 to 3 L; a flow rate of 8 to 10 L is best for a mask; a flow rate of 10 to 15 L is needed for an Ambu bag

**Additional Information:** liter flow is dependent on which vehicle is being used to deliver the oxygen (e.g., cannula, mask, Ambu bag)

**Name:** oxytocin

**Alias:** Pitocin

**Medication Class:** oxytocic

**Use:** induces or stimulates labor; controls postpartum hemorrhage; contracts the uterus after a cesarean section

**Features:** given IM or IV; IV onset of action is 1 minute

**Additional Information:** usual adult dosage is 10 units (IV infusion is infused at 20 to 4 microunits/min)

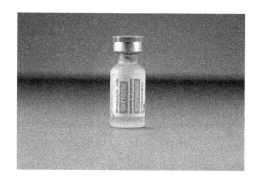

**Name:** papaverine

**Alias:** none

**Medication Class:** peripheral vasodilator

**Use:** treats arterial spasm

**Features:** can be given PO, IM, or IV; should not be used in patients with complete heart block; usual IM/IV dose is 30 to 120 mg every 3 hours as needed

**Additional Information:** none

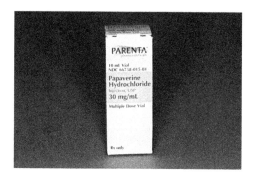

**Name:** Pentothal

**Alias:** thiopental

**Medication Class:** general anesthetic

**Use:** induces anesthesia; short-term general anesthesia

**Features:** given IV; onset is 30 to 40 seconds

**Additional Information:** usual adult induction dose is 210 to 280 mg

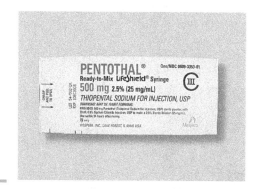

**Name:** pentazocine

**Alias:** Talwin

**Medication Class:** opiate analgesic

**Use:** controls moderate-to-severe pain

**Features:** can be given PO, SC, IM, or IV; may cause drowsiness and respiratory depression; IV onset of action 2 to 3 minutes

**Additional Information:** usual SC, IM, or IV dose is 30 mg every 3 to 4 hours

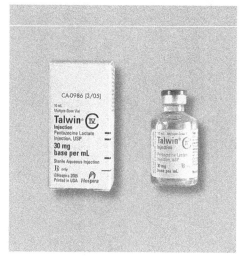

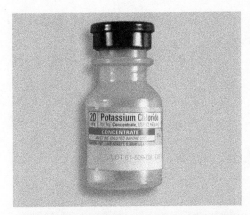

**Name:** potassium chloride

**Alias:** KCl; K-Lor; Micro-K; Slo K

**Medication Class:** electrolyte

**Use:** prevents and treats low serum potassium levels

**Features:** may be given PO or IV; too much may cause cardiac arrhythmias or cardiac arrest; ECG needs to be monitored

**Additional Information:** usual adult IV dosage is 20 mEq/hr

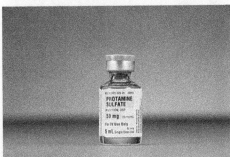

**Name:** protamine

**Alias:** none

**Medication Class:** heparin antagonist

**Use:** reverses effects of heparin

**Features:** given IV

**Additional Information:** usual dose is 1 mg protamine for every 100 U of heparin that was given (not to exceed 50 mg in 10 minutes); administer over 1 to 3 minutes

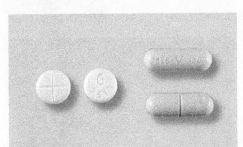

**Name:** pyridostigmine

**Alias:** Regonol

**Medication Class:** anticholinesterase

**Use:** reverses nondepolarizing muscle relaxants

**Features:** can be given PO, IM, or IV; should not be used in patients with bradycardia or hypotension

**Additional Information:** usual IV dose is 10 mg to 30 mg

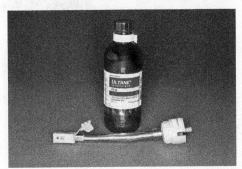

**Name:** sevoflurane

**Alias:** Ultane

**Medication Class:** inhalation anesthetic

**Use:** induces and maintains general anesthesia

**Features:** has a more rapid and smooth onset and recovery than some gases

**Additional Information:** can cause bradycardia and hypotension; reduces cardiac output; may cause postoperative nausea and vomiting

**Name:** scopolamine hydrobromide

**Alias:** hyoscine

**Medication Class:** antiemetic; anticholinergic

**Use:** reduces nausea, vomiting, and dizziness in patients prone to motion sickness

**Features:** most commonly administered via transdermal patch but can be given IV (0.4 mg)

**Additional Information:** not recommended for use in children; should not be used in patients with glaucoma; causes dilation of pupils

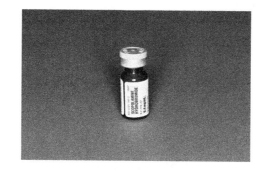

**Name:** scopolamine patch

**Alias:** Transderm Scop

**Medication Class:** antiemetic; anticholinergic

**Use:** reduces nausea in patients prone to motion sickness

**Features:** patch delivers a dose of 0.5 mg over 72 hours; may cause dizziness or drowsiness

**Additional Information:** patch is placed behind the ear; not recommended for use in children; should not be used in patients with glaucoma

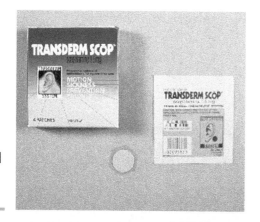

**Name:** sodium bicarbonate 8.4%

**Alias:** bicarb

**Medication Class:** alkalinizer

**Use:** treats documented acidosis

**Features:** given IV; each bristojet contains 50 mEq (50 mL)

**Additional Information:** usual dose is 1 mEq/ kg; blood gases need to be checked frequently to avoid overalkalization

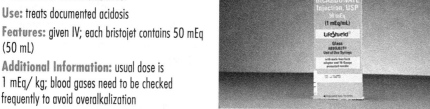

**Name:** succinylcholine

**Alias:** Anectine; Quelicin

**Medication Class:** depolarizing neuromuscular blocker

**Use:** causes skeletal muscle relaxation; facilitates intubation

**Features:** can be given IM or IV; onset of action is 1 minute with a duration of 6 to 10 minutes

**Additional Information:** should not be used in patients with a history of malignant hyperthermia

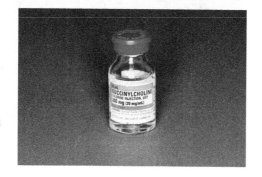

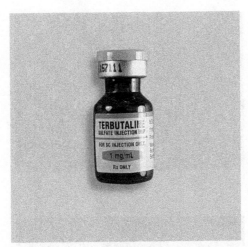

**Name:** terbutaline

**Alias:** Brethine

**Medication Class:** bronchodilator

**Use:** treats bronchospasm, asthma; stops premature labor

**Features:** can be given PO, SC, or by inhaler; may cause tremors, palpitations, and tachycardia

**Additional Information:** PO doses should be given with food; usual adult inhaler dosage is two puffs every 4 to 6 hours; usual SC dosage is 0.25 mg every 8 hours

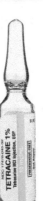

**Name:** tetracaine

**Alias:** Pontocaine

**Medication Class:** local anesthetic

**Use:** used as regional anesthesia, including peripheral nerve blocks, epidural, spinal, and caudal

**Features:** duration of action is 3 hours

**Additional Information:** vital signs and ECG should be monitored during anesthesia; should not be used in patients with severe liver disease

(Akorn Pharmaceuticals)

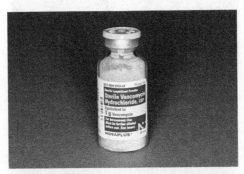

**Name:** vancomycin

**Alias:** Vancocin

**Medication Class:** anti-infective

**Use:** treats organisms resistant to other antibiotics

**Features:** given PO or IV; overdosing can cause ototoxicity and/or nephrotoxicity

**Additional Information:** usual adult IV dose is 500 mg every 6 hours

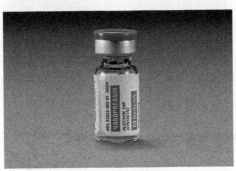

**Name:** vasopressin

**Alias:** Pitressin

**Medication Class:** pituitary hormone

**Use:** treats cardiac arrest; diabetes insipidus; bleeding esophageal varices

**Features:** comes 20 units per vial; need two vials for a dose

**Additional Information:** cardiac arrest dose is 40 units IV one time only

**Name:** vecuronium

**Alias:** Norcuron

**Medication Class:** nondepolarizing neuromuscular blocker

**Use:** causes skeletal muscle relaxation; facilitates intubation

**Features:** given IV; duration of action is 45 to 60 minutes

**Additional Information:** usual dose for patients older than age 9 years is 0.08 to 0.10 mg/kg

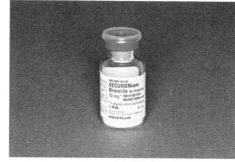

**Name:** Zemuron

**Alias:** rocuronium

**Medication Class:** nondepolarizing neuromuscular blocker

**Use:** causes skeletal muscle relaxation; facilitates intubation

**Features:** given IV; duration of action about 0.5 hour

**Additional Information:** usual dose is 0.6 mg/kg

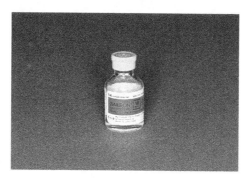

**Name:** Zofran

**Alias:** ondansetron

**Medication Class:** antiemetic

**Use:** prevents nausea and vomiting

**Features:** can be given PO or IV

**Additional Information:** usual adult dose is 4 mg given over 30 seconds

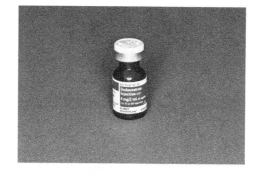

## Surgical Session Review

1) The purpose of _____ is to absorb carbon dioxide in the anesthesia machine breathing circuit.
   a. Soda lime
   b. Limestone
   c. Soap stone
   d. Soda pop

2) _____ is the medication used in the treatment of malignant hyperthermia.
   a. Decadron
   b. Lasix
   c. Dantrolene
   d. Digoxin

3) A reading of below _____ on the BIS monitor means the patient is unconscious.
   a. 80
   b. 90
   c. 70
   d. 60

4) A _____ _____ is a type of blanket that blows warm air over the patient's skin surface to help prevent hypothermia.
   a. Bear Hugger
   b. Bair Hugger
   c. Bare Hugger
   d. Bear Blanket

5) _____ is used to reverse the effects of narcotics.
   a. Digoxin
   b. Decadron
   c. Narcan
   d. Atropine

6) Pediatric defibrillation pads may be used on children weighing up to _____ kg.
   a. 10
   b. 15
   c. 20
   d. 30

7) The strength of epinephrine used in a cardiac arrest situation is
   a. 1:100
   b. 1:1,000
   c. 1:10,000
   d. 1:100,000

8) The strength of epinephrine used to treat an allergic reaction is
   a. 1:100
   b. 1:1,000
   c. 1:10,000
   d. 1:100,000

9) Your patient is feeling nauseous. Which of the following medications might the anesthetist give to the patient?
   a. Narcan
   b. Kytril
   c. Sodium bicarbonate
   d. Lidocaine

10) A setting of 2 to 3 L/min of oxygen would be an appropriate setting for a(n)
    a. Ambu bag
    b. Nonrebreather mask
    c. Oxygen mask
    d. Nasal cannula

11) _____ forceps may be used during intubation to help guide the ETT.
    a. Magill
    b. Maguile
    c. DeBakey
    d. Mayo

12) Isoflurane and sevoflurane are
    a. Antiemetics
    b. Antipyretics
    c. Inhalation anesthetics
    d. IV anesthetics

13) _____ can be used to treat a patient with symptomatic bradycardia.
    a. Lidocaine
    b. Amiodarone
    c. Vasopressin
    d. Atropine

14) The anesthesiologist asks for the TEE. What does TEE stand for?
    a. Transesophageal endoscope
    b. Transendotracheal endoscope
    c. Transesophageal echocardiogram
    d. Transendotracheal echocardiogram

15) Vancomycin is a type of
    a. Antiseptic
    b. Antibiotic
    c. Antiemetic
    d. Anti-inflammatory

16) Which type of airway device is generally used on a conscious patient with an intact gag reflex?
    a. Endotracheal tube
    b. Oral airway
    c. Right-angle endotracheal tube
    d. Nasal airway

17) Hespan is a(n)
    a. Plasma expander
    b. Isotonic IV solution
    c. Electrolyte replacement
    d. Antibiotic

18) The other name for lidocaine is
    a. Xylocaine
    b. Marcaine
    c. Pontocaine
    d. Bupivacaine

19) A Bier block is a type of
    a. General anesthesia
    b. MAC anesthesia
    c. Spinal anesthesia
    d. Nerve block anesthesia

20) An adequate oxygen flow rate for a BVM device is _____ L/min.
    a. 10
    b. 15
    c. 5
    d. 2 to 4

# Answers to Surgical Session Reviews

## CHAPTER 1

1. c
2. b
3. b
4. d
5. d
6. b
7. d
8. c
9. d
10. b
11. a
12. c
13. c
14. d
15. a
16. b
17. c
18. d

## CHAPTER 2

1. b
2. a
3. d
4. c
5. a
6. c
7. d
8. a
9. c
10. c
11. c
12. c
13. c
14. d
15. b
16. d
17. a
18. c
19. d
20. c

## CHAPTER 3

1. a
2. b
3. c
4. b
5. b
6. c
7. d
8. b
9. a
10. b
11. c
12. a
13. c
14. c
15. b
16. c
17. a
18. c
19. d
20. b

## CHAPTER 4

1. c
2. b
3. a
4. d
5. c
6. c
7. b
8. d
9. b
10. c
11. b
12. c

## CHAPTER 5

1. c
2. b
3. b
4. a
5. d
6. d
7. d
8. c
9. b
10. c
11. b
12. c
13. c
14. a
15. d
16. b
17. a
18. a
19. c
20. b

## CHAPTER 6

1. b
2. c
3. d
4. c
5. b
6. a
7. c
8. a
9. b

## CHAPTER 7

1. c
2. d
3. c
4. b
5. d
6. b
7. a
8. c
9. d
10. c
11. c
12. d
13. a
14. d
15. b
16. c
17. c
18. b
19. c
20. b

## CHAPTER 8

1. b
2. c
3. d
4. c
5. a
6. b
7. c
8. b
9. b
10. d
11. d
12. b
13. a
14. d
15. d
16. c
17. a
18. c
19. b
20. d

## CHAPTER 9

1. c
2. b
3. c
4. a
5. d

## CHAPTER 10

1. b
2. a
3. c
4. c
5. d
6. c
7. a
8. c
9. d
10. c
11. d
12. c
13. d
14. c
15. c
16. c
17. a
18. b
19. d

## CHAPTER 11

1. a
2. c
3. d
4. b
5. c
6. b
7. c
8. b
9. b
10. d
11. a
12. c
13. d
14. c
15. b
16. d
17. a
18. a
19. d
20. b

# INDEX

Page references followed by f, t, or b indicate material in figures, tables, or boxes respectively.